This book is to be returned on or before
the last date stamped below.

27 SEP 1993
15 FEB 1994
10 MAR 1995
24 APR 1995
26 MAY 1995
8. FEB. 1996
14 MAR 1996
13 FEB 1997
14 MAR 2000

EVERED, David (ed.)

RESEARCH AND THE AGEING POPULATION

The Ciba Foundation is an international scientific and educational charity. It was established in 1947 by the Swiss chemical and pharmaceutical company of CIBA Limited—now CIBA-GEIGY Limited. The Foundation operates independently in London under English trust law.

The Ciba Foundation exists to promote international cooperation in biological, medical and chemical research. It organizes about eight international multidisciplinary symposia each year on topics that seem ready for discussion by a small group of research workers. The papers and discussions are published in the Ciba Foundation symposium series. The Foundation also holds many shorter meetings (not published), organized by the Foundation itself or by outside scientific organizations. The staff always welcome suggestions for future meetings.

The Foundation's house at 41 Portland Place, London, W1N 4BN, provides facilities for meetings of all kinds. Its Media Resource Service supplies information to journalists on all scientific and technological topics. The library, open seven days a week to any graduate in science or medicine, also provides information on scientific meetings throughout the world and answers general enquiries on biomedical and chemical subjects. Scientists from any part of the world may stay in the house during working visits to London.

Ciba Foundation Symposium 134

RESEARCH AND THE AGEING POPULATION

A Wiley – Interscience Publication

1988

JOHN WILEY & SONS

Chichester · New York · Brisbane · Toronto · Singapore

© Ciba Foundation 1988

Published in 1988 by John Wiley & Sons Ltd, Chichester, UK

Library of Congress Cataloging in Publication Data

Research and the ageing population.
    p. cm. — (Ciba Foundation symposium ; 134)
    Editors: David Evered (organizer) and Julie Whelan.
    "Symposium on Research and the Ageing Population, held at the John
E. Fogarty International Center for Advanced Study in the Health
Sciences, Bethesda, Maryland, USA, 28–30 April 1987"—Contents p.
    "A Wiley–Interscience publication."
    Includes indexes.
    ISBN 0 471 91420 7
    1. Geriatrics—Congresses. 2. Aging—Congresses. 3. Aged—
Diseases—Congresses. 4. Aged—Health and hygiene—Congresses.
I. Evered, David. II. Whelan, Julie. III. Symposium on Research
and the Ageing Population (1987 : John E. Fogarty International
Center for Advanced Study in the Health Sciences) IV. Series.
    [DNLM: 1. Aged—congresses. 2. Aging—congresses. 3. Health—
congresses.   W3 C161F v. 134 / WT 104 R432 1987]
RC952.A2R48   1988
618.97—dc19
DNLM/DLC
for Library of Congress   87-29440
                                                                     CIP

British Library Cataloguing in Publication Data

Research and the ageing population.—
(Ciba Foundation symposium; 134).
1. Aging—Research
I. Series
612′.67′072   QP86

ISBN 0 471 91420 7

Typeset by Inforum Ltd, Portsmouth.
Printed and bound in Great Britain by the Bath Press Ltd., Bath, Avon.

Contents

---

* Dr Brody was unable to attend the symposium, through illness. His paper was presented by
Dr L.R. White.

Participants

G.R. Andrews   Department of Primary Care & Community Medicine, Flinders University of South Australia, Flinders Medical Centre, Bedford Park, SA 5042, Australia

T.H.D. Arie   Department of Health Care of the Elderly, Floor B, Medical School, Queen's Medical Centre, Clifton Boulevard, Nottingham NG7 2UH, UK

J.A. Brody   University of Illinois at Chicago, Office of the Dean (M/C 922), School of Public Health, PO Box 6998, Chicago, Illinois 60680, USA

P.D. Coleman   Department of Neurobiology & Anatomy, University of Rochester School of Medicine & Dentistry, Box 603, Rochester, New York 14642, USA

A.J. Fox   Social Statistics Research Unit, The City University, Northampton Square, London EC1V 0HB, UK

J.F. Fries   Stanford University School of Medicine, Department of Medicine, HRP 109C, Stanford, California 94305, USA

J. Grimley Evans   Nuffield Department of Clinical Medicine, Geriatric Medicine Division, Radcliffe Infirmary, Oxford OX2 6HE, UK

C.F. Hollander   Department of Safety Assessment, Centre de Recherche, Laboratoires MERCK SHARP & DOHME-CHIBRET, Route de Marsat, BP 134, 63203 Riom Cédex, France

R. Katzman   Department of Neurosciences, University of California at San Diego, School of Medicine (M-024), La Jolla, California 92093, USA

T.B.L. Kirkwood   National Institute for Medical Research, The Ridgeway, Mill Hill, London NW7 1AA

F.A. Lints   Université Catholique de Louvain, Faculté des Sciences Agronomiques, Laboratoire de Génétique, Place Croix du Sud 2, B-1348 Louvain-la-Neuve, Belgium

D.M. Macfadyen   Global Programme for Health of the Elderly, World
Health Organization, 8 Scherfigsvej, DK-2100 Copenhagen, Denmark

D. Maeda   Tokyo Metropolitan Institute of Gerontology, Department of
Sociology, 35-2 Sakaecho, Itabashi-ku, Tokyo 173, Japan

V. Mor   Centers for Long Term Care Gerontology & Health Care Research,
Box G, Brown University, Providence, Rhode Island 02912, USA

K. Ostermann   Arbeitsgruppe für ASG, Gesamthochschule Kassel, Postfach
101380, D-3500 Kassel, Federal Republic of Germany

J.P. Phair   Infectious Diseases – Hypersensitivity Section, Department of
Medicine, The Medical School, Northwestern University, Ward Memorial
Building, 303 E Chicago Avenue, Chicago, Illinois 60611, USA

B.L. Riggs   Division of Endocrinology & Metabolism, Mayo Clinic & Mayo
Medical School, 200 First Street SW, Rochester, Minnesota 55905, USA

N. Solomons   CESSAIM (Centre for Studies of Sensory Impairment, Aging
& Metabolism), Hospital de Ojos y Oidos, 'Dr Rodolfo Robles V',
Diagonal 21 y 19 Calle, Zona 11, Guatemala City, Guatemala, Central
America

A. Svanborg   University of Göteborg, Department of Geriatric &
Long-Term Care Medicine, Vasa Hospital, S-411 33 Göteborg, Sweden

S.S. Wallack   Bigel Institute for Health Policy, Heller Graduate School,
Brandeis University, 415 South Street, Waltham, Massachusetts 02254,
USA

N.K. Wenger   Emory University School of Medicine, Department of
Medicine (Cardiology), Thomas K. Glenn Memorial Building, 69 Butler
Street SE, Atlanta, Georgia 30303, USA

A. Williams   Institute for Research in the Social Sciences, University of
York, Heslington, York YO1 5DD, UK

T.F. Williams (*Chairman*)   National Institute on Aging, National Institutes
of Health, Building 31, Room 2CO2, Bethesda, Maryland 20892, USA

L.R. White Epidemiology Office, National Institute on Aging, National Institutes of Health, Federal Building, Room 612, Bethesda, Maryland 20892, USA

P.M. Wise Department of Physiology, The University of Maryland School of Medicine, 655 West Baltimore Street, Baltimore, Maryland 21201, USA

Preface

The 265th Ciba Foundation Symposium (134 in the new series) on Research and the Ageing Population was held at the Stone House, National Institutes of Health, Bethesda on 28–30 April 1987 as one event to mark the centenary of the National Institutes of Health and the long-standing friendship which exists between the Ciba Foundation and many scientists at the NIH. The meeting brought together those engaged in basic biomedical research — epidemiologists, demographers, physicians, health-care planners and economists. The major objective of the symposium was to review progress in research relevant to the elderly and to consider its significance in planning for the provision of care for elderly people, taking demographic, social and economic factors into account. The meeting was chaired throughout by Dr T. Franklin Williams, Director of the National Institute on Aging.

We were pleased to have the opportunity to mark the centenary of the NIH in this way. The occasion also gave us the chance to establish many new scientific contacts and to renew existing ones. We were gratified by the enthusiastic response to the symposium and by the welcome we received at the NIH. We are particularly grateful to Dr James Wyngaarden, the Director, who first extended such a warm invitation to us, and to Dr Williams and Dr Craig K. Wallace (Director of the Fogarty International Center) for their help with the planning and organization of the meeting. We also appreciated the very considerable professional help that we received from Marcia Aaronson and Rita Singer, who both took such pride in ensuring that everything ran smoothly throughout.

David Evered
Director, The Ciba Foundation

Introduction

T. Franklin Williams

National Institute on Aging, National Institutes of Health, Building 31, Room 2C02, Bethesda, Maryland 20892, USA

1988 Research and the ageing population. Wiley, Chichester (Ciba Foundation Symposium 134) p 1–2

The field of ageing research is much indebted to the Ciba Foundation for undertaking this symposium: I am sure the outcome will be an important contribution to our further understanding in this challenging area. The participants are all leaders from scientific arenas closely related to ageing and the common problems of older people, and it is a privilege to have so many disciplines joining in the discussion of such important issues.

Let me suggest what our priorities should be in this symposium and what we may hope to learn from it. My suggestions may be especially important for a topic as broad and multifaceted as ageing and its related disorders. I would first suggest that we try to discard our stereotypes of ageing, and recognize that new knowledge is coming along rapidly and that we must be prepared to change our views. That is a standard principle in science, but I am afraid that, because of the strength of traditional views about ageing, stereotypes still abound, and infect scientists as much as the general public. It is all too often true that most of us in ageing research have not kept up with advances in related fields, and are prone to repeat or use stereotypes in our thinking. We should be prepared to discard these stereotypes and be open to the new ideas that will be presented here by people in different disciplines from our own.

My second suggestion is that we concentrate on what seem to be the most significant new findings and ideas, and that we should—in the formal papers and the discussions—be open to speculation about where we might go in our further research.

Thirdly, and most important of all, we should try to look for potential interactions between the fields represented in the symposium, and for the implications of our own work for that of others—for example, the implications of cardiac findings for the field of dementia, and vice versa; the implications of the common presence of multiple chronic conditions (such as diabetes, chronic lung disease and arthritis) for infection in old age; and so on, across the whole range of topics. We should be looking for ways by which we can inform and stimulate each other, because of the major interactions that are inevitable as part of the complex picture of old age. As an example of this interaction, it is my experience that diabetes and cardiovascular disease both have a very low prevalence in people with dementia of Alzheimer's type, and conversely one rarely sees this type of dementia in older people with diabetes or extensive cardiovascular disease. People with Alzheimer's disease are astonishingly healthy in many other ways; specifically, they rarely if ever have diabetes. That observation may or may not hold up on further investigation: I know of one study (unpublished) which tends to corroborate this clinical observation. All sorts of speculations could arise if this is true, and would call for further investigations.

I offer this as one observation. One of our tasks here is to look at the cross-reactions and cross-implications between our different fields of expertise, not only from one disease to another, but from basic biological approaches to the variety of both biomedical and social problems in older people. This symposium provides the opportunity, through the conjunction of able people from many fields, to contribute a combined impact to ageing research.

The health of the elderly population: results from longitudinal studies with age-cohort comparisons

Alvar Svanborg

Department of Geriatric and Long-Term Care Medicine, University of Göteborg, Vasa Hospital, S-411 33 Göteborg, Sweden

Abstract. In the longitudinal study of 70-year-olds in Göteborg the first age cohort (born 1901–1902) has now been followed for 15 years and the second cohort (born 1906–1907) for nine years; an intervention study has been added to the third age cohort (born 1911–1912). These longitudinal perspectives (derived from studies of samples shown to be representative of the total population) have successively improved the possibilities of distinguishing between ageing manifestations and symptoms caused by definable diseases. In addition to previously reported figures on the proportions of apparently healthy people at age 70 and 75, preliminary conclusions from the follow-up periods from age 79 indicate that at that age at least 20% do not suffer from symptoms of definable diseases. These findings have allowed detailed analyses to be made of the morphological and functional consequences of ageing as well as the calculation of clinical reference values for the age interval 70–79. The improving possibilities for distinguishing between ageing and morbidity have allowed certain conclusions to be drawn on obvious differences between age cohorts relating to the prevalence of disease and manifestations of ageing. These age-cohort differences could not be related to migration and ongoing genetic changes but there is indirect evidence for relationships to lifestyle and certain environmental factors. The reasons for these age-cohort differences in the manifestations of ageing are being analysed retrospectively through information on differences in living conditions between the cohorts and prospectively through the intervention programme (InterVention Elderly in Göteborg, IVEG).

1988 Research and the ageing population. Wiley, Chichester (Ciba Foundation Symposium 134) p 3–16

The longitudinal study of 70-year-olds in Göteborg, Sweden (Rinder et al 1975, Svanborg 1977) now includes three (Fig. 1) different age cohorts (Svanborg et al 1984, Mellström & Svanborg 1987). The first age cohort (born 1901–1902) has been followed for 15 years, up to age 85, and further yearly follow-ups are planned. The second cohort (born 1906–1907) has been followed for nine years. Because of the rather remarkable differences between these two cohorts — differences not only in the state of health, but also in the

3

YEAR OF INVESTIGATION

YEAR OF BIRTH	1971/72	1976/77	1980/81	1981/82	1982/83	1983/84	1984/85	1985/86	1986/87
1901/02 (H70)	70 years	75 years	79 years		81 years	82 years	83 years		85 years
1906/07 (H70)		70 years		75 years				79 years	
1911/12 (IVAG)				70 years	70 years	72 years	72 years		

FIG. 1.   The present design of the longitudinal study of 70-year-olds in Göteborg, Sweden, showing the three age cohorts. IVEG, intervention programme (InterVention Elderly in Göteborg) added to the study of the third cohort.

rate and manifestations of ageing (Berg 1980, Svanborg et al 1984, 1986) — a third age-cohort sample of 70-year-olds (born 1911–1912) has been studied. In order to test certain theories about the reasons for these age-cohort differences, which were also obvious in the comparison of the second and third age cohorts, we added an intervention programme (InterVention Elderly in Göteborg, IVEG) to the study of the third cohort (Svanborg et al 1986, Eriksson et al 1987).

These longitudinal perspectives, derived from a broad and detailed investigation covering many of the basic biological, clinical, behavioural and social perspectives provided by age-related morphological, biochemical, physiological and psychological changes, have successively improved the possibility of distinguishing between the manifestations of ageing and the symptoms produced by definable diseases and disorders. We have given examples of these changes in various reports, on clinical biochemical reference values (Landahl et al 1981, Lindstedt et al 1983, Svanborg 1985a, Larsson et al 1986); on age-related changes in blood pressure (Landahl et al 1986), heart volume (Landahl et al 1984) and lung function (Sixt et al 1984); on body composition (Steen et al 1979); on striated muscle function (Aniansson et al 1983); and on cognitive function (Berg 1980). This information, from studies of groups representative of a defined and characterized population, has considerably modified previous thinking on the nature and manifestations of ageing. An awareness of the complexity of both the morphological and the functional consequences of ageing has replaced previous simplified and stereotyped ideas about human ageing (for reviews of results from our longitudinal study see Svanborg et al 1982, Svanborg 1983, 1985b, 1987).

There are certain functional measures in humans that show only a two-phase curve and start to decline almost directly after the initial phase of growth and maturity. But for many functions the relationships between functional ability and chronological age are more complicated, and a global generalization implies at least four phases (Fig. 2). The beginning of the phase of decline varies considerably over the age period from about 20 to about 75. The previously reported 'terminal phase' of ageing (Svanborg et al 1986) has become more and more obvious, the longer we have followed our sample. This is a period in which in some individuals vitality goes down rapidly, with no obvious medical causes for this functional decline (phase IV in Fig 2). The reasons for an accelerated functional decline might be an ultimate lack of reserve capacities within different functional components.

It has commonly been thought that different components of organ systems, such as the immune system and the cognitive system, should show similar age-related changes. The discrepancy between the rate of functional decline in psychomotor speed (perceptual speed), which starts to go down around the age of 20–30, and the other measurable parameters of intelligence and memory (well preserved at least up to age 70 in the healthy elderly), is one

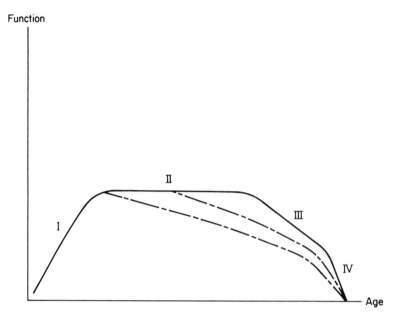

FIG. 2. The relationship between functional performance and chronological age. Some functions (—— – ——) decline earlier than others.

example of the diversity in the rate of ageing within functionally related systems. This particular discrepancy also has clinical implications. From our experience, it is a common reason for the misdiagnosis of dementia/senility in the elderly. This is especially the case when the perceptual speed is further lowered because of sensory deprivation, such as unwanted isolation, bereavement, different forms of somatic injury and disease, or mental depression (Svanborg et al 1984). During phase III (Fig. 2) it has also been fascinating to see longitudinally how the age-related changes over time often imply not only downhill slopes in functional performance, but also periods of levelling-off (Larsson et al 1986) or even certain improvements, although the longer longitudinal perspective obviously must imply a functional decline.

The longer the observation period available, the more we realize that previously reported (Svanborg 1977, Landahl et al 1977) over-diagnosis not only is real but is more common than we previously thought (see, for example, Svanborg et al 1982, Svanborg 1983, Landahl et al 1984, 1986, Svanborg et al 1986). Our present experience suggests that at age 70 at least 30–40% of subjects were without symptoms that could be referred to any definable disease. The preliminary conclusion is that the proportion of 'healthy' people at the age of 79 is still at least 20%. We have therefore been able to study ageing in a group of apparently healthy older people and also to calculate clinical reference values for the age interval 70–79. We have, we hope, therefore also improved our diagnostic criteria for these elderly subjects.

Generally, our studies have shown that under-diagnosis is very common in the elderly. One reason is that elderly people expect to have certain impairments at older ages and do not even mention certain problems to their doctors. This suggests that a more systematic interview technique is urgently needed for examining elderly patients. Another reason is that many symptoms are much more discrete and sometimes also different in the elderly. Chest pain, for example, is relatively uncommon in myocardial infarctions in the elderly, and mental depression is often manifested by symptoms that are more vague and difficult to identify than in younger age groups.

The study shows, however, that over-diagnosis seems to be even more common than under-diagnosis. The reason for this is mainly our limited knowledge of how to distinguish the manifestations of physiological ageing from symptoms of definable disease. Examples of over-diagnosis include hypertension, congestive heart failure and dementia. The studies also show an over-consumption of medical services and of drugs by those experiencing loneliness as an everyday problem in life.

We have also made a detailed investigation of the nature and prevalence of different forms of disability and handicap in the elderly. As an example, at the ages of 70, 75 and 79 years, we found 3%, 5% and 8% respectively to have such advanced handicaps that institutional care is considered to be necessary. On the other hand, at 70 years, 95% of the elderly have thus been shown to be without advanced handicap. Further measurements of functional capability for certain 'activities of daily living' have been made. For example, a standardized test was performed in bathrooms, where older people's ability to look after their own hygiene was assessed. The investigation of arm and hand function included tests of coordination and strength, power capacity in opening jars and bottles, and the basic movements of the arms and hands involved in washing and dressing. We have also investigated walking ability, and have shown, for instance, that only a few 79-year-old people are able to walk at the speed needed for pedestrians to cross street intersections with traffic signals (Lundgren-Lindquist et al 1983).

The dynamics of ageing and of the state of health have been further emphasized in our comparisons of the manifestations of ageing and the prevalence of disease in the three age cohorts studied at age 70, and of the two cohorts for which results are now available for ages 70, 75 and 79. So far as we can judge, from studies of the migration in the Swedish population during this century, these rather marked age-cohort differences do not seem to be explainable by genetic changes. Indirect evidence exists for relationships to lifestyle and to certain environmental factors. A marked change in longevity and further life expectancy has occurred. In 70–79-year-old women, age-adjusted mortality during the years 1970–1979 has decreased by no less than 19%. The age-cohort differences observed also include differences in cognitive ability, dental state, and body mass index, as well as in the occurrence of advanced handicaps in women and the prevalence of certain diseases. We also have indirect evidence for probable future negative age-cohort differences, because both smoking and alcohol abuse, which are becoming more common in female cohorts, have been found to be related to lower muscle strength, lower skeletal density, and altered gonadal function (Mellström et al 1981, 1982a, Mellström & Svanborg 1987).

One example of the dynamics of ageing — an example with practical clinical implications — is age-related changes in blood pressure (Landahl et al 1986). These changes show, first, a difference between men and women; second, a difference between systolic and diastolic pressure; and finally, a two-phase curve for systolic and diastolic pressure in women and for systolic pressure in men. We have also found a three-phase curve for diastolic pressure in men, with an increase up to age 50, a plateau between 50 and 70, and a decline between 70 and 79! The diagnostic criteria for hypertensive disease have become even more difficult to establish, now that we have shown that the heart volume increases with age, apparently for physiological reasons (Landahl et al 1984). The age-related morphological changes seen in the heart seem to be mainly a structural adaptation of the ageing heart in the direction of an increased volume. Our results from echocardiographic measurements (Lernfelt et al 1987) indicate that the ratio between the volume and thickness of the heart wall is astonishingly constant. In the ageing heart there is mainly an eccentric hypertrophy, in contrast to the concentric hypertrophy of essential hypertension.

The clinical problem is illustrated by the fact that the general doctor treating the elderly very seldom has the methodological resources available for distinguishing between these different forms of heart changes. Higher blood pressure and a greater heart volume in elderly people than in younger adults are commonly taken as evidence of hypertension with increased heart load. We know that at present no fewer than 30% of women at the age of 70 are treated because of a blood pressure level considered to be too high. At age 75, close to 40% are receiving such treatment. The percentage of males — the sex that really could be expected to have an increased risk of cardiovascular complications — is considerably lower: 13% are being treated for blood pressure at age 70 and 17% at age 75, in Sweden.

The complexity of these problems is further illustrated by our observations of ongoing age-cohort differences in blood pressure (Table 1). Clinical reference values calculated from studies of present generations might thus not be relevant for the coming generations of elderly people.

We now have both direct and indirect evidence that (1) inter-individual differences commonly increase with age, up to at least age 79; (2) sex differences vary markedly over short periods of time; (3) age-cohort differ-

TABLE 1   Arterial blood pressure in three age cohorts of 70-year-olds in Göteborg

	Women			
	Cohort 1	Cohort 2	Cohort 3	
Systolic blood pressure	168	166	160	P<0.000
Diastolic blood pressure	93	90	185	P<0.000
	Men			
	Cohort 1	Cohort 2	Cohort 3	
Systolic blood pressure	159	160	157	P<0.361
Diastolic blood pressure	96	92	84	P<0.000

Comparisons were made in subjects not receiving treatment for hypertension (β-blockers, diuretics, and/or other anti-hypertensive drugs).

ences arise within periods as short as five years; and (4) differences exist that imply not only the occurrence of different definable disorders, but also the manifestation, and rate, of certain age-related functions. This evidence must stimulate our thinking in the direction of possible measures for postponing or preventing age-related changes. We are now tackling these problems in the intervention programme added to our longitudinal follow-up of the third age cohort of 70-year-old people (Svanborg 1985c) (see Fig. 1).

The three main aims of the intervention study (InterVention Elderly in Göteborg, IVEG) are:

(1) *Early and more correct diagnosis and treatment.* We know from the results of the longitudinal study that both under-diagnosis and over-treatment are common in the elderly. Some examples have been mentioned here. Early diagnosis and treatment become urgent when the reserve capacity is falling.

(2) *Improved options for meaningful lives with a reasonable degree of activity.* The elderly in Göteborg were found to have much greater intellectual and physical capacities than was generally thought. Their 'trainability' seems to persist not only up to age 75, as was previously shown for striated muscle (Aniansson et al 1983), but up to 80 years and beyond, from our present experience.

(3) *Improved possibilities for preventing or postponing the influence of various risk factors.* Accidents are too common in the elderly. Unwanted sudden changes of a psychological and social kind, such as bereavement, are a common cause of a rapid decline in vitality and state of health (for a review see Mellström et al 1982b). We need a better understanding of the

mechanism responsible for this decline and also systematic studies of possible preventive and supportive measures.

An intervention period of two years has now been completed. After a follow-up period of another three years we shall compare this sample, in whom interventions were made, with controls of the same cohort, as well as with the 75-year-olds of the two previously investigated, longitudinally followed age cohorts (see Fig. 1).

Indirectly we thus have many reasons to believe that preventive/postponing measures could influence not only the occurrence of certain definable disorders in the elderly, but also the rate and functional consequences of ageing. In the intervention study we want to see the extent to which such effects might be obtained when the lifestyle and environment are altered, even at such a relatively advanced age as 70 years.

Acknowledgements

The study of 70-year-old people in Göteborg was made possible by grants from the Swedish Ministry of Health and Social Affairs, the Commission for Social Research, the Swedish Medical Research Council, the Göteborg Medical Services Administration and the Göteborg Administration of Social Services.

References

Aniansson A, Sperling L, Rundgren Å, Lehnberg E 1983 Muscle function in 75-year-old men and women. A longitudinal study. Scand J Rehabil Med Suppl 9:92–102
Berg S 1980 Psychological functioning in 70- and 75-year-old people. A study in an industrialized city. Acta Psychiatr Scand 62 Suppl 288
Eriksson BG, Mellström D, Svanborg A 1987 A medical–social intervention in a 70-year-old Swedish population. A general presentation of methodological experiences. Compr Gerontol, in press
Landahl S, Lindblad B, Roupe S, Steen B, Svanborg A 1977 Digitalis therapy in a 70-year-old population. Acta Med Scand 202:437–443
Landahl S, Jagenburg R, Svanborg A 1981 Blood components in a 70-year-old population. Clin Chim Acta 112:301–314
Landahl S, Svanborg A, Åstrand K 1984 Heart volume and the prevalence of certain common cardiovascular disorders at 70 and 75 years of age. Eur Heart J 5:326–331
Landahl S, Bengtsson C, Sigurdsson J, Svanborg A, Svärdsudd K 1986 Age-related changes in blood pressure. Hypertension 8:1044–1049
Larsson M, Jagenburg R, Landahl S 1986 Renal function in an elderly population. Scand J Clin Lab Invest 46:593–598
Lernfelt B, Landahl S, Svanborg A 1987 Coronary heart disease at 70, 75 and 79 years of age. A longitudinal study with special reference to sex differences and mortality. To be published
Lindstedt G, Edén S, Jagenburg R, Lundberg PA, Mellström D, Odén A, Svanborg A 1983 Factors influencing serum free T_4 in 70-year-old men. Implications for reference intervals in the elderly. Scand J Clin Lab Invest 43:401–413

Lundgren-Lindquist B, Aniansson A, Rundgren Å 1983 Functional studies in 79-year-olds. III. Walking performance and climbing capacity. Scand J Rehabil Med 15:125–131

Mellström D, Svanborg A 1987 Tobacco smoking — a major cause of sex differences in health. Compr Gerontol 1:34–39

Mellström D, Rundgren Å, Svanborg A 1981 Previous alcohol consumption and its consequences for ageing, morbidity and mortality in men aged 70–75. Age & Ageing 10:227–286

Mellström D, Rundgren Å, Jagenburg R, Steen B, Svanborg A 1982a Tobacco smoking, ageing and health among the elderly: a longitudinal study of 70-year-old men and an age cohort comparison. Age & Ageing 11:45–58

Mellström D, Nilsson Å, Odén A, Rundgren Å, Svanborg A 1982b Mortality among the widowed in Sweden. Scand J Soc Med 10:33–41

Rinder L, Roupe S, Steen B, Svanborg A 1975 Seventy-year-old people in Gothenburg. A population study in an industrialized Swedish city. I. General presentation of the study. Acta Med Scand 198:397–407

Sixt R, Bake B, Oxhöj H 1984 The single-breath N_2-test and spirometry in healthy non-smoking males. Eur J Respir Dis 65:296–304

Steen B, Isaksson B, Svanborg A 1979 Body composition at 70 and 75 years of age: a longitudinal population study. J Clin Exp Gerontol 1:185–200

Svanborg A 1977 Seventy-year-old people in Gothenburg. A population study in an industrialized Swedish city. II. General presentation of social and medical conditions. Acta Med Scand Suppl 611:5–37

Svanborg A 1983 The physiology of ageing in man — diagnostic and therapeutic aspects. In: Caird FI, Evans JG (eds) Advanced geriatric medicine 3. Pitman, London, p 175–182

Svanborg A 1985a The Gothenburg longitudinal study of 70-year-olds: clinical reference values in the elderly. In: Bergener M et al (eds) Thresholds in aging. Academic Press, London, p 231–239

Svanborg A 1985b Biomedical and environmental influences on aging. In: Butler R, Gleason H (eds) Productive aging: enhancing vitality in later life. Springer-Verlag, New York, p 15–27

Svanborg A 1985c Health, productivity and aging: interventions. In: Butler R, Gleason H (eds) Productive aging: enhancing vitality in later life. Springer-Verlag, New York, p 87–91

Svanborg A 1987 Cohort differences in the Göteborg studies of Swedish 70-year-olds. In: Brody J, Maddox G (eds) Epidemiology of aging. Springer-Verlag, New York

Svanborg A, Landahl S, Mellström D 1982 Basic issues of health care. In: Thomae H, Maddox G (eds) New perspectives on old age: A message to decision makers. Springer-Verlag, New York, p 31–52

Svanborg A, Berg S, Nilsson L, Persson G 1984 A cohort comparison of functional ability and mental disorders in two representative samples of 70-year-olds. In: Wertheimer J, Marois M (eds) Modern aging research, vol 5: Senile dementia: outlook for the future. Alan R. Liss, New York, p 405–409

Svanborg A, Berg S, Mellström D, Nilsson L, Persson G 1986 Possibilities of preserving physical and mental fitness and autonomy in old age. In: Häfner H et al (eds) Mental health in the elderly. A review of the present state of research. Springer-Verlag, Berlin/Heidelberg, p 195–202

DISCUSSION

Katzman: You mentioned the possibility of improvements with ageing during your phase III (Fig. 2) and you also suggested that joint disorders would not lead to selective mortality. Do X-ray changes improve in individuals between the ages of 70 and 79?

Svanborg: These were cross-sectional comparisons. When we started with the first age cohort we unfortunately did not include methods for comparing joint disorders in our programme. We thus simultaneously studied the third cohort at age 70, the second at age 75 and the first at age 79. In the first cohort we have followed the subgroup of probands with joint disorders longitudinally to see to what extent they had a higher mortality between 70 and 79 than those without joint disorders. Although we know that certain forms of malignant rheumatoid arthritis might have an increased mortality, there were generally no statistically proved higher mortality rates in those with joint complaints and joint morbidity than in those without joint problems. Neither did we find any correlation between the density of the skeleton and the prevalence of osteoarthritis.

Fries: We have looked at the methods of assessing radiological progression in osteoarthritis by use of longitudinal study (Altman et al 1987). We studied pairs of X-rays of the same joints taken from two to five years apart, and were unable to find any case of improvement in osteoarthritis when studied longitudinally. But we did find evidence of two populations of individuals, one group who are remarkably stable over a five-year period and a second group of subjects who show progress over this period.

Svanborg: We haven't said that we have found an improvement, longitudinally, in osteoarthritis! I said that, from these cross-sectional comparisons, we have no evidence for an increase in the occurrence of osteoarthritis with age, at ages above 70. The common observation that elderly people often suffer from pain less than younger individuals might explain a difference in current complaints between the ages. We have never claimed any evidence for longitudinal radiological improvement in osteoarthritis—for example, for a disappearance of radiologically observed spurs.

Wenger: When you examined the three cohorts, could you make any comparison of changes in lifestyle? You suggested that lifestyle can exert an important effect. What have you been able to conclude about changes in activity, diet, smoking, or levels of stress (so far as one can determine the latter)?

Svanborg: Epidemiologically the prevalence of tobacco smoking is one of the lifestyle factors that is rather easy to define. In women the first two cohorts had very similar smoking habits (12–13%); the third cohort had only a slightly higher prevalence of women smokers (15%). The real increase in smoking in older women will thus be expected in later cohorts. There were also age-cohort differences in men in smoking (50%, 37% and 34%), but showing a decreasing trend. There were also differences in the known occurrence of alcohol abuse between the cohorts. Changes in the educational system had taken place between the first and third cohorts; exposure to television and other forms of the mass media has obviously been different for these age cohorts. There must also have been differences between the cohorts in nutrition during childhood, especially in the First World War period.

We have tried to measure and estimate most of these differences. There are clearly lifestyle differences, but they are so manifold that we need to add the results from our intervention study before we can talk about causal relationships, aside from these differences related to smoking and alcohol abuse.

Wenger: What was the pattern for alcohol abuse, and was it comparable in men and women?

Svanborg: We found differences in alcohol abuse between men and women. However, it is difficult to identify alcohol abuse in an epidemiological study. We have therefore taken a contrast group of abusers of alcohol that has also caused social problems, and compared this group with all the others. Although we knew that alcohol abuse exists in the other group also, we have found marked differences between the two contrasted groups.

We know that the density of the skeleton at age 70 is about 25% lower in tobacco smokers than in non-smokers. We have also found that muscle strength is lower in smokers. In those whom we can really define as alcohol abusers we also found more loss of skeleton at the age of 70 than in the contrast group. Let me re-emphasize that the women in Göteborg who are smokers had had their menopause two years earlier than non-smoking women. We have also measured gonadal function indirectly and showed differences between smokers and non-smokers in the balance between oestrogenic and androgenic gonadal steroids. This is one reason why we can expect certain negative age-cohort differences, especially in women, when the present age cohorts with a higher prevalence of smokers reach the age of 70.

Arie: You are finding these changes in lifestyle and health-related factors between the three cohorts. Have you any information on deliberate changes made by your subjects, late in life, in part perhaps in response to local awareness of your studies? Is there a spontaneous intervention effect, in other words?

Svanborg: It is difficult to say to what extent our longitudinal study has influenced the behaviour of the elderly, and also the way doctors treat them. We have made very thorough studies to ensure that the age-cohort differences are not due to differences in non-response. Obviously, publications from a study like this have reached not only colleagues in medicine from different specialities, psychologists, sociologists, architects and so on, but also the general public. However, I think it unlikely that the later two cohorts before the age of 70 would have been markedly influenced by our comments on the vitality and health of earlier cohorts aged 70 or more.

In the intervention study we have certainly been aware that the alterations we have suggested for a representative sample have soon been extended to many other people. When we found marked differences in vitality and state of health among those who had lost their spouse compared to those still living with a spouse, we were of course interested to understand the reason for a lower state of health and longevity among widows and widowers. We know, for example, that the mortality rate increases in widowers by 48% and in widows by 22% during the first three months of bereavement. Our interest in helping these widows and widowers has apparently filled a need for these people, and care for the elderly in this situation has therefore become the interest also of other care givers besides those in our research study.

Finally, let me emphasize that if we compare age-cohort differences at age 70, 75 and 79 in the first two cohorts, we find that the differences are approximately the same at these three ages between the first two cohorts.

Andrews: In a ten-year period, many things will change besides an individual's characteristics and behaviour. To what extent in a longitudinal study is it important to monitor changes in socioeconomic conditions in the environment—such as pollution levels or other environmental risk factors, or changes in the provision and efficacy of health services? Perhaps these extrinsic elements have significant effects on your cohorts over that period of time?

Svanborg: There are many implications of those questions. In the comparison of, say, the state of health of different professional groups exposed to different forms of pollutant, one has to consider the possibility of the selection of certain individuals to certain jobs. When we look at specific risk factors, such as the inhalation of asbestos, our study material is too limited to allow any conclusions. In comparisons between Sweden and Japan we found, astonishingly, enhanced longevity in industrial areas of Japan with considerable air pollution—but also a better economy, better schools, better nutrition, better hygienic and medical facilities, and so on. The possibilities of making correlations between state of health and air pollution factors in the Göteborg study are very limited, although we know that there is an interesting age-related difference in mortality between different professional groups.

Solomons: I'd like to speculate about the implications of your data. There is no question that you are demonstrating statistically valid trends, and many of us have been trying to identify the intermediate or proximal causes responsible for the trends. But perhaps there are inherent cycles here—like the business cycle—and you happen to be looking at the down slope, or the improvement slope, of a very long, undulating cycle that may operate over centuries, and that we know nothing about. If this study had been done 50 years earlier or were done 50 years hence, you might see similar differences across time, but in the opposite direction (with increasing systolic pressures with ageing, and so forth). There is no answer to this, but it is something always to consider when we look at longitudinal data.

Svanborg: You are talking about regression towards the mean, and when we look at different variables, such as blood pressure, we have to take that possibility into consideration. As far as we can see now, there must be a risk that the increase in longevity in Swedish women will level off, or maybe even go down, because of the fact that coming generations will have a much higher prevalence of smokers and presumably also of alcohol abusers. Also, future generations of women smokers will have started smoking on an average around the age of 18, rather than at the age of 32 in the first two age cohorts we studied.

Riggs: Going back to your Fig. 2, which showed four phases of the curve relating functional performance to age, I was specially interested in the fourth phase in which there is a rapid deterioration in function, presumably near the expected time of death. To what extent is this a true accelerating deterioration of organ function, and to what extent a gradual loss of organ function over many years, to the point that a lower threshold for the maintenance of organ function is passed? This second possibility appears to be what happens in hip (proximal femur) fracture; the incidence of hip fracture is very low in middle life, even though bone is being lost over many decades, but late in life the bone density falls below the threshold required for skeletal integrity, resulting in an exponential increase in the number of hip fractures.

Svanborg: We believe that the discrepancy between our results and some animal studies is partly due to the fact that in the human it is more difficult to measure total functional ability—most organs have such a remarkable reserve capacity. There is evidence that the dopamine content of the caudate nucleus might fall to about 20% of what it was when we were young before Parkinsonian symptoms develop. We know that we can remove one kidney and half of the other without causing obvious functional decline. This final phase might be the 'naked' or 'basic' rate of ageing, but it goes very fast in some individuals and might therefore not reflect our continuous rate of change over the years. Some of our patients have had good hearing, sight and so on, yet within 1½–2 years they might go downhill in function at a very high rate. So it seems to be difficult to explain this fourth phase solely by the idea that this part of the curve reveals the 'naked' rate of ageing.

Kirkwood: The interesting example of glomerular filtration rate, which you find to decline from the age of 50 and then to level off between 70 and 79 and decline again thereafter, seems to be a good candidate for what Dr Williams mentioned in his Introduction—the importance of interaction between different factors. You also showed that systolic blood pressure rises progressively, levels off, and then starts to fall over a somewhat similar age range. If there are interactions between different factors, quite small changes in one factor can perhaps be amplified through interaction with other factors to produce a significant change over a period of time.

Svanborg: Our data on glomerular filtration rate are longitudinal, but there are cross-sectional comparisons in the literature showing that glomerular filtration rate starts to go down earlier in life, but falls more markedly (in the Swedish population) from around the age of 50. The decline after 50 seems to be approximately 1% per year. In this context it is interesting that my collaborators have been unable to show any further decline between age 75 and 79.

T.F. Williams: In our longitudinal study in Baltimore we found great variation in glomerular filtration rate. About a third of the subjects showed no change with age; in two-thirds there was variable change (Lindeman et al 1985).

Svanborg: It depends of course on one's definition of 'normality'. The definition we are now using is based on a follow-up of close to 15 years. This follow-up period has markedly changed our criteria for definable disease.

References

Altman R, Fries JF, Bloch DA et al 1987 Radiologic assessment of disease progression in osteoarthritis. Arth Rheum, in press
Lindeman RD, Tobin J, Shock N 1985 Longitudinal studies on rate of decline in renal function with age. J Am Geriatr Soc 33:278–285

Health and ageing in the developing world

Gary R. Andrews

Department of Primary Care and Community Medicine, Flinders University of South Australia, Bedford Park, South Australia 5062, Australia

Abstract. Although ageing is not yet a high priority issue for health planners, policy makers and clinicians in most developing countries there will be a growing need in coming years to pay more attention to the important health issues associated with population ageing in the developing world. This paper reports some of the relevant findings of a cross-national study (sponsored by the World Health Organization) of the health and social aspects of ageing in four developing countries — Republic of Korea, the Philippines, Fiji and Malaysia. The key findings are compared and contrasted with those of a similar eleven-country WHO study in Europe. In very broad terms, the overall demographic, physical, mental health and social patterns and trends associated with ageing as demonstrated by age-group and sex differences were consistent throughout the four countries studied. Comparisons with European findings in other similar studies underlined the fundamental universality of age-related changes in biophysical, behavioural and social characteristics. The importance of the family in developing countries was evident, with about three-quarters of those aged 60 and over in the four countries living with children, often in extended family situations. Levels of adverse health-related behaviour and the prospect of changing patterns of morbidity with further increases in the total and proportional numbers of aged persons point to a need for emphasis on preventive health measures and programmes directed to the maintenance of the physical and mental health of the ageing population.

1988 Research and the ageing population. Wiley, Chichester (Ciba Foundation Symposium 134) p 17–37

In Europe, in North America and in the developed world generally, the issues associated with health and population ageing have been increasingly subject to scientific inquiry. Literature on ageing and health has expanded at a rapidly escalating rate and policy makers and health service planners have accepted the importance of taking account of the ageing population in assessing health care needs and priorities. Data collection and research have increasingly been recognized as an essential underpinning of new directions in policy and planning (Maddox 1982).

Only very recently has the developing world been recognized as facing a

TABLE 1   World population projections[a]

Year	Total population (millions)	Population over 65 years (millions)	% over 65 years
Developing countries			
1980	3284	129	3.9
2000	4297	229	4.7
Developed countries			
1980	1131	129	11.4
2000	1272	167	13.2

[a] Source: Age and sex composition by population by country, 1960–2000. United Nations, New York, 1979

challenge in these respects of far greater total dimensions than that of the developed world. Demographers, and social scientists working in developing countries, have generally been overwhelmingly concerned with population growth issues, while policy makers and planners have been preoccupied with the daunting task of absorbing rapidly growing young populations (G. Hugo, unpublished working paper, 13th International Congress of Gerontology, July 1985). Health-care providers in the developing world have focused primarily on the problems of providing primary health care to young and rapidly growing populations, the treatment and prevention of infectious diseases, and health problems associated with poverty and malnutrition. In situations which have for many years been characterized by high infant and maternal mortality, diarrhoeal diseases and limited life expectancy, the health issues associated with ageing and the appearance of chronic disease and disability have only just emerged as matters to which attention should be paid (Schade & Apt 1983).

It is, however, in the future, especially in the developing countries of the world, that the challenge of ageing will be greatest in numerical terms, and where the institutional, financial, economic and manpower resources — already seriously extended — are least likely to be able to respond effectively without significant change in the allocation of resources and the direction of current policies (Binstock et al 1982).

As Jorge Tapia-Videla (1985) has pointed out, the search for solutions to the problems associated with the need to meet the health-care requirements of the elderly with efficiency, effectiveness and equity often reveals a need for the collection of basic data that will allow decision makers to use more rational approaches to dealing with the complex public policy questions involved. Valid, timely and relevant research is clearly required now if future policy and programme directions are to be guided by sound information rather than political rhetoric.

Tapia-Videla (1985) suggests that the range of information relevant to policy makers and administrators dealing with the health care of the elderly should include data collected '. . . for the purposes of:

(a)   Developing a general profile of the elderly population including, but not limited to, its age composition, sex distribution, levels of education, residence, income, and general socioeconomic conditions;

(b)   Describing the problems and needs affecting the target population, with special emphasis on those that influence its health status and general wellbeing;

(c)   Securing a comprehensive overview (listing/description) of available services (public and private) for meeting the problems or needs of the elderly;

(d)   Determining the types and levels of unmet needs (these might be produced by problems that are not met by existing programmes);

(e)   Devising, from the perspective of the elderly, a priority ranking of both needs and problems which may balance the views of the decision-makers and professionals, who tend to define the needs of the elderly population from the 'supply' perspective — too often with paternalistic overtones; and

(f)   Obtaining feedback on the operation, quality and impact of particular policies or programmes pertaining to the elderly population.'

Western Pacific Region Study

The Western Pacific Regional Office of the World Health Organization, in consultation with governments in the region, recognized a need to respond to these requirements for information on health and population ageing. The region is made up largely of developing countries experiencing rapid socioeconomic change. Most of the countries show a pattern of increasing urbanization, industrialization and technological and social change. Patterns of family structure are changing and traditional values, including those related to respect for the ageing and family responsibility for care of the elderly, are under increasing pressure. In these circumstances, in the face of significant proportional and absolute increases in the numbers of ageing in the population, the need for information on the likely impacts on demands for health and social services becomes urgent. In the first instance, and in response to these needs, a study of the social and health aspects of ageing in four countries, namely Malaysia, the Philippines, Republic of Korea (South Korea) and Fiji, was undertaken, sponsored by the Regional Office for the Western Pacific of WHO (Andrews et al 1986).

The demographic characteristics of the countries chosen for study were typical of developing countries generally in that the proportion of elderly is

TABLE 2   The ageing population in Fiji, Korea, Malaysia and the Philippines, 1980 and 2000[a] (in millions)

Age (years)	Fiji		Republic of Korea		Malaysia		Philippines	
	1980	2000	1980	2000	1980	2000	1980	2000
60+	0.03	0.06	2.4	4.8	0.8	1.4	2.2	4.6
Percentage	4.9	7.7	6.3	9.5	5.6	6.7	4.5	6.0
65+	0.02	0.04	1.5	3.1	0.5	0.9	1.4	3.0
Percentage	3.0	4.9	4.0	6.0	3.6	4.3	2.8	3.8
70+	0.01	0.02	0.9	1.8	0.3	0.5	0.7	1.7
Percentage	1.6	2.9	2.0	3.5	2.1	2.5	1.5	2.2

[a] Source: Demographic indicators of countries; estimates and projections as assessed in 1980. New York, United Nations.

still relatively small with significant growth anticipated to the year 2000 and beyond.

Random samples of the elderly population (defined as aged 60 and over) in selected urban and rural locations were obtained in each of the countries. The smallest sample was 796 (Fiji) and the largest 1000 (Malaysia). In the Philippines 927 subjects were interviewed and in Korea a sample of 947 was included.

The objectives determined for the study were as follows:

(1)   To increase awareness among researchers and policy makers of the issues associated with an ageing population;
(2)   To provide a pilot cross-sectional study using largely quantifiable techniques, in order to gain experience in undertaking such research in an Asian setting;
(3)   To generate provisional and indicative quantifiable information on which to base objectives for more intensive and specific investigations;
(4)   To move towards achieving a comprehensive data base on ageing for the Western Pacific region of the World Health Organization; and
(5)   To provide some information that will be relevant in the formulation of policies and provision of programmes to meet the needs of the ageing population.

The key objective was to achieve some concrete recommendations which could govern future action in the area of the health and social care of the elderly.

The questionnaire developed for the study included a total of 140 items. Questions were asked of the randomly selected subjects themselves, and of an informant who knew the subject (usually a close relative) and an assessment was made by the interviewer of the subject's social and economic resources, physical health, mental health and housing. The questions, which were carefully selected to minimize cultural bias, ranged across demographic, social and economic factors, physical health, activities of daily living, health behaviour and mental health.

The results of the surveys in each of the four countries were processed and analysed in Adelaide, under my supervision. A more detailed description of the methodology and results of the study has been published (Andrews et al 1986). The data was also subject to Grade of Membership (GOM) analysis (Manton et al 1987).

In 1979–1980 the Regional Office for Europe of WHO initiated a cross-national study of the elderly in fifteen centres in ten European countries (Heikkinen et al 1983). In addition, Kuwait, which is in another WHO region, joined the study. Approximately 1200 elderly subjects were interviewed. Various sampling designs were used by different study centres, depending upon the resources and the availability of a reasonable sampling frame. The questionnaire covered health, functional ability, living conditions, way of life and the use of services. It was possible, in the case of identical (or nearly so) wording of questionnaire items, to make some comparisons between the European findings, consisting largely of developed countries, and those of the Western Pacific Region study.

I shall focus here on the findings relating to physical and mental health, functional ability, and family support in the four Western Pacific countries and draw attention to the comparison (where results are available) between these findings and those of the study carried out in Europe.

Physical health and functional abilities

In our Western Pacific study we used several approaches to evaluate the health of the study population, including asking respondents to assess their overall health status; inquiring about past accidents or injuries and the presence of chronic illness, and the relationship between these conditions and functional abilities; the application of a standard symptoms list; and an assessment of their ability to perform activities of daily living.

The classically age-related problems of impaired hearing, poor sight, difficulties in chewing and reduced mobility were encountered with increasing prevalence with advanced age, attesting to the universality of the biophysical manifestations of ageing (Table 3).

Overall, however, the impression was one of relatively robust health among the subjects in our study. In terms of activities of daily living, the study revealed that the great majority of subjects were able to undertake the basic tasks effectively. The ability to cope with activities of daily living (ADL) was

TABLE 3 The percentage of people in each country with various health problems, by age and sex

Type of problem/country	Men			Women			Total		
	75	75+	Total	75	75+	Total	75	75+	Total
Hearing problem									
Fiji	21	33	24	19	38	24	20	36	24
Rep. of Korea	18	25	19	14	32	18	16	29	18
Malaysia	15	32	18	10	22	12	12	27	15
Philippines	18	44	23	16	37	20	17	40	21
Sight problem									
Fiji	76	70	75	70	76	72	73	73	73
Rep. of Korea	31	39	32	31	49	35	31	45	33
Malaysia	64	84	67	67	76	69	65	80	68
Philippines	78	83	79	83	82	82	81	82	81
Difficulty walking 300 metres									
Fiji	38	55	42	35	68	43	36	62	42
Rep. of Korea	15	19	15	10	30	14	13	25	15
Malaysia	8	29	12	13	35	17	11	32	15
Philippines	18	44	23	25	52	30	22	48	27
Difficulty chewing									
Fiji	57	58	57	55	66	58	56	62	57
Rep. of Korea	60	63	60	59	76	63	60	71	62
Malaysia	49	56	60	43	64	47	46	60	48
Philippines	29	51	33	32	33	32	31	42	33

assessed by asking twelve questions. The results from two questions (usage of the telephone and ability to prepare meals) were hard to interpret across cultures and so these questions were dropped from the subsequent analysis. The remaining questions fell into two categories. The first category concerned questions relating to basic bodily functions (physical ADL) — eating, dressing and undressing, caring for personal appearance, walking, getting in and out of bed, taking a bath or shower, and getting to the toilet in time. The second group pertained to activities related to independent residence in the community (instrumental ADL) — travelling beyond walking distance, shopping, and handling one's own money. These categories were combined and a simple additive score was created with a value of 10 for those who could perform all ADL activities with help, and zero for those who could perform none of them without help. The internal reliability of the scale (over all countries combined) was high.

Contrary to the stereotyped view that the elderly are incapacitated and therefore unable to control their lives, most subjects were able without help to carry out all of the ten tasks about which they were asked. In the Republic of Korea, 71% of people were able to accomplish all ADL. In Fiji, 82% of subjects said that they were able to accomplish all ADL, 8% had difficulty carrying out one activity, and 10% had trouble with more than one. In particular, personal care, dressing and eating were not common problems. Difficulties with shopping and getting to the toilet were more frequently encountered.

The subjects were asked if they had any disease, injury, accident, or long-term health problem or illness that affected their daily activities. In Fiji, the older respondents were affected more often than younger ones; 55% of men and 52% of women aged 60–64 years stated that they had a health problem that interfered with everyday life, compared with 69% of men and 71% of women aged 80 years or more. Rural residents were more likely to report a health problem than urban residents (68% compared with 47%).

In the Republic of Korea, where just over 40% of respondents reported a health problem which affected activities of daily living, and in Malaysia, where the figure was about 35%, there was no association between this variable and sex or urban/rural distribution. Age trends for these two countries were noted only for Malaysian men; the proportion of men with health problems increased with age, except among the 70–74 years age group.

Although Filipinos reported higher levels of satisfaction with their health status than the other countries, they also had the highest prevalence of health problems. Two-thirds of Filipinos indicated that they had accidents, injuries or chronic illnesses that impinged on their functional ability. The prevalence of these problems increased with age, from 64% for men and 52% for women aged 60–64 years, to about 74% for both men and women over 79 years of age.

In general, these rates were lower than those reported in the European study, though in both studies there was quite wide variation between countries.

Health and wellbeing in any population group are concepts not easily separated from a large set of interacting factors, including economic and social circumstances, environmental conditions and living arrangements, as well as physical and mental health status. The subjective evaluation of an individual's own health is therefore a complex issue and must be interpreted with care. In response to a basic set of questions about self-perceived healthfulness, at least half the subjects in all four countries studied described themselves as healthy. There were no consistent age trends but overall more women than men described themselves as healthy (64% compared with 53%). By contrast, in the European study findings, women reported a poorer view of their health than men at all ages. In general the European subjects had a more negative view of their health at all ages, and for both sexes, than the subjects in our study (Andrews et al 1986). (Fig. 1.)

The impression of better health and fitness, particularly when compared

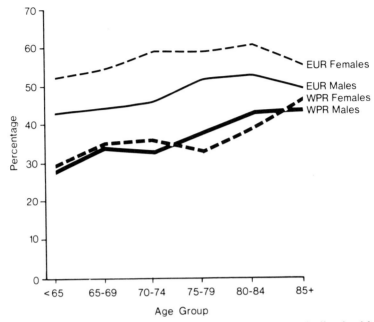

FIG. 1.   The percentage of the population who report not feeling healthy.

with findings in European and North American Surveys, might give rise to optimism about ageing in developing countries. Evans (1986), however, has pointed out that other studies have shown that this is no cause for discounting the impact of ageing in the future. With improved social, environmental and health services, the infirm and disabled among an ageing population can be expected to show a significant improvement in survival, so that among the ageing generally a higher proportion than at present will exhibit disability and accompanying dependence.

In broad terms the classic pattern — decline in physical health and functional abilities — associated with ageing seems to be universal, and the differing prevalence of overt failure in these capacities between countries, and especially between developing and developed countries, seems more likely to reflect differing survival rates rather than any inherent biological or other advantage. The analysis of the data from the Western Pacific study using GOM methods also demonstrates similarities between developed and developing countries in basic age, sex, morbidity and disability associations (Manton et al 1987).

Mental health

Mental health was assessed in this study by applying a simple portable mental health status assessment, including a set of standardized simple tests of cognitive functions, and enquiring about the presence or absence of a range of mental symptoms. In addition, an informant (usually a relative of the responder) was asked about mental functioning and especially any noted change in behaviour. As in the case of physical health, the study population in general showed minimal decline in mental functioning.

The analysis of mental symptoms revealed generally that forgetfulness, feelings of depression, tiredness, worry and anxiety, apathy and sleep difficulties were not uncommon findings, but evidence of any overt mental illness was rarely encountered.

While the findings on cognitive function should be interpreted with care, in general in all four countries consistent patterns emerged which demonstrated an association between age and cognitive function (Table 4).

The findings of our study thus suggest that the developed countries' experience of an increasing incidence of dementia with very advanced age may be duplicated in the developing world. This is an area where more in-depth and specific research would be well justified. Given the demographic projections, the impact of a substantial burden of dementia on family, community and government resources would have major consequences (Andrews & Davidson 1984).

Health-related behaviour

In both the Western Pacific and European studies questions were asked about smoking and drinking habits. Overall rates of smoking were quite high, with Western Pacific subjects being shown to be about twice as likely to smoke as those in the European Study. Men in both studies were found to be about twice as likely to smoke as women. There was some variation between countries in our study. The percentage of males currently smoking were: Fiji (45%), the Republic of Korea (61%), Malaysia (44%) and the Philippines (40%). Comparative figures for women were Fiji (37%), the Republic of Korea (36%), Malaysia (19%) and the Philippines (28%).

Reported alcohol consumption showed great variation between countries in the Western Pacific study, reflecting cultural differences in drinking behaviour and in the social, medicinal and ritual use of alcohol. Men were more likely to drink than women and the overall frequency of drinking among the Western Pacific subjects was comparable with the European findings. In the Western Pacific, drinking rates for men were Fiji (76%), the Republic of Korea (53%), Malaysia (13%) and the Philippines (28%). For females the rates were Fiji (54%), the Republic of Korea (27%), Malaysia (7%) and the Philippines (8%). A small but significant minority of subjects in all countries reported that their families complained that their consumption was excessive.

There is evidently a case in developing countries for emphasizing the promotion of healthy behaviour among the ageing, and for achieving wider

TABLE 4 The percentage of people in each country with good cognitive function (> 10/14), by age and sex

Country	Men				Women				Total			
	70	70–79	80+	Total	70	70–79	80+	Total	70	70–79	80+	Total
Fiji	85	72	64	78	72	66	24	64	79	70	44	72
Republic of Korea	66	59	52	62	58	32	17	44	62	47	30	53
Malaysia	92	84	56	85	83	63	44	72	87	75	50	79
Philippines	94	91	66	91	93	88	63	88	93	89	64	90

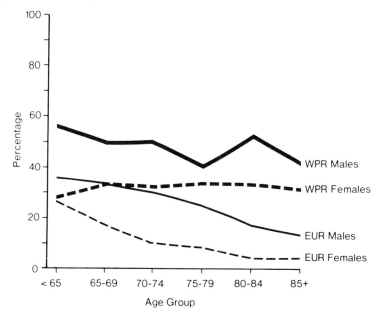

FIG. 2.   The percentage of the population who smoke cigarettes regularly.

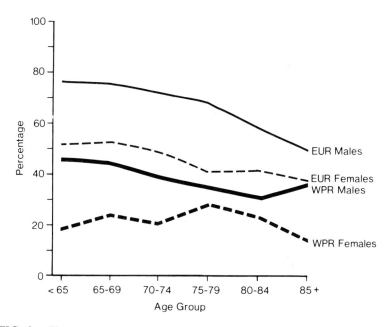

FIG. 3.   The percentage of the population who drink alcohol regularly.

TABLE 5   The percentage of people in each country living with their children, by age and sex

Country	Men			Women			Total		
	<75	75+	Total	<75	75+	Total	<75	75+	Total
Fiji	77	68	75	76	72	75	76	70	75
Republic of Korea	67	74	69	75	76	75	71	75	72
Malaysia	73	67	72	71	62	69	72	64	71
Philippines	80	70	78	78	70	77	79	70	77

recognition of the consequences, even in advanced age, of the adverse health effects associated with smoking and excessive drinking.

Family support

One of the most striking aspects of our findings was the degree to which the elderly are a completely integral part of family structure. Whereas in developed countries a relatively high proportion of those over 60 live alone, this was very uncommon in the Western Pacific countries studied — 5% in the Philippines and 2% in the other countries. Between 70 and 80% of the elderly in the four countries live with their children. In addition, quite a high proportion (more than 50%) were living in households of five or more people (Tables 5 and 6).

Children, and to a lesser extent other family members, are clearly a

TABLE 6   The percentage of people in each country living with others, by sex and urban/rural distribution

Number of people lived with/country	Urban residents			Rural residents		
	Men	Women	Total	Men	Women	Total
Fiji						
0–4	32	27	29	25	32	28
4+	68	3	71	75	68	72
Republic of Korea						
0–4	30	32	31	45	27	40
4+	70	68	69	55	63	60
Malaysia						
0–4	34	33	33	51	49	50
4+	70	68	69	55	63	60
Philippines						
0–4	24	26	25	44	44	44
4+	76	74	75	56	56	56

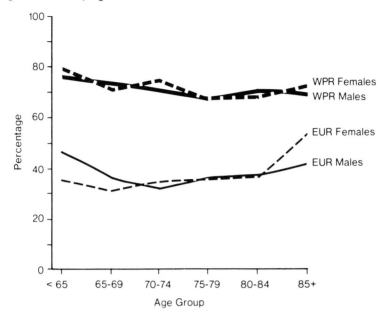

FIG. 4. The percentage of the population who live with their children.

substantial source of support for the ageing in their populations. While this appears to be especially so in developing countries, the same pattern has been demonstrated recently in developed countries (Kendig et al 1983). The importance of the family in developed countries, in contrast to formal non-family-oriented community and institutional care, has been increasingly acknowledged in the development of programmes. More emphasis is now being given in developed countries to the provision of respite services, day care and other arrangements which support the family carers of the elderly in their central role. Much of this change in focus is aimed at correcting the over-emphasis in the past on placing the elderly in institutions when family caring and support arrangements finally broke down under persistent pressure. Often the primary focus was on one person, usually a daughter or daughter-in-law (Kinnear & Graycar 1984). Now the aim is to give greater emphasis to programmes aimed at providing support for the elderly and their families in the community.

There is a real opportunity in developing countries for recognition of the family's central role and for policy and planning decisions to reflect the degree to which the caring role of family members is vital to the wellbeing and independence of the elderly (Chen 1984). These issues become increasingly important with the growing number of the aged in populations as a consequence of increased life expectancy. Apart from supporting services, positive incentives through taxation concessions or other means may be appropriate in

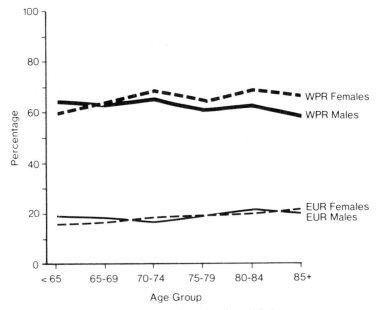

FIG. 5.   The percentage of the population who live with four or more other people.

the future. It should not generally be assumed that all old people in developing countries will have children available to look after them. Smaller families, childless marriages, and an increasing proportion of women going out to work mean that it will not always be possible for the elderly in need of care to be provided for through the family. In addition, urban housing policies are frequently not conducive to multigenerational living arrangements.

Conclusions

Although ageing is still not a very high priority issue for health planners, policy makers and clinicians in developing countries, there will be a growing need in coming years to pay much greater attention to the increasingly important health consequences associated with population ageing in these countries.

If the impact of population ageing on health-care needs is recognized, governments might be able to avoid the mistakes made in the Western developed world, where there is evidence of over-dependence in the past on institutional rather than community solutions to provide support for the aged, and where the importance of the informal family- and community-based support arrangements has been neglected.

To assist planners and others to respond effectively to the emerging requirements of the elderly, there is a need first for basic data collection and research to underpin the development of national policies and programmes. Given the close relationships between physical health, mental health and socioeconomic factors in ageing populations, a multidisciplinary approach seems appropriate. The developing countries of the world provide an extraordinarily rich variety of cultural, political, socioeconomic and geographic characteristics in which to undertake cross-national studies. These could provide information that will be comparable between countries and will allow the exploration of the significance of tradition, culture, ethnicity and other variables in the individual expression of ageing.

The key role played by the family in the care of the aged in developing countries should be acknowledged and programmes should be developed, particularly at local community level, which encourage and support families in their traditional role. There is also a clear need to emphasize preventive health-care measures and programmes directed to the maintenance of physical and mental health of the ageing population. This will minimize the otherwise inevitable burden of disability and handicap that will follow the significant increases in the absolute and proportional numbers of aged in the population.

References

Andrews GR, Esterman AS, Braunack-Mayer AJ, Rungie CM 1986 Ageing in the Western Pacific — A four country study. Western Pacific Reports and Studies No. 1. WHO Regional Office for the Western Pacific, Manila

Andrews GR, Davidson AH 1984 Ageing and dementia in the developing world — a challenge for the future. In: Wertheimer J, Marois M (eds) Senile dementia: outlook for the future. Alan R Liss, New York, p. 479–490 (Modern aging research, vol 5)

Binstock RH, Chow WS, Schulz JH (eds) 1982 International perspectives on ageing: population and policy challenges. United Nations Fund for Population Activities, New York

Chen PCY 1984 Editorial: The elderly Malaysian. Med J Malaysia 39. p 254–256

Evans J 1986 The development of handicap with ageing in Australia and Indonesia. In: Everitt A (ed) Australia in an ageing world. Australian Association of Gerontology (Proc 20th Annual Conference, Melbourne, 1985) p 27–33

Heikkinen E, Waters WE, Brzesinski ZJ (eds) 1983 The elderly in eleven countries — a sociomedical survey. World Health Organization Regional Office for Europe, Copenhagen

Kendig HL, Gibson DM, Rowland DT, Hemer JM 1983 Health, welfare and family in later life. Canberra. Ageing and the Family Project. Australian National University. NSW Council on the Ageing, Sydney

Kinnear D, Graycar A 1984 Ageing and family dependency. Aust J Social Issues 19:13–26

Maddox G 1982 Ageing people and ageing populations. A framework for decision making. In: Thomae H, Maddox G (eds) New perspectives on old age: A message to decision makers. Springer-Verlag, New York

Manton KG, Myers GC, Andrews GR 1987 Morbidity and disability patterns in four developing nations: their implications for social and economic integration of the elderly. J Cross-Cultural Gerontology, in press

Schade B, Apt NA 1983 Ageing in developing countries. In: Bergener M et al (eds) Ageing in the eighties and beyond. (Highlights of the Twelfth International Congress of Gerontology, 1981, Hamburg) Springer-Verlag, New York
Tapia-Videla JI 1985 The use of special surveys of health needs of elderly populations as a basis for establishing policies and plans. Rapp Trimest Statist Sanit Mond 28:76–90

DISCUSSION

A. Williams: I am interested in the relationship between people's self-assessed health (and their perceptions of what aspects of their health are important), and objective measures of their health. I should therefore like to know what it is exactly that your old people express concern about; what their expectations about their health are; and whether some of the features that they report to you are very salient in their health perceptions, whilst others are accepted as not interfering with their lives.

Andrews: Self-assessments of health appear to correlate highly with objective measures of health and physical activities of daily living, in most studies, in developed and developing countries. We asked a series of questions in relation to self-perceived health, including direct questions, such as 'do you feel healthy or unhealthy?', 'how do you rate your health compared with others of your age?', and so on. There was an extremely high correlation between the answers on all variations of this question, so there seems to be no need to ask more than one question of this kind. Just what the answers mean in terms of what the individuals consider important is a question that deserves more study. I have no answer, from our findings; but you are right that there might be surprises in terms of what the elderly individuals will accept as good and poor health in themselves.

Mor: It has been my experience, from the literature on health-services research, that the most important correlates of self-assessed perception of health are functional parameters, such as the activities of daily living; that is, the performance of those activities that people define as essential to their quality of life. There is a much lower correlation between self-assessed health and the ratings of physicians (and/or the presence of specific diseases).

T.F. Williams: From your results, Dr Andrews, it seems that older people in the Philippines reported less loss of function in the activities of daily living than in the other three countries, even out to the very late years of life.

Andrews: Some of the flaws in our survey become apparent here. The sampling approach used in the Philippines meant that the results there were biased towards the fitter elderly population. That was in part a result of the difficulties of doing such an exercise in the Philippines at a time of some political turmoil, and partly difficulties in the approach taken by the project team to the sampling exercise. This was better in the other three countries. So the apparent difference here may be due to the methodological problems of doing the survey.

Wenger: Were you able to ascertain any different expectations of health among elderly people when you compared the European and Western Pacific populations? What was it that they expected to be able to do if they were healthy? And did these expectations relate to the availability or accessibility of health care to the populations?

Andrews: We had the general impression that older people in these four countries were more accepting of the hazards and problems of life—including the acceptance of some degree of failure of health in old age—than are people in Europe; but it was only an impression. Perhaps we can look at the data and find support for this impression.

On your second question, there was much variation, particularly between urban and rural areas, in the provision and utilization of health care, but we couldn't show that the provision of medical services in particular related to health status. There is evidence of a significant degree of undetected and untreated impairment, particularly in sight, hearing, chewing difficulties, and perhaps mobility. It seems that most of the medical services that are provided to these elderly populations don't focus on these problems. This raises questions about future directions for health services in developing countries, particularly as populations age.

Wenger: Different societal attitudes toward physical and mental health obviously influence people's perceptions of their personal health. Were there any major differences, in the four countries you studied, in attitudes toward illness, mental or physical, and did that alter health perceptions?

Andrews: We didn't ask those general attitudinal questions; it is something we should do. I think there are likely to be expressed differences cross-nationally, given the cultural, religious and traditional value systems of these countries, but it would require an in-depth investigation to establish the significance of such different responses.

Solomons: It is perhaps hard to think of the Republic of Korea as a developing country now, and a better definition of the First and Third Worlds might be based on a distinction between agrarian countries and urbanized, industrialized countries. Another possible analysis would be to do some tracking of individuals with regard to changes between rural and urban life by your subjects, or absence of such change, to see whether the microenvironment in which a person lives within a country is more influential than the overall national character. It is interesting that the highest per capita income in the world is still in Saudi Arabia; there is a lot of money per capita, but most of those heads are still on bedouins in rural areas!

Andrews: We recorded the information that would allow us to do that kind of analysis. We did not find such striking differences in findings when we did urban/rural comparisons as we might have expected.

Solomons: Perhaps all your older people in these countries were actually in rural environments in their formative years. This might limit the differences to be expected.

Andrews: That is partly true. South Korea is certainly a fascinating country to study, because it's on the same development course as Japan, and in fact is probably becoming Japan's major if not only competitor in economic development terms.

Solomons: You estimated the percentage of people over 60 in 1980 in the four countries of the Western Pacific as between 5 and 6%. In Guatemala we estimate that about 6% of the population are over 60 years.

A point to remember is that people in these developing countries have experienced all sorts of violence from themselves and others over the years, and that has helped to eliminate sectors of the population that died from unnatural causes during the lifespans of the people now being studied.

It is conventional to compare people of 80–90 years in one society with persons of the same *chronological* age in another, in terms of health and morbidity. One wonders whether this is a legitimate strategy. It might be that comparisons are best made in comparable phases of the lifespan in terms of expected mortality. If 30% of the cumulative mortality of a given birth cohort is between 40 and 60 years in one society and between 60 and 80 years in another, perhaps we should not compare the status of octagenarians between societies. We might better compare the 60-year-olds in the former group with the 80-year-olds in the latter.

Finally, thinking of comparative studies, there is much to be learned where the 'ecological systems' over a lifetime are quite different. In Guatemala, for instance, the intake of calcium is about 2–4 grams per day over a life time. The diseases that are presumably related to calcium intake, such as colon cancer (Newmark et al 1984), hypertension (Villar et al 1986), and bone disease (Recker & Hearney 1985), might be interesting to look at in elderly people in different ecological systems over a life time.

Andrews: Elderly populations in developing countries are changing enormously and very rapidly. In our 'old old' groups in particular we are looking at an elite group of survivors.

Riggs: A three-day diet record, either by recall or by keeping a diary, would be a reasonable way of assessing nutritional state in these developing countries.

Solomons: Another interesting nutritional investigation is suggested by the following. In the USA there is still a generation reared very largely by bottle-feeding; we now seem to have reverted to breast-feeding again. But in Guatemala, and most parts of the Third World, women have never left breast-feeding. That is potentially a very major nutritional variable. We have in the USA an ageing cohort with artificial feeding as the early dietary practice in which we can dissect, perhaps, the influence of bottle-feeding as a determinant of the later ageing process, morbidity pattern and mortality.

This leads to another consideration, namely the differential risk of a specific dietary practice at different ages. Take meat-eating and anaemia. We have societies in the world that consume huge amounts of meat, giving their people plenty of available iron. This protects them in early life from the anaemia that is frequently found in societies that are largely vegetarian in their dietary practices. Iron from plant foods is poorly utilized. Over a certain period of the lifespan there will be a great difference between omnivorous and vegetarian individuals, in favour of the meat-eaters being less anaemic. If we accept the indications that consumption of meat, and its fat, helps to initiate colon cancer, we shall eventually find a cross-over with increasing age in which colon cancer will begin to emerge in the meat-eaters. The formerly anaemic vegetarians— but now non-anaemic older people—will now be being relatively protected from colonic neoplasia by their life-long dietary practices. Thus, the different countries might not be found to be equally afflicted with specific age-related diseases, when compared cross-nationally, and early dietary influences are one possible factor.

White: In looking at cross-sectional data like yours, Dr Andrews, one wonders what the results would be like if it had been a longitudinal survey. Is it feasible to do longitudinal studies in elderly populations in developing countries?

Andrews: If the resources were there, I think one could mount a longitudinal study with no more difficulty than anywhere else.

Solomons: It is overly optimistic to think that doing effective longitudinal studies of the health of older people in Third World countries is purely a matter of more money. Thinking of the migration of people from the countryside into urban areas, and of following up people after they have migrated, in Guatemala City most poorer people do not even have an address, because streets and houses are not numbered. The logistics of following those people would be impossible.

White: An important question is that of selective survival. Because a smaller proportion of people have survived the forces of mortality in childhood and adult life, the older people that you questioned may be much more highly 'selected' than most of the older people that we study in more developed countries. Yet it is surprising to find little evidence of that selectivity in differential health and functioning at older ages.

Andrews: It's not entirely true that in these developing countries populations at various ages show the same degree of decline in function that is found in studies of the elderly in developed countries. They show the same pattern; but when we compare our results with the European findings, for instance, our older Asian populations were significantly fitter and healthier. They showed the same picture with increasing age, but less severely.

White: Have you considered comparing selective survival among these countries, perhaps by studying patterns of age and cause of death of siblings? This approach might allow one to postulate differences among countries with regard to the differential impact of selective survival in determining the characteristics of older people.

Andrews: We haven't done that. Jeremy Evans in Canberra has done a similar type of study in Indonesia, comparing Australian and Indonesian populations. I don't think he has looked at siblings, but he has used the available census data, mortality and morbidity data, and survey data, to try to analyse the question of differential longevity in these populations. His results suggest that those who demonstrate various disabilities earlier on have higher mortality rates. As these populations show increased life expectancy, the survival of those with disability may be proportionally greater.

Katzman: I have recently consulted with a group of psychiatrists in Shanghai who are doing a very similar study to yours. They have now surveyed 4500 individuals over the age of 55, including 1500 over 75. Something that concerns me is the interpretation of the mental status examination; I think you use a variant of the Mini Mental Status (MMS), which they use also. The Shanghai study intended to go on to clinical diagnosis of those with impaired functions, as shown by the MMS score. They ran into a problem which you also pointed out, namely that the results of the mental status test are confounded by the complete lack of education in a significant number of the elderly. Many of the uneducated subjects could not read a simple phrase 'close your eyes', or copy intersecting pentagons, whereas they were well oriented to time and place and did well on memory tests. Can one do anything other than divide up the population into those who are educated and those who are not, and look at the question of dementia in each group separately? If we do that in Shanghai, we may find that cognitive impairment in those with some education is lower than in the West.

Andrews: We found quite a high correlation between cognitive performance and years of education in all four countries, for all the subjects interviewed. The women did significantly less well than men on cognitive tests, and this may be related to their lower level of education than that of men in those countries. We tried to correct for educational level in the analysis and still found some cognitive decline with age, but it was less than appeared at first to be the case.

Arie: I'd like to take up Dr Katzman's point and generalize it a little. As someone inexperienced in work in the Third World, I would expect the difficulties in eliciting uniform information in such diverse cultures to be massive. When I think of the problems that we had, in making our Nottingham survey, of looking at life satisfaction and social engagement in a community with which we are very familiar, the difficulties in these Third World countries seem immense. Dr Katzman spoke about measuring cognitive function. We know the pitfalls that can result from variations in educational level in relation to the tests of that. Can you say more about this? Evidently you surmounted many of these problems.

Andrews: We felt eventually that although the problems were substantial they were no more or no less so than the problems of doing this sort of work in developed countries; the methodological problems of knowing exactly what you are dealing with are of the same general order.

Arie: How did you set about conferring with local people about the sort of questions you should be asking?

Andrews: We used local people to do the surveys, in fact, in each of the four countries. The questionnaire was worked over very thoroughly by those people, almost all of whom had good postgraduate Western training. Nonetheless, they had evidently retained a feeling for and sensitivity to the local circumstances. There were also field supervisors recruited locally with direct experience of working in their local settings. It was certainly difficult to define social interaction, and so on, and many of our questions were, I suspect, inappropriate. Yet we found much the same patterns as have been reported in developed countries. The answers to many of the attitudinal questions followed precisely the patterns found in the Western literature of an association between various attitudes, the involvement of elderly people in decision making within the family, and so on, and age.

Arie: I was interested to see that your figures for people who describe themselves as lonely seem to be just about the same in your four developing countries (15–20%) as they are in Nottingham. In our sample of old people, just over 17% described themselves as lonely. You found no relationship between being lonely and whether people were actually living on their own (only 2–5% in your four countries over the age of 60). The great majority of our 'lonely' old people do live alone, in Nottingham. That difference is interesting, and it raises all sorts of questions. Does 'feeling lonely' mean the same to your Third World people as it does to ours? Why did so many more of your people who weren't living alone feel lonely? It would be interesting to discover the answers.

References

Evans J 1986 The development of handicap with ageing in Australia and Indonesia. In: Everitt A (ed) Australia in an ageing world. Australian Association of Gerontology (Proc 20th Annual Conference, Melbourne, 1985) p 27–33

Newmark HL, Wargovich MJ, Bruce WR 1984 Colon cancer and dietary fat, phosphate, and calcium: a hypothesis. J Natl Cancer Inst 72:1323–1325

Recker RR, Heaney RP 1985 The effect of milk supplements on calcium metabolism, bone metabolism and calcium balance. Am J Clin Nutr 41:254–263

Villar J, Repke J, Belizan JM 1986 Calcium and blood pressure. Clin Nutr 5:153–160

Ageing and disease

J. Grimley Evans

Nuffield Department of Clinical Medicine, Geriatric Medicine Division, Radcliffe Infirmary, Oxford OX2 8HE, UK

Abstract. The concept of disease has a long and changing history, and has accumulated implications that can be unhelpful. The traditional distinction made between 'normal ageing' and 'disease' identifies research into the impact of an ageing population as having arisen within clinical medicine with its tradition of dichotomous thinking. The model is inappropriate for clinical practice among the elderly where diseases should be relegated to the role of mechanisms producing functional problems, and where interventions may not be of the traditional medical form. In this context the concept of 'normal ageing' can act as an excuse for inaction. For gerontological research the basic model is of the interaction between extrinsic and intrinsic factors. We lack the means at present to identify intrinsic processes, although they may be found among the residual ageing effects when extrinsic processes have been excluded. Intrinsic ageing processes may ultimatedly be identifiable on the basis of biological theory. Until this is possible we should study age-associated phenomena without prematurely conceived notions about their origins.

1988 Research and the ageing population. Wiley, Chichester (Ciba Foundation Symposium 134) p 38–57

The relationship between 'ageing' and 'disease' is both a practical and a philosophical issue. At a practical level 'disease' is accepted as comprising phenomena that are the proper and indeed obligatory concern of the doctor, and a 'disease' entitles its victim to sympathy and social support, subject to the constraints of his fulfilling the sundry obligations of the 'sick role'. 'Ageing', to the common mind, is the universal ineluctable and unameliorable lot of mankind, entitling its victim to no particular sympathy and not qualifying him or her for medical attention. Indeed, those victims who attempt to conceal or prevent the ravages of ageing may bring onto their heads the obloquy reserved for those who exhibit pretensions to qualities — in this case, youth — that they do not possess. Those who struggle to overcome the impairments of disease, in contrast, are admired for their courage in adversity.

At a philosophical level the issue is complex. The doctor's rejection of the ravages of ageing as his proper concern is derived from his concepts of disease and of his social role. Both these concepts merit examination. But there are as many philosophies as there are philosophers, who are in general little better than ordinary mortals in declaring the premises from which they argue. In empiricism we can fuse the world of the practical with that of philosophy. In the specific context of the medical sciences, words should be used as labels for concepts that are defined in such a way as to be heuristically useful. Confusion is inevitable if we use words that do not refer to definable concepts or refer ambiguously to several different concepts.

Whatever its ancient implications, the modern concept of disease began with systematic clinical descriptions and autopsy findings relating symptoms to specific pathological findings. Diseases could be differentiated and named in terms of their pathological correlates. Later, nosology put down its roots in aetiology rather than pathology and grew in the fertile context of the nineteenth-century discoveries of infectious agents. The resulting model of a disease definable and diagnosable in terms of a single necessary and sufficient cause was clearly of immense heuristic value, but its fruit has been the persistent idea that a human condition which lacks such a characterizing agent is a phenomenon of a fundamentally different nature from a disease and invites a different response from doctors who encounter it.

By the end of the nineteenth century the doctrine of single necessary and sufficient causes had to be modified because of the observation that not everyone exposed to a necessary agent contracted disease. This was the era of the 'seed and ground' model which retained the concept of the single necessary cause but recognized that this was not always sufficient to cause disease unless it encountered an individual rendered susceptible by other factors. A virtue of this model was that it identified the possibilities for preventing disease by attacking the factors determining susceptibility, as well as by removing the necessary cause.

In economically advanced nations, the twentieth century has seen the rout of the ancient infections and the emergence of chronic diseases as the main preoccupation of medical practice. For many of these, particularly cardiovascular diseases, attempts to identify a single necessary cause have failed. We now work to a multifactorial model of such diseases in which specific pathological mechanisms of symptoms and impairments are seen as the final common pathway of a wide variety of possible causal chains. The 'disease' — for example, coronary heart disease or stroke — is defined in terms of its pathology, as it would have been in the early nineteenth century. But the concept of disease has changed, for we now recognize that not everyone who has the pathologically defined disease has any symptom or impairment. We have also been forced to concede that the distinction between the 'diseased' and the 'healthy' may be quantitative rather than qualitative. This issue was first raised in its most explicit form in the notorious debate between Sir George Pickering and Sir Robert Platt over the nature of hypertension. The idea of continuous distributions of physiopathological variables, with associated risk functions, is now one of the basic modes of epidemiological thought, and although introduced into clinical medicine by Pickering has not flourished there. The reason perhaps has to do with the exigencies of clinical practice, in which, however complex the reasoning and data appraisal, the final output has to be a dichotomous decision — do something or do nothing. These two options are rationalized in the traditional medical formula so that 'do something' corresponds to 'the patient has a disease' whereas 'do nothing' is rationalized as 'the patient is normal'. This equation opens the way to a further aspect of the clinical concept of disease, which now comes to comprise, to quote a United Kingdom Mental Health Act, 'that which requires or is susceptible to medical treatment'.

For historical reasons the study of human ageing grew out of clinical rather than scientific medicine. An anonymous editorialist in *The Lancet* (Editorial 1985) has declared that geriatric medicine came into the world because of the hardness of men's hearts and the unwillingness of the medical establishment to accept responsibility for the inmates of the Workhouse Hospitals that the British National Health Service inherited in 1948. Because geriatric medicine began as a clinical speciality it adopted clinical modes of thought. With a few recent exceptions, textbooks of geriatric medicine exhort their readers to distinguish 'disease' from 'normal' ageing. Without exception, textbooks then fail to offer any definition of normal ageing that bears scrutiny. Indeed it is not difficult to detect in the literature of geriatric medicine a glorious confusion between at least three different meanings of 'normal'. There is, for example, no reason to suppose that what occurs normally in the sense of frequently is necessarily normal in the sense of being optimal for health, and even less reason to suppose that whatever is normal will be distributed normally, in the sense of a Gaussian function around the population mean. In fact, to draw a distinction between disease and normal ageing is to attempt to separate the undefined from the indefinable.

There are inadequacies in traditional clinical thought and organization revealed by the challenge of an ageing population. The 'disease model', in which a single diagnosis implies a treatment of conventional medical form, will not produce the best outcome for a patient with several impairments whose effects in terms of disability are determined by complex social and economic modulators (Jette & Branch 1985). Rather than regarding the diagnosis of disease as the first aim of care, the clinician dealing with an elderly patient has to give primacy to identifying, in functional terms, the patient's problems and analysing how they have been produced. Typically these problems relate to discrepancies between what the physical and social environment demands of an individual and what he or she is able to do, or between what an individual wants to do and what he or she is able to do. In the context of this approach, which requires the specification of objectives of care and the identification of intervention options in order to determine a management plan, 'diseases' are displaced from their traditional dominant

TABLE 1   Sources of differences between young and old individuals

True ageing	Primary	Intrinsic
		Extrinsic
	Secondary	Individual
		Species
Non-ageing	Selective survival	
	Cohort effects	
	Differential challenge	

role in clinical thought. Very often, medical treatment of an impairment or symptom is part of an approach designed to ease a patient's difficulties, but it is rarely the only action necessary and a disease should rarely appear on a primary problem list. Words can be our masters as well as our servants, and as long as medical students are taught to try to distinguish between 'disease', which is a medical responsibility, and 'normal ageing', which by implication is not, so long will elderly people continue to suffer unnecessary hardship.

Health services research, which can be defined, if somewhat restrictively, as concerned with the efficiency and effectiveness in a particular mode of delivery of interventions that have been shown to be effective in other modes, is clearly one important aspect of our response to an ageing population. But research into ageing itself is also crucial. For this we need a model of ageing that retains a relevance to clinical problems, is intellectually coherent and is heuristically valuable. One model is set out in Table 1. It starts, as most gerontological research does, from a comparison of young and old individuals. The basic concept of ageing is loss of adaptability with time, and the first step in deriving the model is to distinguish the effects of true ageing — that is to say, those differences between young and old that have come about because the old people have changed as they grew older — from those differences due to measurement bias or to the particular old people under study having always been different from the young people in the comparison.

Three of the processes that can be identified as possible contributors to non-ageing differences between young and old contemporaries are listed in Table 1. *Differential survival* is a phenomenon that has been widely suspected but is difficult to detect in the human. Barrett (1985, 1986) has found evidence of selective survival of the very fit among men in the eleventh decade of life when mortality rates fall rather than continuing their inexorable rise, characteristic of ageing. In order to identify specific factors undergoing selection by differential survival, we would wish to compare those members of a birth cohort who survive beyond the ninth decade, say, with those who die before then. For obvious reasons such a study design is impracticable and researchers have to fall back on comparisons of the very old with those from younger cohorts who have been less well winnowed by survival selection, or between short- and long-lived kindreds. The need to assume that successive cohorts were originally similarly equipped to meet the challenges of survival restricts the first method to the study of genetic factors and the more interesting, and perhaps more important, effects of behavioural variables on survival cannot be examined. There have been some claims in the literature of evidence for survival advantage associated with lipoprotein patterns (Glueck et al 1977) and with heterozygosity at HLA gene loci, but these findings either have been contested by later studies or have not been replicated (Yarnell et al 1979).

Cohort effects causing differences between young and old that are easily mistaken for ageing have been well recognized since the cross-sequential study by Schaie & Strother (1968) demonstrating that cultural differences between successive cohorts in rapidly changing societies may lead to cross-sectional age-associated differences being very different in form from the true longitudinal pattern of ageing. Although most obtrusive in the sphere of psychological function, cohort effects undoubtedly contribute to cross-sectional estimates of age-associated change in some physical variables, such as serum lipid levels and obesity. The cross-sequential study of ageing Swedes in Göteborg suggests that cohort differences in bone density (Svanborg 1983) and mental function (Berg 1980), even over periods as short as five years, may be comparable in magnitude to age-associated changes over the same period. The importance of such studies for identifying the environmental determinants of disability and for the prediction of future needs for health services is obvious.

The phenomenon of *differential challenge* should concern us as citizens as well as researchers. If ageing is loss of adaptability, we can assess it only by presenting people at different ages with the same challenge and measuring their response. In some ways we organize society so as to present elderly people with more severe challenges than face the young, and this will exaggerate the effects of ageing. The high frequency of hypothermia among the elderly in Britain is partly due to age-associated impairment of homeostatic mechanisms of body temperature maintenance (Collins et al 1977) but is exaggerated by the old tending to live in colder houses than the young (Fox et al 1973). This is in turn partly due to the way social policy discriminates against old people in the allocation of modern, adequately heated housing. Another important way in which the dice may be loaded against the elderly is in the provision of health care. Keeler et al (1982) have shown that doctors tend to spend less time with old people than with younger patients, and the standard of hospital accommodation and facilities provided for geriatric patients in Britain is notoriously inferior to that provided for younger patients. The insidiousness of differential challenge in the health services is that, because old people are expected to do badly, one may not notice that they are doing worse than necessary because of the second-rate care they are given.

The term 'secondary ageing' has been used by some American writers to designate environmentally induced ageing, or extrinsic ageing in the terminology of Table 1. The disadvantage in this American use is that it then leaves no term for secondary ageing in the useful sense of adaptive responses to ageing. In the individual, these are most easily recognized in the field of psychological function in which some age-associated changes, for example obsessionalism and cautiousness, seem to be adaptations to impairments in memory and information-processing capacity. Adaptations in physical structure and function are less easy to identify. Indeed, one of the traditional enigmas of ageing is why its assaults are not recognized and repaired by the body; there is a circularity here, since we can only recognize those assaults of ageing that are not successfully repaired. There may however be recognizable adaptations: increased glomerular filtration fraction may be seen as an adaptation to diminishing renal plasma flow, and Hayes & Ruff (1986) have suggested that changes in the anatomical configuration of bones may maintain strength in the face of age-associated decrease in mineral content.

At a species level, the female menopause is widely thought to be an evolved response to the age-associated decline in the probability of a successful outcome to pregnancy which is universally found among mammals. In the unique context of a species with a family-based social structure and a cumulative culture transmitted through speech there will come a time in a woman's life when in terms of the probability of survival of her genes it will be a better strategy for her to give up increasingly unsuccessful, and biologically expensive, efforts to produce children of her own, even though each would contain 50% of her genes, and instead to foster the survival and success of her grandchildren, each of which contains 25% of her genes. For the male with so much less of an investment, biologically speaking, in unsuccessful pregnancies, the best strategy for his genes is for him to stay sexually active so long as life shall last. The significance of recognizing the menopause as secondary rather than primary ageing is that it should not be recruited as a paradigm for programmed ageing in the human. The secondary ageing theory of the menopause could be disproved if an example could be found of a menopausal phenomenon occurring in a mammalian species without a cumulative culture. For the purposes of this search, a 'menopause' could be defined as a genetically determined species-characteristic of total infertility in the female occurring with little age-variance in onset, at an age approximately half that of the maximum lifespan of the species.

It has been argued that the theory of the origin of the menopause in secondary ageing is untenable because, at the time of high selective pressure on the hominid ancestry, individuals did not live long enough for their phenotype to come under selective pressure at the age of the menopause.

This objection is based on estimates of lifespan derived from palaeogerontology, which is a less precise art than is always appreciated (Molleson 1986), and we do not know at what age the menopause originally developed. If, as Cutler (1975) has proposed, the hominid lifespan expanded rapidly about 200 000 years ago, it could be that female fertility came under selective pressure at that time not to lengthen *pari passu* with maximum age. We may have underestimated the lifespan of those of our ancestors who survived into adult life. Sophocles died at 91, while Aeschylus and Euripides died of accidents at the ages of 71 and 78. Death interrupted Plato's writing at the age of 87. That formidable monarch Agesilaus II of Sparta died at the age of 84 on his way home from Egypt where he had been conducting an active military campaign in the field. Our ideas of the survival of our ancestors at the time they were under evolutionary pressure may have been too much influenced by the experience of the urbanized Romans, with their high rates of infectious disease and, perhaps, endemic lead poisoning.

The main issues in the disease and ageing controversy concern the genesis of true ageing, which is conceptualized in Table 1 as arising through the interaction of extrinsic (environmental) influences with intrinsic (genetic) factors. Extrinsic influences can be detected and ultimately identified by traditional epidemiological methods; intrinsic ageing lies among what remains when extrinsic factors cannot be detected. In practice, what is not demonstrably extrinsic should provisionally be designated 'residual ageing', since in addition to intrinsic processes it will include effects due to yet unidentified or ubiquitous extrinsic factors. The direct and specific identification of intrinsic ageing processes can be hoped for from biological research. Kirkwood (1981) has developed the most convincing explanation of intrinsic ageing by postulating that it arises from constraints on the organism's abilities to repair random environmental damage. An organism could potentially completely repair such damage but, despite the evolutionary value of a long life of continued reproduction, subject to termination by accident or predation, the energy cost of a faultless repair programme is such as to put that organism at an evolutionary disadvantage compared with one that devotes somewhat less energy to repair and more to fuelling a higher rate of reproduction. This balance, struck in terms of the probability of transmission of genes to the next generation, is a dynamic one and the selection pressure in favour of prolonged longevity rather than higher reproduction rate will vary with the dangerousness of the environment and the complexity of the organism. The development of social structures that affect the survival of the next generations will also modulate the basic equation. Kirkwood's theory focuses the search for intrinsic ageing processes on the repair systems of the organism. Some at least of these will be intracellular. The limited reproductive capacity of isolated fibroblasts (Hayflick 1976) seemed at one time to offer insight into ageing-related phenomena at a cellular level. However, James Smith and colleagues have produced some evidence that the Hayflick limit may be caused by a specifically secreted gene product which could have the biological function of stopping the indefinite proliferation of cell clones and thus acting in effect as an anti-oncogene (Lumpkin et al 1986). If this is so, the Hayflick phenomenon may have only limited direct relevance to gerontology, although the question of how the dividing cells 'know' how many times they have divided may well be important, through its implications for the processes of gene control and how this may be damaged (Fairweather et al 1985).

There have also been epidemiological approaches to the direct identification of extrinsic and intrinsic ageing. It has been assumed for many years that the exponential form of the total mortality curve against age must in some way reflect the underlying progression of intrinsic ageing. Gerontologists have perhaps been mesmerized by the apparent regularity of the mortality function, which in fact departs from classic Gompertz-Makeham form at high ages (Economos 1982). Nonetheless, Brody & Schneider (1986) suggest that diseases that are 'age dependent', in the sense of being at least in part a consequence of intrinsic ageing, will show exponential increases in incidence with age, and Kurtzke (1969) proposed the exponential function of stroke mortality against age as evidence that stroke was a direct consequence of intrinsic ageing. In fact, age-specific mortality rates of particular diseases are compounded of age-specific incidence and age-specific fatality, and the incidence of stroke probably follows a power law rather than an exponential function of age (Evans & Caird 1982). This might be regarded as evidence of the extrinsic nature of the age-associated processes causing stroke. Most adult cancers follow a power-law function of incidence against age (Doll 1970) and the majority of cancers are extrinsically caused (Doll & Peto 1981). Peto and colleagues (1975) showed that for production of skin cancers by benzpyrene in rodents, age was not a factor, and the power-law function of incidence was simply a reflection of age being an index of time of cumulative exposure to carcinogen (Peto et al 1986). It would however not be justifiable to assume that all power-law functions necessarily reflect the same underlying mechanism, any more than to assume that exponential functions reflect some unspecified intrinsic ageing process.

Thus we have at present no way of identifying those processes which constitute intrinsic ageing whose effects it might even be reasonable to designate as 'normal', should one insist on this term as a synonym. The premature designation, on speculative grounds, of some selection of age-associated phenomena as intrinsic or normal will have as deleterious effect on gerontological research as on the care of patients and the design of health services. It is surely better, in such a state of ignorance, to sustain a unifying concept of ageing as the sum total of the age-associated loss of adaptability, and at the level of both the individual and the population to tease out, without preconceived notions, such causes and mechanisms as can lead to prevention and amelioration. Let us avoid a terminology whose historical roots and semantic resonances distort the logic of action.

References

Barrett JC 1985 The mortality of centenarians. Arch Gerontol Geriatr 4:211–8
Barrett JC 1986 The mortality of centenarians: a correction. Arch Gerontol Geriatr 5:81
Berg S 1980 Psychological functioning in 70- and 75-year-old people. A study in an industrialized city. Acta Psychiatr Scand (Suppl) 62 Suppl 288:1–47
Brody JA, Schneider EL 1986 Diseases and disorders of aging: an hypothesis. J Chronic Dis 39:871–876
Collins KJ, Dore C, Exton-Smith AN, Fox RH, MacDonald IC, Woodward PM 1977 Accidental hypothermia and impaired temperature homeostasis in the elderly. Br Med J 1:353–356
Cutler RG 1975 Evolution of human longevity and the genetic complexity governing ageing rate. Proc Natl Acad Sci USA 72:4664–4668
Doll R 1970 The age distribution of cancer: implications for models of carcinogenesis. J R Stat Soc (A) 134:133–155
Doll R, Peto R 1981 The causes of cancer. Oxford University Press, Oxford, UK
Economos AC 1982 Rate of aging, rate of dying and the mechanisms of mortality. Arch Gerontol Geriatr 1:3–27
Editorial 1985 Geriatrics for all? Lancet 1:674–675
Evans JG, Caird FI 1982 Epidemiology of neurological disorders in old age. In: Caird FI (ed) Neurological disorders in the elderly. John Wright & Sons, Bristol, p 1–16
Fairweather DS, Fox M, Margison G 1985 DNA-hypomethylation: a new theory of ageing. Clin Sci 69:53–54
Fox RH, Woodward PM, Exton-Smith AN, Green MF, Donnison DV, Wilks MG 1973 Body temperatures in the elderly: a national study of physiological, social and environmental conditions. Br Med J 1:200–206
Glueck CJ, Gartside PS, Steiner PM et al 1977 Hyperalpha- and hypobetalipo-proteinaemia in octogenarian kindreds. Atherosclerosis 27:376–406
Hayes WC, Ruff CB 1986 Biomechanical compensation mechanisms for age-related changes in cortical bone. In: Uhtoff HK (ed) Current concepts of bone fragility. Springer-Verlag, Berlin, p 371–377
Hayflick L 1976 The cell biology of human aging. N Engl J Med 295:1302–1308
Jette AM, Branch LG 1985 Impairment and disability in the aged. J Chronic Dis 38:59–66
Keeler EH, Solomon DH, Beck JC, Mendenhall RC, Kane RL 1982 Effect of patient age on duration of medical encounters with physicians. Med Care 20:1101–1108
Kirkwood TBL 1981 Repair and its evolution: survival versus reproduction. In: Townsend CR, Callow P (eds) Physiological ecology: an evolutionary approach to resource use. Blackwell Scientific, Oxford, p 165–189
Kurtzke JF 1969 The epidemiology of cerebrovascular disease. Springer-Verlag, Berlin
Lumpkin CK, Knepper JE, Butel JS, Smith JR, Pereira-Smith OM 1986 Mitogenic effects of the proto-oncogene and oncogene forms of c-H-*ras* DNA in human diploid fibroblasts. Mol Cell Biol 6:2990–2993
Molleson TI 1986 Skeletal age and palaeodemography. In: Bittles AH, Collins KJ (eds) The biology of human ageing. Cambridge University Press, Cambridge, UK, p 95–118

Peto R, Roe FJL, Lee EN, Levy I, Clack J 1975 Cancer and ageing in mice and men. Br J Cancer 32:411–426

Peto R, Parish SE, Gray RG 1986 There is no such thing as aging and cancer is not related to it. In: Likhachev A et al (eds) Age-related factors in carcinogenesis. International Agency for Research on Cancer, Lyons, p 43–53

Schaie KW, Strother CR 1968 A cross-sequential study of age changes in cognitive behavior. Psychol Bull 70:671–678

Svanborg A 1983 The physiology of ageing in man: diagnostic and therapeutic aspects. In: Caird FI, Evans JG (eds) Advanced geriatric medicine 3. Pitman, London, p 175–182

Yarnell JWG, St Leger AS, Balfour IC, Russell RB 1979 The distribution, age effects and disease associations of HLA antigens and other blood group markers in a random sample of an elderly population. J Chron Dis 32:555–561

DISCUSSION

Katzman: Let me challenge your view that the traditional distinction between the concepts of 'disease' and 'normal ageing' is misguided. I have spent a number of years trying to persuade people that Alzheimer's disease *is* a disease, and not simply what used to be called 'senility' or 'senile dementia': and there has been marvellous progress in research. In my view, this is because people now consider Alzheimer's as a disease. Clearly, environmental factors contribute, but I have been unable to establish that any change after the disease begins, related to any obvious environmental factor, has anything to do with the course of Alzheimer's. It seems to be biologically driven. The rate of progression, measured by psychological tests, in the four geographically separate studies with which I have been associated in the USA, has been exactly the same. The evidence is that genes and environment are both playing a role in this disease.

I agree fully that the care we give to an Alzheimer patient determines how long he or she will live. An interesting comparison in Southern Sweden showed that the life expectancy of demented patients had almost doubled over the past 20 years—an article entitled 'the failures of success', incidentally (Gruenberg 1977).

Grimley Evans: This smacks of politics rather than of science! Translating 'senile dementia' into Alzheimer's disease has undoubtedly produced public and financial support for research that would not otherwise have been forthcoming. But this is merely an example of the terminology being used to solve a problem that it created in the first place. If dementia had not been for so many years categorized as 'normal ageing' the relevant research might have been started decades ago.

You are sceptical of the effect of environmental factors on mental function in patients with Alzheimer's disease. We may be thinking of different things. I find the clinical evidence that the behaviour of affected patients may be modified by environmental factors incontrovertible, and behaviour is a manifestation of mental function. On the other hand, I know of no evidence that environmental factors can retard the development of the pathology of the disease or the decline in the maximal mental capacity of the victim.

Katzman: I have never seen improvement by orientation programmes, although I have used these methods.

T.F. Williams: The advantage in trying to make a distinction between ageing and disease is, as Bob Katzman is saying, that if one can identify a change in older people which is not universal or inevitable, there must be extrinsic causes, and these may be preventable or modifiable. If they are inevitable, on the other hand, that is 'ageing'. The only truly inevitable and well-documented change with age is the racemization from L-aspartic acid to D-aspartic acid that occurs at body temperature, very predictably with the passage of time, in 'protected' tissues such as tendons, lenses, and possibly also brain tissue, which have slow metabolic turnover. You can in fact date a body by its racemic mixture of D- and L-aspartic acid. This may prove to have some pathological meaning, in the brain for example, but it still might be intrinsic 'ageing' and we probably won't be able to do anything about it. It all depends how we use the word 'disease'. You are critical of the way we have used this term, and there may be a better word, but I prefer to use it and then to try to dissect out the characteristics of what I am calling 'disease'. Disease could well include (for, say, Alzheimer's disease) the social and environmental impact as well as the genetic contribution. This may be semantics, but the question does come down to how we approach what we do.

Grimley Evans: I agree. Philosophy is largely, perhaps entirely, a matter of semantics, and philosophy determines action. In Alzheimer's disease we are basically interested in the social disintegration that is the final impact of the condition on the patient. I differ from Dr Katzman about whether there are environmental factors mediating in the transition between Alzheimer's pathology and impairment of mental function, but I imagine there will be no controversy over the involvement of environmental factors in the transition between mental impairment and social disintegration.

There is a problem if you try to equate my 'extrinsic ageing' with 'disease', since there are clearly conditions which are apparently purely genetic—that is, 'intrinsic'—which are classified as diseases. Huntington's chorea is an obvious example. We also do not know which of those conditions appearing late in life, currently classified as diseases, may turn out to be intrinsic in origin—perhaps even Alzheimer's disease itself.

Fries: I have been struggling with the same problems, because of the strong parallelism between 'normal ageing' and 'chronic disease'. Many chronic diseases are nearly universal, if one looks for subclinical forms (Fries 1983). I don't know that every person dying at age 90 has neurofibrillary tangles, but there are pathological elements of osteoarthritis, of cataract, of high tone deafness, of stiffening of the aorta, and of atherosclerotic plaques in essentially every person over that age. Like you, I don't like to talk about either 'ageing' or 'chronic disease' without talking about both intrinsic and extrinsic factors and about complex multifactorial models, because these are so important in determining the variable rate of progression of chronic diseases, as well as their symptomatic incidence. The same factors hold with regard to ageing. The hopeful point about the variability of ageing phenomena between individuals is the possibility of reducing it by managing the relevant extrinsic forces, even though these are not the entire story. There surely need be no collision course between those interested in understanding the intrinsic mechanisms that are outside the control of the individual and of society, and those people interested in making maximal use of the positive potential actions to which the individual and society might contribute.

A. Williams: The common ground between us all is an interest in age-related changes in health and what can be done to improve the health of the elderly. Difficulty arises because we have different notions of the important attributes of health. One part of the biomedical model of disease is that these age-related changes in health are related to morbidity, or to pathologically recognizable elements in someone's situation. Others may be more concerned with seeing health in terms of physical functioning, distress, social integration and so on. What is coming to the surface here is a difference of view about the terms in which we discuss what being healthy, or more healthy, is all about.

Solomons: Like God, the concept of 'disease' seems to be something that if it had not existed, man would have had to invent it! Professor Grimley Evans referred to the Gaussian (normal) distribution of age-related changes. We can't easily discard it as a basic tool in our conceptual analysis. That is to say, there may well be an 'aberrant distribution pattern' of bodily performance with a marked skewing or even a *bimodal* distribution. One could look at the functional consequences of this poorer performance for the society and make the value judgement: 'that is aberrant'. That would be one approach to defining the concept of 'disease'.

Such an approach is open to manipulation. An elegant study was done in Sweden on anaemia. It sought to determine the haemoglobin concentration that represents anaemia (Garby et al 1969). Women of menstruating age were studied. The distribution of haemoglobin was measured, then all were given oral iron for a determined period, and the distribution of haemoglobin was remeasured, to see what subpopulation had been susceptible to change. This seems to be a good model for defining what disease is. Not all diseases, however, are responsive to such easy manipulation. If we could begin to describe bimodal or multimodal distributions of human performance, abnormality of distribution might give us an approach to defining what is 'illness' and what is 'normal ageing'.

Grimley Evans: Among the more theoretical objections to the use of the normal distribution in biology is that strictly it refers to repeated independent measurements on the same object. If applied to biological variables it carries the dubious implication that there is an Ideal Man of which we are all imperfect copies. Moreover, we know that many of the homeostatic mechanisms of the body work on a scale closer to logarithmic than to absolute values, and we might therefore expect a log normal rather than normal distribution to be appropriate. The essence of the controversy is brought out by the example of anaemia. I am not directly interested in the distribution of haemoglobin values in the population; I am principally concerned with the consequences for a person of being in one part of the distribution rather than another. The study by Elwood et al (1967) showed that the common symptoms alleged to be associated with anaemia were not associated with haemoglobin level until it fell to 8 g per decilitre. We should not therefore be preoccupied with some theoretical distribution from which we have to recognize deviance, but rather with establishing, empirically, values of variables that are associated with specifiable outcome probabilities.

Arie: The consequences of correcting the anaemia were also not reliably related to the disappearance of symptoms or to a greater sense of well-being, in that study. In other words, you can push people up into normalcy in terms of their haemoglobin, but they don't necessarily feel better!

Mor: The standard or criterion that you suggest using is the individual's expression of their functioning and sense of well-being: that is surely the criterion against which to assess the physiological variables. However, there may not be a direct correspondence between expressed well-being and physiology. Changing one does not necessarily alter the other.

Grimley Evans: To go back to Alan Williams' point here, the question of the definition of health is so important. A paper by Hunt & Macleod (1987) has discussed how the way patients, or the general public, use the concept 'health' differs from the medical perception of 'health'. This difference undoubtedly contributes to the failure of health education programmes.

Kirkwood: If one focuses on the concept of a statistical distribution of age-related changes, which Dr Solomons referred to, perhaps one can gain insight into the distinction, and relationship, between the concepts of 'ageing' and 'disease'. Consider, for simplicity, only genetic factors and suppose that through our genetic endowment each of us begins life with a certain value of some measure that can be related to an aspect of health. The initial values of this measure in a population define some statistical distribution. As a cohort grows older the measure changes in an age-related way for each individual.

We can consider two possibilities. One is that through chance variation the initial distribution becomes broader as the measure generally declines, but it remains essentially a single distribution. This fits with the concept of 'normal ageing' and the variation that we see among normal individuals in the rates at which age-related deteriorations take place.

A second possibility is that the initial distribution is made up of a mixture of two or more distinct sub-distributions, each of which undergoes a different age-related pattern of change, so that over time we see a separation of the sub-distributions rather than the spreading of a single distribution. A sub-distribution showing a fast decline in the specific aspect of health might be regarded as exhibiting an age-related 'disease'. In the present instance, where we are considering only genetic factors, this would be a disease with a genetic basis or predisposition, of which Alzheimer's disease might be an example.

The two possibilities can, of course, arise together to give a combined picture of both normal ageing, as an overall decline and gradual spreading of measures of health, and age-related disease, as the emergence of specific subgroups.

*T.F. Williams:*That idea has some appeal. Another factor that Grimley Evans mentioned is adaptation—the adaptive factors that enter into adjustments with age, in the cardiovascular system strikingly and in other systems too. There are adaptations that seem to compensate for what might be a true ageing change, such as the declining response of the cardiovascular system to circulating catecholamines, for example. We make a good adaptive response, so we see no resulting physiological defects in most instances in older people.

Solomons: If genetics and the environment are to be contrasted, the classical studies are those on the migration of Japanese people from Japan to Hawaii and on to California: their rates for various diseases have been looked at at given age-adjusted points. Colon cancer and cardiovascular disease rates differ at the same ages, in people with similar early life exposure and of common racial stock (Yano et al 1977, Heilbrun et al 1986). This is another argument for the divergence of nature and nurture, and for a definite environmental component in the expression of what is functional at a given chronological point.

Wise: Studies in human populations that have tried to separate disease-related changes from age-related changes have had repercussions on the work of basic scientists. We have been encouraged to use virus-free and pathogen-free animals, in order to distinguish the two kinds of change. Although this has some value, I question the validity of the results obtained with these artificially reared animals: I am not sure that we are studying any more pure 'age-related' phenomena than we are with healthy but not pathogen-free animals.

T.F. Williams: I agree. Let me give an example relating to this. One problem in doing ageing research in rodents is that many strains of rats and mice develop renal disease late in life. Strains that do not develop it have been searched for. One is presented with a problem when trying to interpret changes in other organ systems with age when renal disease is present, because it produces changes in circulating levels of phosphate and parathyroid hormone, and one may attribute this to age when it may be secondary to the renal disease. It depends on the questions you are asking, whether you want to exclude all other factors and focus on just one. If so, you may want to use pathogen-free and disease-free animals that have lived to a late age. But if we are interested in the phenomenon of ageing in the social world of rats or humans (and we want to come back eventually in humans to the need to develop approaches which recognize the highly multifactorial nature of 'typical' or 'usual' ageing), we need other methods for dealing with multifactorial issues. I don't think we know how to do this.

Hollander: There is a misconception, anyway, about the specific pathogen-free animal. If you want to extrapolate to man you have to realize that people living in industrialized parts of the world have a very different pattern of disease from people in developing countries. The specific pathogen-free animal can be compared to the situation in the Western world, with all our vaccination programmes and so on. Recent studies have shown, however, that even the specific pathogen-free animal has as complicated a system of ageing as man in the developed world, with multiple pathology and multifactorially produced lesions (Hollander et al 1984).

As a more general comment, in discussions of this type I have the impression (and I am a physician myself) that a distinction is made in the medical profession between those giving *care*, and those interested in producing *cure*. If, as I do, you take the view that care is important but cannot be dissociated from cure, and cure has to be related to basic research, you need an integrated model and you cannot separate normal ageing from disease—from Alzheimer's disease or any other condition.

Grimley Evans: I agree with you, and that is a point I was trying to make. I do not accept that there is any fundamental difference between care and cure; and I would also assert that care is as susceptible to evaluation by research as is cure.

Andrews: You reminded us that we are discussing science rather than politics here, but one cannot entirely avoid politics. One reason for trying to develop a new model by which to understand ageing and ill-health is that a movement is gaining support around the world that rejects the traditional model of disease and health, and would also abandon the medical model as an effective basis for intervening. The political rhetoric around this development would move us towards a so-called social view of health, which would suggest that social class, economic circumstances, environmental factors, public policies in areas such as education and agriculture, and social opportunities, are far more important in determining an individual's health and well-being than any notion of pathology in the sense of the traditional medical model. The problem is that if this view gains credence, and is out of phase with the biomedical view of the world shared by many of us, resources are likely to be significantly shifted in that direction—resources in terms of research and of the development of forms of intervention and programmes in health care. We therefore need to understand what this movement is saying and to try to integrate it with existing notions of ill-health and disease. In an area like Alzheimer's, for example, the interface between what we understand about the genetics and the pathology and the social consequences and environmental factors becomes at least as important as our understanding of what is going on in brain cells.

Katzman: This is correct, but there are in the world infectious agents that change people's opinions about these things! An instance that tends to be forgotten is the position in the USA in the 1950s with regard to polio. Vast amounts of money were being spent on care and improvements in care. The Salk vaccine wiped out the epidemic and changed major parts of our environment in the USA; for example, it became possible to have community swimming pools again. In the USA, and elsewhere, we are now faced with the acquired immune deficiency syndrome (AIDS) epidemic, which in some areas takes up a quarter of the hospital beds. Here is a disease which could be prevented entirely by 'social' means; yet one is left with an obvious medical problem. To some extent the reason that the medical model has not been found to be as acceptable for chronic diseases as for the infectious diseases is that we have not made much progress, despite the amount of effort put in, towards an understanding of the processes underlying the chronic conditions and an ability to deal with them—the major exception being atherosclerosis and heart disease. When one has to treat AIDS patients one quickly puts aside this other approach and has to recognize the existence of the medical problem.

Wenger: One problem is that the association of 'health' and 'well-being' that has been made over the years is not characterized by a one-to-one relationship. A variety of features have an impact on well-being but have nothing to do with health. If we consider a disease model, 'health' is probably the more important component. But, having said that, I am concerned that we may be causing some features of disease to be attributed to ageing. Many signs and symptoms either are attributed to 'age', or are described because people expect them to develop with increasing age. We learned a great deal about what 'labelling' someone as having hypertension will do; it may produce an entire complex of signs and symptoms. Some of what we see with ageing may reflect the expectations of a particular society of the concomitants of ageing. This attitude may limit the search for disease; it may also limit access to care; and it may limit both the medical perceptions and the patient's perception of what degree of improvement can be obtained if treatment is undertaken. One place to examine this issue is in societies that have different attitudes toward ageing; these differing attitudes may affect what people think should happen with increasing age.

Fries: I want to comment on the 'compression of morbidity', and by this means perhaps help to unify and clarify points that have been discussed already. Alvar Svanborg brought this subject up, and Grimley Evans has also made relevant comments. I define the 'compression of morbidity' as an increase in the age-specific incidence of ageing or chronic disease markers which is more rapid than the increase in life expectancy (Fries 1987). Therefore, the age at onset of disease gains on the age at death, granted that they are both moving targets and that the relative rates of the two are what we need to determine. It is my view that increases in morbidity were the rule up to at least 1975. This came about as we exchanged the acute diseases previously prevalent for the chronic diseases. That exchange inevitably increased the overall morbidity in an average life, even though age-specific morbidity was probably slowly decreasing.

At some time in the past ten years we entered a phase where a plateau in lifetime morbidity is being reached. We are pushing out the limits—the age of onset of disease is moving up; life expectancy is also moving up. The rates of change in individual areas of morbidity are not necessarily the same. Professor Svanborg noted the several areas of advanced handicap, decreased intellectual activity, and congestive heart failure in which his cohorts were showing a 50% decrease in morbidity over ten years. By contrast he noted at most a 19% change in mortality rates over that period, so for some areas he can see compression of morbidity. In the USA (and, I suspect, other developed countries) we see such compression in cardiovascular disease and in lung cancer in men.

The main issue is not so much where we are now, but where we can go in the future. This will depend on our ability to use improvements of both lifestyle and environment to bring about improvements in the health and the 'productive' ageing of a society.

A major question is whether it is possible, experimentally, to compress morbidity. Three large randomized controlled trials in the USA have demonstrated our ability to reduce morbidity by interventions affecting lifestyle (see Rose 1985). These are the Veterans Administration study on hypertension, the MRFIT study, and the Lipid Research Clinics trial. The aim of the MRFIT study was to reduce cigarette smoking, cholesterol levels and body weight. But there was a 2% *increase* in overall mortality in the 'intervention' group, so there was only a small effect on death rates. However, there was a 23% decrease in all the morbidity measures—angina, congestive heart failure and intermittent claudication among them—so the intervention actually had a major effect on morbidity. In the LRC trial, there was a 3% fall in mortality, again not statistically significant, in the intervention group (cholestyramine was taken, to reduce serum levels of cholesterol). However, there was a major (23%) decrease in morbid events. Similarly, the VA hypertension study reduced congestive heart failure but not mortality. So the experimental evidence is that interventions in people's lifestyles will have far greater effects on morbidity than on mortality (Fries 1987). Thus, perhaps we can suggest some more positive scenarios for future health than those gloomy predictions so frequently made.

Mor: What attracted me most in Dr Svanborg's evidence on the compression of morbidity was not so much the delayed incidence of disease, but the fact that people are able to enter into exercise and other kinds of activity-enhancing programmes and thereby either increase, or sustain, their level of physical activity before they reach the functional decline associated with what he called the fourth stage. From the patient's point of view, that may be even more important than the reduced incidence of disease. What matters to patients is what happens to their lives in terms of their daily function.

T.F. Williams: At some point we need to make explicit our ideas about what ageing means. One knows examples of people who remain healthy into their eighties and nineties and are still very active physically. There seems to be no evolutionary reason for further change in our human make-up, beyond the period of reproduction and the nurturing of offspring to maturity: there is no obvious selective pressure for us to go one way or another and we might equally well live for ever. So what are the factors that we define as 'ageing'? We must face the issue of how to account for an event that seems to be ageing *per se* (and each of us has a certain genetic endowment) as compared to some influence imposed by external events in the course of our lives.

Phair: I wanted to ask Professor Grimley Evans whether Dr Svanborg's fourth stage of 'accelerated mortality' is inherent, or a cumulative effect of extrinsic impacts on the organism. One can derive ideas on this from findings such as the observation that certain elderly people, instead of increasing levels of circulating immunoglobulins, show a decrease (Buckley et al 1974). This subgroup has an increased mortality. This might be a marker for entry into the accelerated decline stage. Similar studies in Australia on delayed hypersensitivity showed that mortality rates are unusually high over the two years after the demonstration of anergy (Roberts-Thomson et al 1974). I don't know whether these two studies have been confirmed by longitudinal studies, but declining immunoglobulin levels and anergy might be markers for accelerated decline. If so, are they intrinsic? Is that 'normal ageing' or does this represent the impact of innumerable (possibly immunological) insults?

Grimley Evans: I would like to see people concentrating on specific questions such as this. One would anticipate that if there were no extrinsic ageing, an individual who escaped accidental death would finally meet some limiting factor within his or her genetic programme that would precipitate death. But until the relevant research has been done we must not assume that all examples of terminal decline represent the emergence of such intrinsic processes.

A. Williams: The bridge between what we have been talking about so far, and the topics that the Chairman was encouraging us to talk about, lies in the implicit criteria by which we judge success in providing health care. These implicit criteria seem to be that we are concerned with enhancing both the length and quality of life, and that if we have to choose between putting resources into one treatment or another, those would be the criteria used to establish priorities. But the discussion is now shifting to a more ecological or demographic point, namely, that supposing we were successful in enhancing people's capacities from a biological point of view, we might find ourselves constrained by the capacity of our habitat to support us in the numbers that would then be generated. The question that Grimley Evans is posing is that if we look beyond the aspects we are now considering, to look at their demographic implications, is there a notion of optimum population that we ought also to be thinking about? Might we find ourselves increasing our life expectancy so much that our quality of life declines sharply because we are fighting for the last crumb of sustenance?

Fries: I am not positive that one should argue for natural selection beyond the reproductive age, but two arguments frequently made by students of evolution are that, first, evolution is designed to protect the species, and a species which doesn't change its genetic material becomes very non-adaptive over time, so the species needs some finite period of turnover. And second, there is the 'grandmother' theory, which says that, particularly in primitive cultures, having a family unit through which experience of the world and its diseases and problems can be transmitted culturally is important to the survival of the young. So, it is not just the parents that are important but the preceding generation as well.

On the mechanism of the terminal drop phenomenon, I have based my thoughts on Strehler & Mildvan's (1960) hypothesis, which anticipates 'terminal drop' as a logarithmic rate of loss of total body homeostatic reserve as a result of linear rates of failure in many constituent parts. This is of course an oversimplified model, and some of the reasons for that have been noted here already.

Wenger: In terms of improving lifestyle characteristics in an elderly population, we shall soon face a population reaching older adult life that has been exposed to the same preventive features from early middle age. With our 30- and 40-year-old population of today, assuming they have adopted health-conscious behaviour such as smoking cessation, reasonable diet, moderate physical activity, limitation of alcohol use—all the changes that we have been advocating—what will happen to them as they reach the elderly years? Will that elderly population be the same? Will there be preventive interventions suitable for that population? Some of our projections about disease prevalence and health- care needs 20–30 years from now may not be correct if they are based on a group exposed to long-term preventive care—a group that has had a very different lifestyle—reaching the older age ranges.

References

Buckley CE III, Buckley EG, Dorsey ER 1974 Longitudinal changes in serum immunoglobulin levels in older humans. Fed Proc 33:2036
Elwood PC, Waters WE, Greene WJ, Wood MM 1967 Evaluation of a screening survey for anaemia in adult non-pregnant women. Br Med J 4:714–717
Fries JF 1983 The compression of morbidity. Milbank Mem Fund Q 61:397–419
Fries JF 1987 Aging, illness, and health policy: implications of the compression of morbidity. Perspect Biol Med, in press

Garby L, Irnell L, Werner I 1969 Iron deficiency in women of fertile age in a Swedish community. III. Estimation of prevalence based on response to iron supplementation. Acta Med Scand 185:113–119

Gruenberg EM 1977 The failures of success. Milbank Mem Fund Q 55:3–24

Heilbrun LK, Hankin JH, Nomura AMY, Stemmermann GN 1986 Colon cancer and dietary fat, phosphorus and calcium in Hawaiian Japanese men. Am J Clin Nutr 43:306–309

Hollander CF, Solleveld HA, Zurcher C, Nooteboom AL, Van Zwieten MJ 1984 Biological and clinical consequences of longitudinal studies in rodents: their possibilities and limitations. An overview. Mech Ageing Dev 28:249–260

Hunt SM, Macleod M 1987 Health and behavioural change: some lay perspectives. Community Med 9:68–76

Roberts-Thomson IC, Whittingham S, Youngchaiyud U, Mackay IR 1974 Ageing, immune response, and mortality. Lancet 2:368–370

Rose G 1985 Role of controlled trials in evaluating preventive medicine procedures. In: The value of preventive medicine. Pitman, London (Ciba Found Symp 110) p 183–202

Strehler BL, Mildvan AS 1960 General theory of mortality and aging. Science (Wash DC) 132:14–21

Yano K, Rhoads GG, Kagan A 1977 Coffee, alcohol and risk of coronary heart disease among Japanese men living in Hawaii. N Engl J Med 297:405–409

Cerebrovascular disease and the elderly

Klaus Ostermann and Brigitte Sprung-Ostermann

Arbeitsgruppe für Angewandte Soziale Gerontologie (ASG), Gesamthochschule Kassel, Postfach 101380, D-3500 Kassel, Federal Republic of Germany

Abstract. A three-year follow-up study in Kassel (Federal Republic of Germany) has shown that (1) the incidence of stroke rises with increasing age, (2) the incidence is higher for men than for women, and (3) the survival rate is 37% three years after the attack. The survivors differ significantly from those who died in their Barthel index scores on discharge from hospital and in age (chi-square test). Only a small subgroup (15% of the survivors) received treatment in a residential rehabilitation centre in the year after discharge from hospital.

1988 Research and the ageing population. Wiley, Chichester (Ciba Foundation Symposium 134) p 58–68

We initiated a prospective study of stroke during 1983–1984 (in this paper 'stroke' includes all ICD numbers from 430 to 438). Stroke is an illness in which death is a frequent outcome. We have analysed stroke patients who died and those who survived as two independent groups. We were interested in the question of who are the patients who have survived the critical acute phase of the disease, and have then died in the subsequent years. Are there particular conditions that are connected with the probability of death or survival, and with the quality of life of the survivors?

The epidemiological part of our study (cf. Karl 1986) has shown that stroke is a disease of the highest age groups, the incidence rising from an average of 308 per 100 000 for the 60- to 64-year-olds to 1305 for those over 75 years. By comparison with international studies such as those done in the USA (Robins & Baum 1981), our Kassel investigation shows the following (see Table 1):

1. The incidence of stroke rises with increasing age.
2. The incidence rates are substantially higher for men than for women.
3. The survival rate three years after the attack is 37%.

In what follows we shall consider 311 patients who were discharged from hospital care: 91 patients who died in the first year (U_1); 43 who died before the second examination, at three years (U_2); and 177 who were alive after that examination, three years after their stroke. The causes of death of those patients who died at home are not usually known to us for reasons of protecting personal information.

TABLE 1 The incidence of stroke in the district around Kassel per 100 000 persons, according to age and sex

Age group	Women	Men	Average incidence
60–64 years	278	436	308
65–69 years	383	567	454
70–74 years	496	990	684
Over 75 years	1263	1391	1305
Average incidence	675	877	749

We asked a number of questions. Do the 177 patients surviving after three years represent a group who also differ in other ways from those who died? What state can these patients achieve after their illness? Can they return to their state before the illness? And are there connections between social and physical activities, and the need for help and care, in relation to the activities of daily living, sociodemographic variables, and those risk factors and diseases that cause and accompany the illness? We used the chi-square test to assess the statistical significance of the differences between the groups (with significance values of 5% and 1% as significant and highly significant, respectively).

Comparison of the two groups of deceased patients

There was no difference in the proportions by age of the two groups of deceased patients (91 dying in the first year and 43 dying before the third year). In the first year, 8% of those under 70 years of age died; twice as many (16%) died in the period up to the second examination, after three years. The proportion of women is in each case slightly higher than that of men (U_1, 53%; U_2, 56%).

If the patients need help, it is supplied by a partner or by their children. Whereas 57% of the first group were still married, 42% of the second group were. There was a difference in the frequency of visits by the children. Of those asked after one year (U_1), 40% were visited daily and 46% at least once a week. Of those asked after three years (U_2), the figures were 61% and 32%. With very slight deviations, these values agree with those in the average population of a town in the Federal Republic of Germany (cf. Voltenauer-Lagemann 1986), representing a well-developed network of contact and relationships which emphasizes the assistance given by children when the husband or wife is not there to help.

This assistance was in fact necessary even before their illness, because almost half the patients (43% for $n = 91$ and 47% for $n = 43$) were already unable to walk properly and, for example, every tenth patient (10% for $n = 91$ and 9% for $n = 43$) could not carry out his or her personal toilet without help. Rather lower percentages were found for dressing and undressing, eating independently, and going to the toilet — restrictions which are undoubtedly related to the fact that 40% of those who died in the first year (U_1) and 29% of those who died later (U_2) had suffered at least one previous stroke.

Questions to the patients on their social and physical activities before the illness told us about their previous state of activity. Physical activities such as 'going for walks' or 'gardening' were carried out regularly only by a third of the patients; this also holds good for 'reading' and 'receiving visitors'. Only 'watching television' was mentioned by more than three-quarters of the stroke patients as being a regular pursuit, before their stroke.

Apart from their previous strokes, the deceased patients had been burdened with 'risk factors': more than half suffered from hypertension (59% of $n = 91$ and 54% of $n = 43$); three-quarters had cardiac or coronary artery insufficiency (of $n = 91$; and 70% of $n = 43$); every seventh patient had had a heart attack; every fifth, cardiac arrhythmia; and more than a third suffered from diabetes mellitus.

During their stay in hospital (the length of stay was on average 4.3 weeks) improvements were noted in both their mental and physical condition. To compare their physical status on admission and discharge we used the Barthel index, a system of scoring the activities of daily living, with a range from zero to 100 points (Kane & Kane 1981). A high score indicates a better condition than a lower one, and the scale is generally used to evaluate the effects of rehabilitation. At discharge, those patients who died within the year (U_1: $n = 91$) achieved an average of 30 points and those who lived two years longer, 55 points; the latter had a better original score of 30 points on admission (d% = -10 of $n = 91$). A significantly higher proportion of those who died earlier failed to achieve more than 60 points on the Barthel index, as compared with those who died later ($\chi = 11.86$, $\phi = 0.31$; $P = 0.001$).

Once they were at home, only 5% of the discharged patients went shopping for themselves; a partner, and their children, helped half of the patients; and every fifth patient had help with the housework. All regular everyday activities became fewer from the time before the attack until the time of the check-up: between 28% for 'gardening', 14% for 'handwork' (needlework and other handicrafts), and 9% for 'going for walks' and 'watching television'.

Comparison of survivors and deceased patients

There was relatively little difference in the proportion of men and women among the survivors who were checked up on at home and among those who died ($n = 91$ deceased, 53% women, 47% men; $n = 43$ deceased, 56 to 44%; $n = 177$ survivors, 58 to 42%). The groups differed considerably in age; the older stroke patients (above 70) were significantly more likely to die and those below 70 to survive ($\chi = 23.332$, $\phi = 0.27$, $P = 0.001$ for $n = 91$; $\chi = 8.233$, $\phi = 0.193$, $P = 0.004$ for $n = 43$).

The younger patients receive statistically highly significantly more help from their partners in coping with everyday life ($\chi = 8.958$, $\phi = 0.238$, $P = 0.002$). This support is predominantly related to sex: the men receive help from their wives (highly significant: $\chi = 39.185$, $\phi = 0.499$, $P = 0.001$), whereas the women are looked after by their children ($\chi = 10.595$, $\phi = 0.259$, $P = 0.001$).

Among the surviving 177 patients we found no statistically different frequency of risk diseases or risk factors dependent on age, when the older and younger patients (above and below 70 years) were examined for the frequency of high blood pressure, cardiac and coronary artery insufficiency and diabetes. However, cardiac and coronary artery insufficiency divide the survivors from the deceased highly significantly ($\chi = 11.166$, $\phi = 0.196$, $P = 0.003$); only a few of the deceased had stated that they had no medically treated cardiac insufficiency. Added to this is the fact that the deceased had a significantly higher rate of diabetes mellitus requiring insulin ($\chi = 10.190$, $\phi = 0.184$; $P = 0.006$). No connection could be proved with other risk factors or diseases.

Lastly, in our comparison of survivors and deceased, the diagnosis on admission is more favourable according to the state of consciousness rather than to the frequency and distribution of hemiplegia: 7% of the survivors were classified as presomnolent or somnolent, whereas 12% of those who died later (U_2) and 25% of those who died within the first year (U_1) were initially in a state of limited consciousness.

When arm and leg function were tested on admission we found limited function less frequently in the survivors, whereas almost identical values were found for all groups for 'buttoning clothes' and 'using the hand when eating'. If the results of the initial diagnoses are combined in an index in which lameness, inability to walk, incontinence of bladder and bowels, loss of speech and unconsciousness are all included, a marked accumulation of diagnoses in the women stroke patients is seen — they are predominantly the older patients — which is statistically significant ($\chi = 5.883$; $\phi = 0.188$; $P = 0.015$).

When the 177 patients who were alive after three years were grouped according to their Barthel scores (Table 2), on admission 29% scored over 65 points, 9% scored 45–60 points, but 62% scored only 0–40 points. Stroke is thus a disease that creates a great need for help and care in the initial stages (Granger et al 1979). At the time of discharge the picture has reversed: 10% scored in the middle group, there are still 33% scoring only up to 45 points, but 57% have already reached 65 or more points and are in a better physical condition. These changes during the stay in hospital are highly significant when the Barthel scores at discharge are compared between the survivors and

TABLE 2   Barthel scores achieved by 177 patients surviving for three years, on admission and discharge

Barthel scores	Admission	Discharge
0–40 points	62%	33%
45–60 points	9%	10%
65–100 points	29%	57%

the deceased in the various groups ($\chi = 19.196$; Cramers' $V = 0.259$; $P = 0.001$), showing that the scores of those who died hardly changed at all during their stay in hospital.

Condition of survivors before and after their illness

The physical and social activities of stroke patients before their illness do not differ from those of the average population in the Federal Republic of Germany (cf. Voltenauer-Lagemann 1986). When their activities were compared for six physical or social activities, we found that a large number of patients increase their activities after their stroke, or at least maintain their former level (Table 3). These differences in the activities of stroke patients were looked at in the context of sociodemographic data and risk factors or diseases on admission; rehabilitation in hospital and/or out-patients' exercises at home; Barthel score groups; and the occurrence of another attack in the intervals between check-ups. A statistically significant decrease in 'handwork' after a second attack ($\chi = 5.757$; $\phi = 0.192$; $P = 0.016$) occurred more often in the younger (under 70) patients ($\chi = 5.026$; $\phi = 0.168$; $P = 0.025$), and in the men. There was a trend towards a decrease in social activities after a second attack ($\chi = 3.304$; $\phi = 0.159$; $P = 0.069$). We found a trend towards the level of activity staying high when help from a partner or children is not available at home.

TABLE 3   The frequency of social and physical activities: individual differences from before the stroke until the second check-up in 177 patients surviving for three years

Activities	Frequency		
	Decrease	The same	Increase
Going for walks	33%	49%	18%
Handwork	33%	57%	10%
Gardening	36%	59%	5%
Reading books	28%	59%	13%
Watching television	14%	75%	11%
Receiving visitors	31%	40%	29%

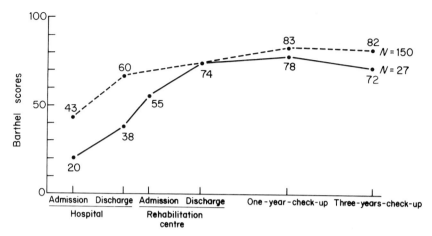

FIG. 1.   Average Barthel scores of 150 non-rehabilitated (– – –) and 27 rehabilitated
(——) stroke patients at different time intervals.

Only some of the patients received further rehabilitation in a residential
rehabilitation centre during the year after the stay in hospital. This group of
27 patients, representing 15% of the survivors, when compared to average
values on the Barthel scale (Fig. 1), is a group which is initially relatively
impaired but then improves. However, long-term rehabilitative support at
home is needed to keep up the level of function attained, and this is unfortunately not available.

Summary

From our analysis we are able to conclude that (1) the existing international
epidemiological results on stroke patients have been substantiated in our
study; (2) the survivors and the deceased differ from one another in age and
in the Barthel index values reached on discharge from hospital; (3) the
survivors and the deceased form two distinct groups, in terms of the frequency of 'risk diseases' such as cardiac and coronary artery insufficiency and
diabetes mellitus; (4) assistance in everyday life comes predominantly from
wives or children, and only seldom from social institutions; and (5) a group
which is initially very badly off can be improved by rehabilitation in hospital.
The follow-up examinations show, however, that out-patient rehabilitation
after discharge from hospital is in general not adequate to stabilize the
progress previously achieved by stroke patients.

Acknowledgements

Our study (Rehabilitation in Geriatrics) was sponsored by the Volkswagen Foundation.

Discussion

References

Granger CV, Dewis LS, Peters NC, Sherwood CC, Barrett JE 1979 Stroke rehabilitation: analysis of repeated Barthel index measures. Arch Phys Med Rehabil 60:14–17

Karl F 1986 Epidemiologische Aspekte des apoplektischen Syndroms. In: Schütz RM (ed) Praktische Geriatrie. HRSG, Lübeck, p 232–247

Kane RA, Kane RL 1981 Assessing the elderly. Lexington Books, Lexington, Massachusetts

Robins M, Baum HM 1981 The national survey of stroke incidence. Stroke 12 (2 Pt 2 Suppl 1):45–47

Voltenauer-Lagemann M 1986 Ältere Menschen in Grosstädten. Hrsg von Ministerium für Arbeit, Gesundheit und Sozialordnung, Stuttgart

DISCUSSION

T.F. Williams: You find that the level of activity of the patients stays high even when no partners or children are in the home. One of my colleagues in Rochester, New York (Carol Podgovsky, unpublished) made similar observations on people with stroke and other conditions who were assessed to be disabled enough to need nursing-home care, yet went home instead of entering a nursing home. Among that group, at one-year follow-up, those who lived alone had maintained a higher functional status than those who were living with family members. You might say that they had to; but it is interesting that you also saw that in your group of stroke patients.

Mor: In a recently completed study (to be published), Lois Monteiro has looked at the effects of myocardial infarction on older women (age 65+) and found something similar. The women in general were very debilitated after the infarction but, in the follow-up for one year, those with more dependency-inducing support networks—that is, whose families did more for them than might be desirable—remained at a lower level of functioning than did those who lived alone or whose families did less for them.

T.F. Williams: These are speculations about a 'dependency-inducing' environment. Do you have any more analysis on that feature, Dr Ostermann?

Ostermann: Not directly; however, we did a study in two rehabilitation centres with 770 women stroke patients, and if we divided them into groups according to their Barthel index level, those who initially had a lower score could be seen as the learners; they developed a higher degree of function than those starting with a higher score.

Grimley Evans: Trials of rehabilitation among older patients suggest that there may be only a small proportion, perhaps as low as 10% to 15%, who are susceptible to rehabilitation (Sheikh et al 1981, Rubenstein et al 1984). The rest, presumably, follow the natural history of their illness. If true, this obviously has important implications for the cost and provision of health services. It would be interesting to know if the shift in scores in your group was produced by a small subgroup who responded. (Your Fig. 1 showed *average* scores.) Yours was a retrospective analysis, of course. One really wants to identify predictors of response to rehabilitation in stroke, as in many other conditions.

Wenger: In other settings, such as residential rehabilitation after myocardial infarction, as practised in some European countries, one predictor of response is the consideration for admission to a rehabilitation facility. By and large, patients with almost any disorder who have a reasonable functional capacity will probably be sent home; this group will tend to live independently. Patients who are thought to be significantly impaired, but who have a potential for recovery, are sent to the rehabilitation facility. So there is some self-selection. That selection also applies to the people who continue to live independently, as compared with those who agree to live with children or family; sometimes that is not a spontaneous decision, but one that either is occasioned when patients can't cope alone at home, or is engendered by the placement plans at discharge from hospital. I am not sure that the fact that people who live alone at home function better than those who live with children or other relatives is the result of their being 'independent'. It may reflect the initial selection, namely that they were allowed to go home, to continue living alone.

Ostermann: I have asked myself the same question about the reason for this result. We do sometimes see over-protection from the family. Therefore if they go home and we see them there later, the scores may depend on 'mothering' by their children, or by their wives, for the male patients.

White: You observed a higher risk of dying within the follow-up period for those with a lower Barthel score. My question concerns those who received rehabilitation and those who didn't—the solid and dotted lines in Fig. 1. If a low score is associated with going to a rehabilitation unit, and a low score is also being associated with an increased risk of dying in the follow-up interval, I wonder if the people represented in the solid line of Fig. 1 include only those who survived the whole three-year follow-up, or whether it includes, at the beginning, some who then died. We need to know whether the individuals who scored poorly at first nevertheless survived the whole period of follow-up.

Ostermann: The total group who survived the three-year follow-up were examined retrospectively for their changing scores from the time of the stroke.

White: So, thinking of Grimley Evans' question, those represented in the solid line are a surviving subset of the people who had strokes.

Solomons: Your Fig. 1 makes me wonder whether in fact there is a 'ceiling' (or maximum) score—that is, a restrictive, upper limit—which both groups are approaching, so that one would not expect, with any amount of continued observation or intervention, to bring the patients above that level. They might reach it quicker with interventions, but it could not go higher. In other words, is the Barthel score that your patients achieved the same score that all stroke victims would achieve (if they lived long enough), no matter what their pathway to that achievement—be it at home or with rehabilitation—because they can't get any higher? So you actually have maximum recovery in both groups. If we knew the distribution of individual scores and what the upper individual levels in the distribution are at the end of three years, it would help us to know whether there is also a narrowing of the distribution at that point (three-year check-up), as if the population were reaching a ceiling, or whether there really is a distribution which allowed certain patients to go still higher.

Mor: The Barthel score goes up to 100, and it is certainly possible for stroke patients to reach 100, with or without rehabilitation.

Ostermann: The distribution of the values of the individual patients was narrow; there was no appreciable range. I don't know whether these patients have reached their highest possible scores. They stayed only a short time in the rehabilitation centre (on average, nine weeks). If we spent more money and time on them, perhaps we could increase their performance.

Solomons: The patients seem to be 'saturating' at a score of 75 in this study. If the distribution of values showed that some did reach 100, we could ask why all individuals in both groups do not reach that level. If the distribution was narrow, as you report, that might represent a biological phenomenon, related to stroke specifically in Germany in this particular birth cohort; and despite the potential recovery score of 100 that is possible in others, one might be reaching saturation level for this German population around 75 years.

T.F. Williams: I rather doubt that. The question is whether some of your patients score very highly through spontaneous recovery.

Ostermann: I don't think there is a definable limitation on rehabilitation. In both groups (those with and without rehabilitation) we saw high scores and recovery from stroke.

Fries: It looks to me as if the most steeply rising part of either curve in Fig. 1 was the period after discharge from hospital and before admission to the rehabilitation unit, which reinforces Dr Wenger's point about self-selection for rehabilitation.

Ostermann: It perhaps is spontaneous recovery during this time, but it could be a problem of institutional behaviour, too, and the method of evaluation of the Barthel index. In hospital the patients normally stay in bed during the early phase of their illness, whereas at home, and in rehabilitation centres, they are out of bed, which raises the level of the index.

Arie: You mentioned a differential outcome for men and women and related it to the possibility that women stroke patients did better because they were often living alone and simply had to manage. There are other fields where there seems to be a relationship between gender and the care given. Studies of the care of people with dementia (e.g. Horowitz 1985, Fitting et al 1986, Zarit et al 1986) suggest there may be important differences in the way that the care of demented people impinges on men and on women, with different implications for the way in which care is given, and for levels of stress on carers. A factor might be that when women are the main carers, they have a tradition of self-sufficiency, and of feeling that this is their role and they must cope. Often they go on 'coping' inadequately, but they feel obliged to try; whereas men, feeling that it is not the male role to cope, are quicker to bring or buy in help, or to attract help as being men. Alternatively, men sometimes appear to tackle the task of caring with new energy, because it is new to them. To return to stroke, this is a physical condition, but we know how important are psychological factors in recovery from stroke; such considerations as the drive of simply having to be self-sufficient on the part of women could be important.

Wenger: How sure are you of your role stereotypes, Dr Arie? Does the picture you describe apply universally? Do you have evidence that your characterizations are valid? Gender stereotypes may be like some age stereotypes; they may reflect what we have been told, what we expect, rather than what actually happens.

Arie: It could be so! These are hypotheses for investigation.

Ostermann: When we found that the care givers are mostly the women, we visited both men and women patients at home and asked for their coping strategies in extended interviews, including questions about help and care by women and children. We hope to be able to say something more about these questions when this new study is completed.

Fox: Of the patients who went home, you separated those who lived alone from those who were cared for by family. A woman stroke patient who went back to live with her husband might be looked after by him or she might be looked after by her children. These are two different types of family relationship. It is likely that the traditional role for this woman has been to look after her husband, rather than the reverse. There may therefore be more incentive for that woman to try to take up her original role again, on returning home from hospital to her husband. A woman who is a widow, going to live with her children, would behave quite differently. It would be interesting to separate these two groups out for further study.

Ostermann: You are right. I recall only one instance when a man was caring for his ill wife. We found that older wives are in fact mostly widows, living on small incomes, so they cannot buy professional help. This may be one reason why they have to cope better than men. Also, in our study we found that the women as patients are usually older, because normally in Germany a man is married to a younger wife. By the time they get strokes, the women have been widowed: therefore they depend on the help of their children, and this is connected with ambivalent feelings.

A. Williams: Thinking of the psychological barriers to recovery from stroke during rehabilitation, has anyone tried to use as a predictive factor the social psychological tests on people's beliefs about the 'locus of control'? Strong beliefs about one's level of health being one's own responsibility, rather than the responsibility of professionals (or being a matter of chance), should be a good predictor of whether people will benefit from rehabilitation regimes.

Secondly, and more conjecturally, suppose that a stroke victim, or any other ill person of this kind, is happy to be dependent, and has carers who are happy to have them dependent: should they really be persuaded into any other regime?

Ostermann: One can question whether people like to be dependent in their old age. I don't think they do. But the prediction of the outcome from stroke supported by rehabilitation is difficult. I recall two women: one had a family and enough money, and a social network, and was supported by it; a year after returning home she was writing a book, doing the cooking, and so on. Yet I remember her in the rehabilitation centre, where I evaluated her and expected that she would be dead a year later. An opposite case was a woman who looked forward to her future at home, doing the gardening and so on. When I saw her a year later she was very ill. She was alone at home and felt lonely because her children were out at work. She had a further stroke and died some days later. We have started to look at these questions of coping.

T.F. Williams: When studying diabetic patients and their response to efforts to help them control their disease we looked at the 'locus of control' among other variables. We expected that those who saw control as lying outside themselves (literally beyond their own control) would not be as much concerned in managing their illness as those who saw themselves as being in control. We actually didn't find any difference in that. One interesting point was that patients who had compulsive personalities, and a compulsive doctor, managing their diabetes best. Those who were compulsive themselves, but whose doctor told them not to worry too much about their diabetic management, didn't carry out recommended measures effectively. Patients who were not themselves compulsive did this even less effectively. This was the only personality factor that could be related to the level of performance of recommended measures for the control of diabetes (Williams et al 1967).

References

Fitting M, Rabins P, Lucas MJ, Eastham J 1986 Caregivers for dementia patients: a comparison of husbands and wives. Gerontologist 3:348–352

Horowitz A 1985 Sons and daughters as caregivers to older parents: difference in role performance and consequences. Gerontologist 6:612–617

Rubenstein LZ, Josephson KR, Wieland GD, English PA, Sayre JA, Kane RL 1984 Effectiveness of a geriatric evaluation unit: a randomized clinical trial. N Engl J Med 311:1664–1670

Sheikh K, Meade TW, Brennan PJ, Goldberg E, Smith DS 1981 Intensive rehabilitation after stroke: service implications. Community Med 3:210–216

Williams TF, Martin DA, Hogan MD, Watkins JD, Ellis EV, Coyle V, Lyle IK, Whittinghill M 1967 The clinical picture of diabetic control, studied in four settings. Am J Publ Health 57:441

Zarit SH, Todd PA, Zarit JM 1986 Subjective burden of husbands and wives as caregivers: a longitudinal study. Gerontologist 3:260–266

Alzheimer's disease as an age-dependent disorder

Robert Katzman

Department of Neurosciences, School of Medicine (M-024), University of California, San Diego, La Jolla, California 92093, USA

Abstract. Alzheimer's disease is the most significant of the age-related diseases of the brain. The incidence of Alzheimer's at age 80 is twenty-fold that at age 60 years. In one study the incidence at age 80 surpassed that of stroke. Three major advances have occurred in regard to Alzheimer's disease: (1) clinical diagnosis has markedly improved and now approaches 90% accuracy; (2) understanding of the biology of Alzheimer's has increased with delineation of specific fibrous protein abnormalities and identification of the amyloid precursor gene and the gene linked to familial Alzheimer's, both genes being located on chromosome 21; and (3) there have been advances in the correlation of specific nerve cell involvement and neurotransmitter changes with physiological (positron emission tomography), behavioural and neuropsychological manifestations.

1988 Research and the ageing population. Wiley, Chichester (Ciba Foundation Symposium 134) p 69–85

Alzheimer's disease is an example par excellence of an age-dependent disorder. Recent advances in research on this disease suggest that it may be one of the first age-dependent diseases whose pathophysiology will be understood.

Dementia and its two major causes, Alzheimer's disease and strokes, meet the criteria proposed by J.A. Brody for age-dependent diseases — namely, diseases whose incidence continues to rise in a geometric or exponential fashion as a function of age. The statistical data relating to stroke have been discussed elsewhere in this symposium (see Ostermann & Sprung-Ostermann 1988). The incidence of dementia and Alzheimer's disease increases with age in an exponential fashion (Fig. 1), even more strikingly than that of stroke. In two population studies, one in New York State and the other in Denmark, investigators found that at age 65 less than 1% of the population suffer from severe dementia, whereas at age 80 or 85, some 15–20% suffer from severe dementia. By 'severe dementia' these investigators meant individuals who were no longer able to live independently but either were in chronic-care hospitals or nursing homes, or were being cared for full time by their family.

Recent incidence data are based on ongoing longitudinal studies in which the initial cohorts were volunteers and perhaps, therefore, subject to some

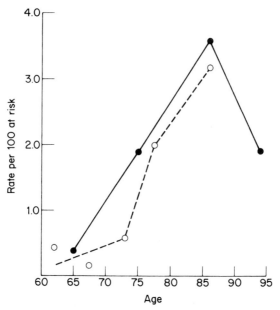

FIG. 1. The incidence of development of dementia per 100 individuals at risk per year. ● – ●, data for women in the Lundby study (Hagnell et al 1981). ○ – – – ○, data for men in the Baltimore longitudinal study (Sluss et al 1981). (Reproduced with permission, Fig. 2, p 137 in *America's Aging: Health in an Older Society*. © 1985 by the National Academy of Sciences.)

selection bias. Nevertheless, there is excellent congruence between available incidence studies. One study, by Hagnell and co-workers (1981), in southern Sweden, the Lundby study, has followed a cohort for well over 25 years; many of the individuals are now above age 75. As indicated in Fig. 1, there is a sharp rise in the incidence of dementia between ages 60 and 85, with an apparent falling-off after age 85. In these and other studies in which a plateau in incidence in subjects in their 90s has been reported, the total number of individuals in this advanced age group has been so small that no conclusion can be reached. The second study shown in Fig. 1 is that of the incidence of Alzheimer's disease that developed in the Baltimore longitudinal study (Sluss et al 1981). This almost exactly parallels the results of the Lundby study. We have had the opportunity to study the development of dementia in a volunteer cohort of more than four hundred 80-year-olds in New York City whom we have now followed for approximately five years. In this cohort the incidence of dementia has been greater than 3% per year; during the first three years 56 cases of dementia developed, 32 with Alzheimer's disease, 15 with multi-infarct dementia, and nine with other diagnoses. In the same time period there were 35 new cases of myocardial infarcts and 17 cases of stroke.

Thus, the incidence of Alzheimer's disease starts to pass the incidence of stroke at age 80, at least in this particular sample.

From these figures one can begin to project what might happen if the entire population lived to the age of 90 (Fig. 2). We would predict that about one-third of the population would remain intact intellectually, about one-third would develop Alzheimer's disease, and the other one-third would have a mixture of what has been called 'benign senescence forgetfulness' and a variety of other diseases (which number more than 70) that can produce the dementia syndrome, the most important of which is multi-infarct (vascular) dementia. Other causes include other neurodegenerative diseases such as Huntington's; structural changes such as brain tumours and hydrocephalus; metabolic, such as electrolyte abnormalities; nutritional, such as thiamine deficiency or vitamin B_{12} deficiency; toxic, including alcoholism — the most treatable condition being iatrogenic cognitive impairment occurring as a side-effect of medication (Katzman 1986a).

Alzheimer's disease, however, is not an epidemiological abstraction, but rather a very specific process biologically, with characteristic pathological and neurochemical changes in the brain (Katzman 1986b). The hallmarks of Alzheimer's disease include atrophy of brain tissue with loss of specific nerve cells and the presence of neuritic plaques and neurofibrillary tangles. To consider the issues in regard to the relationship of Alzheimer's disease and ageing, and to understand the significance of the very recent findings on the molecular biology of this disorder, we need to be aware of the current state of knowledge on the brain alterations in Alzheimer's disease.

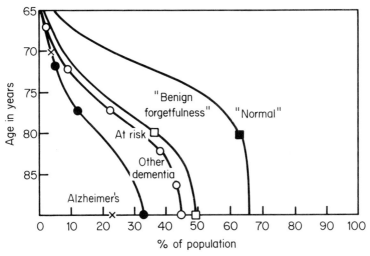

FIG. 2.   Changing patterns of cognitive abilities as a function of age. (Modified from Fig. 1, p 130 in *America's Aging: Health in an Older Society*, National Academy Press, Washington, D.C.)

A primary characteristic of the brain in Alzheimer patients is the selective loss of neurons. The brains of these patients lose substance, as is reflected in a loss of weight by comparison with brains of age-matched controls. However, because of the degree of variability in brain weight in both normal and Alzheimer patients, the weights of individual diseased and age-matched normal brains overlap. On gross inspection there is usually atrophy of the outer surface of the cerebral cortex, especially pronounced in the association cortex. Quantitative computer-assisted counts of neurons in the association cortex, however, show that the loss of neurons in the cerebral cortex is confined to the largest class size of neurons (Terry et al 1981), especially the pyramidal neurons — nerve cells that are believed to connect one area of association cortex with another (Morrison et al 1986). Specific groups of large cells are affected in amygdala and hippocampus (a region of the brain important for memory processing).

Similarly, a group of very large neurons present in clusters in the entorhinal cortex — neurons that act as a relay between hippocampus and association cortex — are markedly affected, whereas surrounding nerve cells in this structure appear intact (Hyman et al 1984). Cell involvement in deeper nuclei in the cerebral hemispheres is also relatively specific, involving neurons that project to cerebral cortex or hippocampus; that is, the cholinergic neurons in the basal nuclei of the forebrain, the serotoninergic neurons in the midbrain, and the noradrenergic neurons in the locus ceruleus.

This selective loss is observed anatomically but is most apparent when neurotransmitters are studied (Table 1). The marker of the cholinergic neurons, the biosynthetic enzyme choline acetyltransferase (ChAT), is markedly reduced in the basal nucleus, the locus of the neuronal cell bodies, and in the cerebral cortex and hippocampus, where the endings terminate. In contrast, ChAT levels and ChAT-containing neurons in other regions of the brain are normal in the brains of Alzheimer patients. The specificity is also shown in neurons that are located within the cerebral cortex; cortical concentrations of the neuropeptide somatostatin are markedly reduced, whereas cortical concentrations of the neuropeptides cholecystokinin (CCK) and vasoactive intestinal peptide (VIP), present in adjacent cells, are not reduced. It has been estimated that fewer than 15% of the nerve cells in the cerebral hemisphere of Alzheimer patients are affected in the disease process; if this estimate is correct, these cells must play a special role in cognitive processing.

Neuritic plaques and neurofibrillary tangles, the other two hallmarks of this disease, were identified in 1907 by Alois Alzheimer, a psychiatrist interested in discovering neuroanatomical changes that might be associated with mental disorders. Alzheimer (1907) applied newly synthesized organic silver dyes to the brain of a patient with a progressive dementia who died after a five-year course; he observed the presence of structures staining intensely with the silver dye, namely the neuritic plaque and the neurofibrillary tangle. The

TABLE 1   Chemical pathology of Alzheimer's disease

		Pathological correlates	
Neurotransmitter change		Cells of origin (cell loss and NFT)	Terminal field (NP)
Cholinergic	↓ 40–90% (15 labs.)	Basal nucleus of Meynert	Cerebral cortex
Somatostatin	↓ 49–90% (4 labs.)	Cerebral cortex, ?hippocampus	Cerebral cortex, hippocampus
CRF	↓ 40+% (2 labs.)	Cerebral cortex	Cerebral cortex
Noradrenaline	Variable	Locus ceruleus	Cerebral cortex, hippocampus
Serotonin	Variable	Dorsal raphe	Cerebral cortex, hippocampus
Substance P	Variable	?	Cerebral cortex

Probably unchanged:
   γ-aminobutyric acid (GABA)
   Dopamine
   Vasopressin
   Oxytocin
   Enkephalin
   Neurotensin
   Cholecystokinin (CCK)
   Vasoactive intestinal peptide (VIP)
   Neuropeptide Y (NPY)

NFT, neurofibrillary tangles; NP, neuritic plaques; CRF, corticotropin-releasing factor.

neuritic plaque consists of a cluster of degenerating nerve endings surrounding a core which is an accumulation of extracellular amyloid protein fibrils. The neurofibrillary tangle is an abnormal nerve cell body filled with an accumulation of an atypical fibril, the paired helical filament.

Important information on the amyloid peptide, its precursor protein and gene, and the possible role of this gene in the aetiology of Alzheimer's has recently been reported. Glenner & Wong (1984) had been successful in isolating and solubilizing amyloid from the meningeal blood vessels of patients with Alzheimer's disease and were able to obtain a partial sequence of the peptide; the same sequence subsequently proved to be present in neuritic plaque amyloid. The gene coding for the precursor protein of the Alzheimer amyloid has now been identified and sequenced (Kang et al 1987). The precursor protein coded by this gene has a relative molecular mass (M_r) of about 79 000 and resembles a membrane surface protein, with the major part of the protein in the extracellular domain and with the 42 or 43 amino acid amyloid sequence embedded within the transmembrane portion.

Whether the function of this molecule is that of a receptor or whether it is a structural protein is not known; it may well be a metal-binding protein.

Advances have also been made in understanding the molecular chemistry of the filaments that accumulate to form neurofibrillary tangles, but this story is far from complete. The abnormal filaments in neurofibrillary tangles appear to be made up of two 10 nm-thick fibrils that are wound around each other (with a hemiperiod of about 80 nm) and therefore termed paired helical filaments (PHF). PHF have a unique structure on X-ray crystallography, differing from all other known biological fibrils (Wischik & Crowther 1986). PHF are found only in human disease and have not been observed in other species. These fibrils had been especially difficult to study because of their insolubility (Selkoe et al 1982). However, partial solubilization has been achieved using formic acid and other techniques. Purified samples of this material have proven to be very antigenic; antibodies obtained interact with phosphorylated, high-molecular-weight neurofilaments and microtubule-associated protein (MAP)-2 but especially with tau protein. Tau protein (a family of $\approx M_r$ 45 000–60 000 phosphoproteins [$\approx$ four isoforms] associated exclusively with axonal microtubules in normal brain tissue) in neurofibrillary tangles appears to be abnormally phosphorylated (Grundke-Iqbal et al 1986). It is not at all clear yet whether the PHF is composed solely of these known proteins or whether an additional protein or peptide is present that accounts for the unique molecular structure.

Investigators have been interested in the question of whether a specific component of the Alzheimer process is particularly related to the presence of dementia. In the classic study of Blessed et al (1968) there was a quantitative correlation between the number of neuritic plaques in the cerebral cortex of dementia patients and the degree of cognitive deficit measured by mental status examination during life, a finding that has been confirmed (Katzman et al 1983). There is also an excellent correlation between the degree of dementia measured during life and the loss of the cholinergic marker ChAT (Perry et al 1978, Katzman et al 1986). As degenerating cholinergic endings are a major component of neuritic plaques (Armstrong et al 1986), there is, as expected, a strong intercorrelation of these two markers of the Alzheimer process. The correlation of the loss of the cholinergic marker with the degree of dementia has been specially interesting because replacement therapy is theoretically possible, but cholinomimetic agents have not proved to be as therapeutically effective as had been hoped, although greater success has been attributed to the cholinesterase inhibitor THA (tetrahydroaminoacridine), a finding that has yet to be replicated (Summers et al 1986).

A problem that had led to controversy has been the existence of a small number of individuals who showed Alzheimer-like changes in the brain but were apparently normal during life. We have had the opportunity to look at a large series of human brains for which we have extensive neurochemical and morphometric data. What has distinguished the brains of those who have neuritic plaques and loss of ChAT, but relatively normal mentation during life, has been the continued survival of the large nerve cells in the association cortex normally lost in the Alzheimer brain. Apparently the retention of these cellular elements has been sufficient to maintain cognitive function, even in the presence of neuritic plaques and neurotransmitter loss.

Individuals with Down's syndrome typically develop Alzheimer-type changes in their brains if they live beyond the age of 40. The gene for the amyloid precursor protein (a gene present in normal individuals) proved to be located on chromosome 21 (Goldgaber et al 1987, Kang et al 1987, Robakis et al 1987, Tanzi et al 1987). A marker linked to the presence of familial Alzheimer's disease in pedigrees with many Alzheimer cases in several generations is located on chromosome 21 (St George-Hyslop et al 1987). Down's syndrome patients of course have a third copy of each gene on chromosome 21. An intriguing preliminary finding is that in (three cases of) sporadic Alzheimer's disease, DNA from peripheral leucocytes shows a 50% increase in DNA coded for the amyloid gene, as if a third copy of this gene were present (Delebar et al 1987). If sporadic Alzheimer's disease results from a gene dosage effect resulting from triplication of the amyloid precursor gene, part of the puzzle of this disorder will have been solved and a new set of questions related to the age effect can be directly addressed.

Thus, modern pathological, neurochemical and molecular biological methods are beginning to clarify the pathogenesis of Alzheimer's disease. But we are still far from understanding its aetiology. In the risk factor studies done so far, the two most important factors predicting the development of Alzheimer's disease have been family history and age. Studies have shown that first-degree relatives of Alzheimer probands are at several times increased risk for Alzheimer's disease (Heston et al 1981) and, in a few large pedigrees, the inheritance appears to be dominant. The new familial linkage studies described above point to a locus on chromosome 21 for the familial Alzheimer gene. The preliminary report of an increase in the gene dosage of the chromosome 21 amyloid protein precursor gene in sporadic cases strongly suggests that the family history factor is indeed genetic (rather than familial transmission of a virus, for example). However, in only a few families and in Down's syndrome is the genetic effect so strong that the disease begins at a typical age. The more common event is that the genetic abnormality predisposes toward the disease with age and another factor or factors determining the time of onset. For example, in the pair of identical twins reported by Cook et al (1981) the age of onset of autopsy-proven Alzheimer's disease in one twin preceded that of the other twin by more than 13 years. Thus, even when genetic factors appear overriding, unknown risk factors or endogenous events determine the age of onset. And these factors must act in such a way that the outcome is an age-dependent disorder.

I shall now consider several working hypotheses relating to the interaction between Alzheimer's disease and age:

(1) *Functional reserve hypothesis*. During normal ageing there is atrophy of the brain. This is observed directly in computed tomography (CT) scans of the brain; indeed the degree of atrophy as observed on scans during normal ageing overlaps the atrophy observed in age-matched Alzheimer patients, although if the degree of atrophy is quantitatively estimated, the means of the two groups are significantly different. The loss of brain substance as measured by brain weight is about 10% between ages 30 and 80. It had long been thought that the loss of brain substance was due to neuronal loss; a classical study by Brody (1955) reported over a 50% loss of large neurons during normal ageing. The most recent quantitative computerized counts of neurons indicate, however, that the number of neurons present in the cerebral cortex does not change with age; rather, the neurons shrink in size, perhaps simultaneously with the loss of their dendritic arborizations.

Loss of large neurons, together with their dendritic arborizations, is a major feature of Alzheimer's disease. One can postulate that early in the course of Alzheimer's disease, when neuronal changes are still very mild and a younger patient would not show symptoms, an older patient with age-related neuronal changes might develop cognitive loss. However, it is unlikely that this mechanism is the primary basis of the age effect since the rate of progression of clinical symptoms is independent of age in Alzheimer patients aged 55 to 90 and the correlation of psychological changes with plaque count and neurochemical changes is altered only slightly during ageing.

(2) *Gene interaction with exogenous substance*. An excellent example of a genetic degenerative disease of the brain in which an exogenous substance is the major risk factor is Wilson's disease. Here a genetic alteration in the mechanisms of copper metabolism leads to eventual accumulation of copper in the brain and consequent changes, both motor and cognitive. Elimination of copper-containing foods from the diet can delay the onset of Wilson's disease. The use of chelating agents to remove copper can stop the progression and sometimes produce an improvement in symptoms. In Alzheimer's patients' brain there is accumulation of aluminium, especially in areas of cerebral cortex with many neurofibrillary tangles. Although the ingestion of aluminium-containing antacids has not been shown to be a risk factor in Alzheimer's disease, other sources of exogenous aluminium still need to be ruled out as contributors to the disease.

(3) *The MPTP model*. The designer drug, 1-methyl-4-phenyl-1,2,3,6-tetrahydropyridine (MPTP), produces an almost exact clinical and pathological model of Parkinson's disease, both in patients exposed to the drug and in susceptible animals. Experimentally, the disorder can be produced with

much lower doses of MPTP in older animals. It has been shown that the toxic effect of MPTP in destroying substantia nigra neurons is due to a metabolite, 1-methyl-4-phenylpyridinium (MPP⁻), produced by the action of monoamine oxidase B on MPTP. Monoamine oxidase B is present in glial cells in the brain. The concentration of this enzyme *rises* with age, as the number of glial cells increases. Although no equivalent molecule has been implicated in Alzheimer's disease, it is conceivable that the increase in glial cells with age may alter another toxic precursor molecule which acts to initiate the series of events leading to neuritic plaque formation or neurofibrillary tangles.

(4) *Disease interaction with age-dependent changes in blood–brain barrier*. Hardy et al (1986) have argued that the primary lesion in the Alzheimer brain is the neuritic plaque. Hardy postulates that neuritic plaque formation is incited by local breakdown of the blood–brain barrier with entry into the brain of one or more toxic substances or proteins (e.g., the amyloid peptide) which then serve(s) as the focus for development of the neuritic plaque. In turn, the microvascular changes leading to the blood–brain barrier changes are postulated to be age dependent and the result of normal alterations with age in neurochemical systems that project to cerebral cortex — for example, the noradrenergic, serotoninergic and cholinergic systems, projection systems whose neurotransmitters may affect vascular permeability.

(5) *Virus interaction with age-dependent changes in the immune system*. The classical example here is shingles, an eruption due to infection of dorsal root ganglia by herpes zoster, the same virus that produces chickenpox in childhood under the name of varicella, remains dormant for decades, and is activated by a change in the immune system later in life. However, so far there is no evidence of the presence of any known virus in the brains of Alzheimer patients.

(6) *Excitatory amino acids as endogenous toxins*. An interesting recent finding has been that excitatory amino acids (glutamic and aspartic acids) can be neurotoxic. Very recent experiments indicate that the destructive effects of ischaemia and injury can be ameliorated in part by drugs that block the action of these amino acids. Certainly glutaminergic neurons, such as the pyramidal cells in association cortex and in entorhinal cortex, are among the cell groups vulnerable to the Alzheimer process. Could the neurotransmitter in these very cells be contributing to the pathogenesis of cell loss in Alzheimer's disease?

(7) *Programmed cell death and neurotrophic factors*. An interesting discovery of modern neuroscience is that only half the neurons that are formed in the brain at the time of birth survive to adult life. This phenomenon has been called programmed cell death; how long it continues into adult life is a matter of controversy. One of the major mechanisms that keeps surviving

neurons alive is the presence of very small amounts of potent trophic peptides. The best known and characterized of the neurotrophic peptides is nerve growth factor (NGF), but there is evidence that there are dozens of other such factors. One hypothesis relating ageing to Alzheimer's disease assumes that there is a trophic factor needed for the survival of the types of neurons vulnerable to the Alzheimer process, a trophic factor that normally decreases during ageing. No such factor has yet been identified. One group of susceptible neurons, the basal forebrain cholinergic neurons, do depend on NGF for survival. However, NGF is present in normal amounts in the cerebral cortex of Alzheimer's disease brain. Perhaps the need for NGF adds to the Alzheimer process, in that NGF is usually transported from the nerve terminals down the axon to the nucleus of the cell. In Alzheimer's disease it is likely that the presence of neurofibrillary tangles will interrupt this transport and thus contribute to further degeneration of the neurons. There is some evidence to suggest that NGF supplied directly to the cell body might slow this degenerative process. But it seems unlikely that changes in NGF can explain the age dependence of Alzheimer's disease.

Acknowlededgments

I thank Robert W. Davignon for his assistance in preparing and editing this manuscript. Support for this project was provided by National Institute on Aging grant AG05131 and by the Florence Riford Chair in Alzheimer's Research.

References

Alzheimer A 1907 Uber eine eigenartige Erkrankung der Hirnrinde. Allg Z Psychiatr 64:146–148

Armstrong DM, Bruce G, Hersh LB, Terry RD 1986 Choline acetyltransferase immunoreactivity in neuritic plaques of Alzheimer brain. Neurosci Lett 71:229–234

Blessed G, Tomlinson BE, Roth M 1968 The association between quantitative measures of dementia and of senile change in the cerebral grey matter of elderly subjects. Br J Psychiatry 114:797–811

Brody H 1955 Organization of the cerebral cortex. III. A study of aging in the human cerebral cortex. J Comp Neurol 102:511–556

Cook RH, Bard BE, Austin JH 1981 Twins with Alzheimer's disease. Arch Neurol 38:300–301

Delabar J-M, Goldgaber S, Lamour Y et al 1987 β Amyloid gene duplication in Alzheimer's disease and karyotypically normal Down syndrome. Science (Wash DC) 235:1390–1392

Glenner GC, Wong CW 1984 Alzheimer's disease: initial report of the purification and characterization of a novel cerebrovascular amyloid protein. Biochem Biophys Res Commun 120:885–890

Goldgaber D, Lerman MI, McBride OW, Saffiotti U, Gajdusek DC 1987 Characterization and chromosomal localization of a cDNA encoding brain amyloid of Alzheimer's disease. Science (Wash DC) 235:877–880

Grundke-Iqbal I, Iqbal K, Quinlan M, Tung Y-C, Zaidi MS, Wisniewski HM 1986 Microtubule-associated protein tau. J Biol Chem 261:6084–6089

Hagnell O, Lanke J, Rorsman B, Ojesjo L 1981 Does the incidence of age psychosis decrease? Neuropsychobiology 7:201–211

Hardy JA, Mann DMA, Wester P, Winblad B 1986 An integrative hypothesis concerning the pathogenesis and progression of Alzheimer's disease. Neurobiol Aging 7:489–502

Heston LL, Mastri AR, Anderson VE, White J 1981 Dementia of the Alzheimer type: genetics, natural history, and associated conditions. Arch Gen Psychiatry 38:1085

Hyman BT, Van Hoesen GW, Damasio AR, Barnes CL 1984 Alzheimer's disease: cell-specific pathology isolates the hippocampal formation. Science 225:1168–1170

Kang J, Lemaire H-G, Unterbeck A et al 1987 The precursor of Alzheimer's disease amyloid A4 protein resembles a cell-surface receptor. Nature (Lond) 325:733–736

Katzman R 1985 Aging and age-dependent disease: cognition and dementia. In: America's aging: health in an older society. Committee on an Aging Society, Institute of Medicine/National Research Council. National Academy Press, Washington, DC, p 129–152

Katzman R 1986a Differential diagnosis of dementing illnesses. In: Hutton JT (ed) Neurologic clinics. Saunders, Philadelphia, p 329–340

Katzman R 1986b Alzheimer's disease. N Engl J Med 314:964–973

Katzman R, Brown T, Fuld P, Peck A, Schechter R, Schimmel H 1983 Validation of a short orientation-memory-concentration test of cognitive impairment. Am J Psychiatry 140:734–739

Katzman R, Brown T, Fuld P, Thal L, Davies P, Terry RD 1986 Significance of neurotransmitter abnormalities in Alzheimer's disease. In: Martin JB, Barchas J (eds) Neuropeptides in neurologic and psychiatric disease. New York: Raven Press (A.R.N.M.D. Vol 64), Chap 14, p 279–286

Morrison JH, Scherr S, Lewis DA, Campbell MJ, Bloom FE 1986 In: Scheibel AB, Wechsler AF (eds) The biological substrates of Alzheimer's disease. Academic Press, Orlando, p 115–131

Ostermann K, Sprung-Ostermann B 1988 Cerebrovascular disease and the elderly. In: Research and the ageing population. Wiley, Chichester (Ciba Found Symp 134) p 58–68

Perry EK, Tomlinson BE, Blessed G, Bergmann K, Gibson PH, Perry RH 1978 Correlation of cholinergic abnormalities with senile plaques and mental test scores in senile dementia. Br Med J 2:1457–1459

Robakis N, Wisniewski HM, Jenkins EC et al 1987 Chromosome 21q21 sublocalisation of gene beta-amyloid peptide in cerebral vessels and neuritic (senile) plaques of people with Alzheimer disease and Down syndrome. Lancet 1:384–385

Selkoe DJ, Ihara Y, Salazar FJ 1982 Alzheimer's disease: insolubility of partially-purified paired helical filaments in sodium dodecyl sulfate and urea. Science (Wash DC) 215:1243–1245

Sluss TK, Gruenberg EM, Kramer M 1981 The use of longitudinal studies in the investigation of risk factors for senile dementia-Alzheimer type. In: Mortimer JA, Schuman LM (eds) The epidemiology of dementia. Oxford University Press, London, p 132–154

St George-Hyslop PH, Tanzi RE, Polinsky RJ et al. 1987 The genetic defect causing familial Alzheimer's disease maps on chromosome 21. Science (Wash DC) 235:885–890

Summers WJ, Majovski LV, Marsh GM, Tachiki K, Kling A 1986 Oral tetrahydroaminoacridine in long-term treatment of dementia. Alzheimer type. N Engl J Med 315:1241–1245

Tanzi RE, Gusella JF, Watkins PC et al 1987 Amyloid β protein gene: cDNA, mRNA
    distribution, and genetic linkage near the Alzheimer locus. Science (Wash DC)
    235:880–884
Terry RD, Peck A, DeTeresa R, Schecter R, Horoupian DS 1981 Some mor-
    phometric aspects of the brain in senile dementia of the Alzheimer type. Ann
    Neurol 10:184–192
Wischik CM, Crowther RA 1986 Subunit structure of the Alzheimer tangle. Br Med
    Bull 42:51–56

DISCUSSION

T.F. Williams: If the presence of a third copy of the amyloid polypeptide
precursor gene is correct, this should, as you suggest, give us the opportunity of
identifying a susceptible subpopulation where we can look for the other con-
tributory factors.

Katzman: This is so. It has been frustrating looking for risk factors that
haven't been found! These factors could be obscured if one-third of the population is susceptible to Alzheimer's disease and two-thirds are not; looking at the
entire elderly population would not reveal the risk factors.

Fries: Maternal age at birth has been implicated as a risk factor in Down's
syndrome; has anyone looked at maternal age in Alzheimer's disease?

Katzman: Maternal age was a positive risk factor for Alzheimer's disease in a
study in Seattle: that correlation has been confirmed by two other studies but
not found in three or four more.

Fries: What about cigarette smoking as a risk factor?

Katzman: In our prospective study of the development of dementia in four
hundred 80-year-old volunteers we had almost no cigarette smokers among the
32 subjects who developed Alzheimer's disease.

Fries: Perhaps the smokers had died already.

Coleman: If one accepts the central dogma of molecular biology, which
states that DNA makes RNA which makes protein, it is interesting that Jerry
Higgins and his colleagues (personal communication) found the messenger
RNA for the amyloid protein in approximately equal amounts in brains of
Alzheimer patients and in control brains. The mRNA level in Alzheimer brains
was increased over normal only in the entorhinal cortex and the parasubicu-
lum, and not very markedly. If the amyloid gene is closely related to Alzheimer's disease there may be processes at work which complicate the basic, central
dogma.

Katzman: One cannot infer a direct relationship between gene copies and
mRNA: there is a reduction in the numbers of the large nerve cells in the
Alzheimer's brain, which may normally produce the amyloid precursor protein, and also a reduction in total messenger RNA in Alzheimer brains examined at *post mortem*. One could imagine that if the amyloid precursor
molecule were important, its degradation might be one of the first steps in the

Alzheimer process, with the remaining hydrophobic portion of the molecule being accumulated as amyloid.

Coleman: You are right to bring in the possibility of modification of the amyloid protein after it has been made.

Kirkwood: The suggestion in the third gene copy hypothesis is that one chromosome carries a duplication of the amyloid gene. If this duplication were common in the population, one might expect some individuals to be homozygous for the duplicated gene, in which case they would be carrying four copies. It would be interesting to know if people with a family history of Alzheimer's disease on both sides are at risk of developing a more severe form of the disease.

Riggs: What do you think about the prion hypothesis of the pathogenesis of Alzheimer's disease, Dr Katzman?

Katzman: There is a certain analogy, in that the prion of scrapie (a neurological disease of sheep) accumulates in brain extracellular space as a rod-like, amyloid-like protein. The prion is produced by a gene which is normally present in the host genome. It is similar to Alzheimer's only in that the amyloid in Alzheimer's is produced by a gene normally present. However, Stanley Prusiner has claimed but not yet demonstrated that the prion is infectious; he has not been able to put prions into an animal and produce scrapie. One cannot rule out an infectious agent, but there is no evidence for it either, yet.

Arie: The Cambridge group believe that there are two syndromes of Alzheimer's disease, the late and the early (Roth & Wischik 1985, Bondareff 1983). The late form has fewer of the stigmata (both structural and biochemical) of the disease: the early form has a more rapid course and is a more virulent form of the disease. Do you think that work is valid? If it is, this is important from the point of view of further studies, because one may be looking at heterogeneous groups of patients suffering from rather different syndromes, and this may confound the findings. Even if one is not confident that the two syndromes exist, it is perhaps wise to segregate these different groups so that one is studying homogeneous populations.

Katzman: It may resemble the lipidoses: the same phenotype of some of the childhood lipidoses was shown to be produced by many genotypes, with many different biochemical pathways producing the same end result. That could happen in Alzheimer's; the problem is that we do not have an adequate basis for subdividing the disease. With regard to age, there is one clear-cut difference between older and younger Alzheimer patients. We looked at a very elderly population, where the average age was around 87 years. In that group a number of Alzheimer patients had neuritic plaques in the cerebral cortex without neurofibrillary tangles. In the hippocampus and elsewhere in the brain there were tangles, but not in the neocortex. Dr Robert Terry recently contrasted all the brains with plaques only in neocortex with those with plaques and tangles (excluding patients with other diseases). There was an age difference between the two groups; those with plaques alone were older. But there was no difference in the rate of progression of dementia, or in somatostatin or choline acetyltransferase activity in the neocortex or hippocampus, or in neuron counts in neocortex.

We recently studied the rate of change of clinically diagnosed Alzheimer's in the nursing home in New York, in our San Diego population, and in the Bronx ageing study. We found no difference between the three geographical sites, and there were no differences as a function of age in the rate of change of mental status. I have no doubt that there is heterogeneity, but it is not as straightforward as just an age marker.

Coleman: The definition of two classes of Alzheimer's disease used by Bondareff et al (1981) was based on brains examined at autopsy. The early-onset cases probably survived longer than the late-onset ones after the apparent onset of the disease, so the disease process had had longer, on average, to do its work in the brain.

Arie: My impression is that the cumulative evidence withstands that criticism.

Wenger: I was intrigued by the dissociation, suggested by Dr Williams in his Introduction, between the occurrence of coronary artery disease or diabetes mellitus and Alzheimer's disease, despite the common occurrence of all of them in an elderly population. Have the patients whose brains were examined at autopsy had their coronary arteries examined equally carefully, or had blood glucose levels determined during life? Because, as one looks at clinical manifestations of disease, they are dependent on the reporting of the problem. With diabetes, particularly maturity-onset diabetes, the manifestations of the disease often decrease as people lose weight and approach ideal body weight; weight loss is also characteristic of the aged population. Do we have blood sugar levels at a younger age on the Alzheimer population, or autopsy findings describing their coronary arteries?

Katzman: In the Bronx ageing study we unfortunately did not have that information, but it would be accessible in the Framingham study and in the Baltimore longitudinal study.

The other issue is a difficult one. Many patients in nursing homes lose weight in the last few months of the Alzheimer process. They deteriorate, and I have never known whether that is due to the Alzheimer process affecting the hypothalamus and its control of body metabolism, or because the Alzheimer patients are not being cared for or fed adequately. Dr John Blass thinks that it is an important systemic component of the Alzheimer process. So at autopsy you have subjects who have been losing weight for months. Dr Terry thinks there is less atherosclerosis in the large vessels of the brains of those patients. Again, that might be secondary to malnutrition; you can reduce the amount of atherosclerosis by a very restricted diet. We would need to examine the blood vessels by angiography earlier in the course of these patients.

T.F. Williams: I raised this question of the rarity of diabetes in Alzheimer's because a cardiologist commented to me that that is also true of atherosclerotic cardiovascular disease: when an elderly patient comes into their heart station and proves to have a normal electrocardiogram, they have come to expect to find Alzheimer's disease. They compared patients from their heart clinic population (a selected population, therefore) who had a diagnosis of Alzheimer's disease with an age- and sex-matched group with other psychiatric diagnoses, largely schizophrenia or affective disorders, and a third group of patients who had neither. In the Alzheimer group only one of 40 patients had a diagnosis of diabetes, and that was questionable; about 10% in each of the other two groups had diagnosed diabetes. They found roughly the same differences with coronary artery disease; only two or three Alzheimer patients carried that diagnosis, compared to 15% or so in the other two groups. The same prevalence of osteoarthritis was found across the whole group, which reassured them somewhat about the overall comparability of their subgroups.

Solomons: You spoke earlier in defence of the older 'medical' concept of disease, Dr Katzman, but the new evidence on Alzheimer's does not seem to support that view! If one could find individuals who could be identified by some chromosomal damage at birth, constituting a third of the population, I would have to support Grimley Evans' point that, at least for that group, Alzheimer's is a normal part of ageing; if these people live long enough they will all get it. I was also interested that you find Alzheimer changes pathologically in a small proportion of subjects who retain normal cognitive function.

Katzman: I would certainly like to know some way of preventing the onset of the disease if I had the third gene copy!

On the maintenance of normal cognitive function with mild Alzheimer's changes (e.g. small numbers of neuritic plaques), these patients had not lost their large nerve cells in the neocortex. Some of the patients with intact cognitive function had in fact more large neurons in the frontal, parietal and temporal brain regions than age-matched normals. It may be the retention of nerve cells, or their dendritic connections, or both, which is important, rather than neurotransmitter activity levels as such.

Coleman: I would add that whatever single marker you choose for Alzheimer's disease you find at least some overlap between apparently normal older people and Alzheimer cases. This led us to think that we need to use multivariate descriptors, or a combination of morphological and biochemical measures, to give a more adequate post-mortem correlation with clinical status. Indeed, we have found this to be so (Hamill et al 1987).

Ostermann: Can you say anything about interventions that can be made in the normal daily care of these patients, after the diagnosis of Alzheimer's disease is established?

Katzman: In my own practice, and in studies on our patients by people interested in this aspect, it seems that what helps Alzheimer patients is to maintain their interactions with others. We have had occasions where patients were given psychological retraining designed to improve memory, but this tended to produce increased stress within the family without any improvement in cognition. So far, no way has been found of decreasing the cognitive loss. What can be improved is the patients' behaviour, by maintaining full social activity, and by using their existing strengths, such as musical ability. Some abilities remain; if one can build on them, this helps the Alzheimer patient and keeps his or her behaviour from deteriorating.

Andrews: What is the current state of the epidemiology of Alzheimer's disease? The methods used in population studies are often not very refined; the populations studied have not always been representative, and good incidence studies, as opposed to studies of prevalence in various places, are rare. Are any clues emerging from what we understand to be the epidemiological picture? As a corollary to that, is there a case for an international collaborative prospective approach to Alzheimer's disease?

Katzman: Such a study is important, particularly if there is an interaction between events during life and genetic predisposition; one might expect this to vary in different populations. If one could look at risk factors as well as incidence and prevalence in your kinds of populations in developing countries—and I am involved in a study in Shanghai, and we have been talking to Frank Williams about doing similar studies in Africa and India—those would be important investigations. One problem with cross-cultural studies is the lack of methods for assessing cognitive change in people with essentially no education, who are completely illiterate, as we mentioned before (p 36). We simply don't know how to test for cognitive impairment. We would need to devise cross-culturally valid methods. Perhaps the Fuld object-memory test that we used in the New York nursing home, which has also been tried in Japan, will be useful. (There are 10 items, such as a ball, a key, and so on; one can use any kind of common object for the person to touch, feel and name, and then remember. That test seems to work both in Japan and the USA.)

One of the problems in the Alzheimer patient's brain is difficulty with visuospatial relationships. If a person has never used a pencil and doesn't draw, how does one assess this capacity? Perhaps something like the object assembly or block design in the Wechsler Intelligence Scale for Children (WISC) can be used in different cultures. We shall need to know this, before we can do such studies in societies with high illiteracy rates. I understand that the NIH is interested in sponsoring cross-cultural epidemiological studies. The NIH currently supports population-based epidemiological studies of dementia in at least six different communities in the USA (East Boston, Framingham, New Haven, Baltimore, Durham, Iowa City), as well as several prospective longitudinal studies, such as the Bronx ageing study.

References

Bondareff W 1983 Age and Alzheimer disease. Lancet 1:1447

Bondareff W, Mountjoy CQ, Roth M 1981 Selective loss of neurones of origin of adrenergic projection to cerebral cortex (nucleus locus coerulus) in senile dementia. Lancet 1:783–784

Hamill RW, Caine E, Coleman P et al 1987 Multiple morphological and biochemical measures completely distinguish patients with Alzheimer's disease. Abstracts, 1987 Meeting of the Society for Neuroscience, in press

Roth M, Wischik CM 1985 The heterogeneity of Alzheimer's disease and its implications for scientific investigations of the disorder. In: Arie T (ed) Recent advances in psychogeriatrics. Churchill Livingstone, Edinburgh

Questions in the psychiatry of old age

Tom Arie

Department of Health Care of the Elderly, University of Nottingham Medical School, Queen's Medical Centre, Nottingham NG7 2UH, UK

Abstract. The last ten to fifteen years have been a time of rapid development in the psychiatry of old age. Biological research on the dementias has moved forward impressively, but significant too has been the development in many countries of local services specially designed to meet the needs of old people with mental disorders, and of those who look after them. Such services are built on the experience both of psychiatry and of geriatrics, but have also broken new ground: the UK experience is described. The facts have belied earlier misgivings about the potential of this field of work to attract and satisfy able staff in the health professions; indeed, this work has developed with style and enthusiasm, and with widespread educational programmes and growing research activity.

This paper reviews briefly these developments and considers some broader issues of policy as they bear on the care of mentally ill old people. Considered also is tentative evidence that the dementias of old age may be becoming less prevalent. Finally, current studies in Nottingham which look at the social associations of old age mental disorders are briefly described and the implications are considered of the broadening of the base of 'psychogeriatrics' which such studies represent.

1988 Research and the ageing population. Wiley, Chichester (Ciba Foundation Symposium 134) p 86–105

Dr Katzman has described recent exciting advances in our knowledge of the biology of dementia. Certainly this is among the fields of activity relating to my subject that have lately been cultivated most fruitfully. In this brief paper I shall try to give some taste of questions which currently preoccupy us in Britain, not in the biological field, but in regard to social and epidemiological aspects of the psychiatry of old age. I have chosen three topics: first, the development of specialized psychiatric services for the elderly, which are a new feature of our National Health Service; next, some 'straws in the wind' which suggest that it is possible that the dementias of old age may be becoming less common, or at least that they may be less common than previous surveys have reported; and, third, I shall report some aspects of recent studies in Nottingham of the lives of old people living at home. I am deliberately raising topics which I suspect will recur in later contributions to our symposium.

'Psychogeriatrics' as a branch of psychiatry

The growth of psychogeriatric services into what is now a major branch of psychiatry has been a remarkable development in Britain, and in several other countries, over little more than a decade.

In the late 1960s the pressures of changing demography were becoming keenly felt within the workload of psychiatric services and in the populations of mental illness hospitals — and this indeed had been forecast by Sir Aubrey Lewis as far back as 1946 (Lewis 1946). Stimulated by the achievements both of psychiatry and of geriatrics, a small group of psychiatrists applied themselves to developing within local psychiatric services a component shaped to meet the needs of old people.

I started to work in this field at the beginning of 1969. There were few signposts — one had to find one's own way. Only some half-a-dozen people were then devoting themselves specifically to this work.

Nearly twenty years later one remembers the astonishment of colleagues: why, they asked, was one choosing to work not only in the field of old age, but in a mental hospital which was not itself connected with a teaching centre? Implicit in people's incredulity, and sometimes made explicit, were a series of assumptions: first, that work with mentally ill old people could not be sufficiently interesting, nor could it give sufficient professional satisfaction, to make it likely that it could become a distinct branch of psychiatry, capable of attracting its share of able staff; next, that even if people could be persuaded to work in this field, they would not wish to give more than part of their time to it. A third assumption was that if anyone chose to do this work, he or she would do so for only a limited time, at worst until a better job came up, at best by way of an altruistic contribution akin to, say, voluntary service in the Third World. The history of the developments which I shall describe is thus the history of an experiment — the testing of these hypotheses.

When it began to be clear that things were working out very differently (Arie 1970) a new explanation was put forward — namely, that whilst the work might be to the taste of a few eccentrics, or (this was the more flattering version) of a few 'charismatic' figures, the enterprises built around these people would wither if ever they were themselves to move elsewhere.

Events have not borne out these misgivings, and the rest of the first part of this piece briefly describes those events. Table 1 sets out the growth in the number of consultants, who are now commonly, if not euphoniously, called 'psychogeriatricians'.

Table 1 shows how from a very small beginning — little more than a 'coffee-house' group — the number of psychogeriatricians accelerated through the 1970s so that, by 1980, there were 120 psychiatrists (along with associated staff) running 'clearly defined' local psychiatric services for the elderly (Wattis et al 1981). By 1985 this figure had risen to 200 (Arie et al

TABLE 1   Growth in numbers of psychogeriatricians in the UK, 1969–1987

Year	Numbers
1969	'Half-a-dozen'
1973	20
1977	First professorial department
1980	120
1983	150
1984	170
1987	250
	Four professorial departments

(Source: Wattis et al 1981; Wattis & Arie 1984; Arie et al 1985; J. Wattis, unpublished data).

1985) and it is now estimated at some 250, or nearly one in four of all consultants in general psychiatry; over two-thirds (68%) of all UK health districts now have such specialized services (J. Wattis, unpublished data). Along with these developments, programmes of training have been established; psychiatrists who do not plan to specialize in this field are now able to acquire more skill in working with the aged; and those advanced trainees who intend to specialize in old age psychiatry have available to them planned training programmes (Arie et al 1985), though such programmes are still too few in relation to the demand (Wattis & Arie 1984).

The prediction that people would choose to devote only a part, perhaps a minor part, of their time to this work has not been borne out either. On the contrary, more people are giving it more time; of 93 consultants identified in a 1980 survey (Wattis et al 1981) and re-surveyed in 1983 (Wattis & Arie 1984), 58 had not changed the amount of time given to this work by more than one session either way, eight were working an average of two sessions fewer than in 1980, whilst 27 were working an average of 3.5 sessions more than previously. In 1986 no less than 87 consultants were working full-time in this field and nearly half of all those identified were giving at least nine out of their 11 weekly sessions to it (J. Wattis, unpublished data).

A target of two psychogeriatricians in each health district matches well some US targets (themselves in part derived from the British experience) recommended by James Birren and Bruce Sloane when they reported ten years ago to the then Secretary for Health Education and Welfare (Birren & Sloane 1977). Applying their assumptions of needs for the United States to the UK, we should aim at 440 psychiatrists specializing in old age disorders — which means that we are halfway there.

Along with these developments there has evolved a body of guidance about levels of resources and the *modus operandi* of services, originating partly from our Royal College of Psychiatrists, but also from government bodies (NHS Health Advisory Service 1982) and individuals (Arie & Jolley 1982).

Happily, the emphasis has been on flexibility and variety, services tending to capitalize on what is historically available in their locality. But there is agreement on basic principles: that local services should be unselective, in the sense that they cope with all mental disorders associated with old age in a defined population; that there should be a base in the general hospital, so that the service can respond appropriately to the intimate and complex relationship between physical and mental elements in the disorders of old age; that there should be the closest collaboration with related services and agencies, both statutory and non-statutory; and that great emphasis be given to hospital outreach, and to collaboration with primary care, enabling old people to remain at home whenever possible, and supporting them and those who look after them.

There are now four psychogeriatrician-professors. The first appointment was my own in Nottingham, in 1977, and lately there have been three more, all in London University. In Nottingham all medical students spend one month in full-time attachment to our Department of Health Care of the Elderly. I described these developments recently in New York, and they are reported in some detail in the Bulletin of the New York Academy of Medicine (Arie 1985).

As regards the prediction that this field would not prove capable of attracting able staff, suffice it to say that 'psychogeriatrics', like any other field of work, has its more and its less impressive practitioners, but there would certainly be agreement among British psychiatrists that the psychogeriatricians include some of the ablest, liveliest, and most estimable of our colleagues, and that staff are of at least comparable quality to those working in any other branch of psychiatry. That this should be so in a new field, the image of which is never likely to be glamorous, is remarkable and reassuring. In a relatively short time it has been possible also to establish and develop a series of university departments and a respectable volume of research work. The vigour and initiative of the Specialist Section on Old Age in the Royal College of Psychiatrists (the professional focus for the psychogeriatricians) would hardly be disputed by anyone who knows it.

And as regards the prediction that such services would not survive the loss of their central figure, the following can be said: first, that certainly these enterprises, as many others, originate often from the enthusiasm and drive of a particular individual, but organizational principles for such services (Arie & Jolley 1982, National Health Service Health Advisory Service 1982) are now well established; changes of leadership may indeed change style and emphasis, but the services have their own momentum and stability. I am aware of less than half a dozen instances of psychiatrists who, having taken up this work, have later given it up in favour of other branches of the specialty; and whilst there are many instances of key people having moved from one post to another, I know of nowhere where the service has subsequently withered. In short, geriatric psychiatry as a branch of the Health Service has now become 'part of the furniture' — no longer dependent, if it ever was, on leaders with missionary zeal, but simply on the sensible and effective deployment of skill and resources on the part of staff of many different professions working together, and with voluntary organizations and the public.

In Nottingham the development of services for the elderly has been taken a stage further (Arie 1985). Here we have constructed a combined department which brings together old age psychiatry and old age medicine. This is still the only wholly joint department of this sort in Britain, but others seem set to follow. Our academic staff consist of psychiatrists and physicians, along with the other professions involved. Although the components of the service are well-differentiated, there is a common base in the University Hospital, which includes specialized units for stroke, for orthopaedics, and for problems of continence. Thus with easy access for the users, and a common focus of loyalty for the providers, services can be made available according to the assessed need of patients rather than, as so often happens, being confined merely to what is available in that compartment of the system in which the patient happens (often by chance) to find himself or herself. The service aims, in short, to match the intricate and complex mixture of mental and physical disabilities which is characteristic of the aged, and it is also a prime resource for our educational programmes.

I have very briefly summarized the still-evolving British scene, which is reflected in greater or lesser degree, and in different styles, in many countries. Issues that arise are beginning to be tackled by systematic studies. For instance, long ago it became clear that, as in psychiatry in general, so in our field, and especially in regard to dementia, there are limits to the feasibility and indeed the desirability of 'community care' (Hawks 1975, Arie 1987) — that is, to the extent to which people with serious disabilities of the mind can be looked after in their own homes, especially when they live alone. Attention has also been directed to the tricky issues of the design and quality of care in institutions (Norman 1987), including the 'morale' and job satisfaction of staff. Similarly, approaches are now being made towards defining with much greater precision the ways in which professional inputs can most effectively enhance the capacity of patients and of informal carers to cope (e.g. Gilleard 1985, Zarit et al 1986).

With this background in mind I shall now turn to the 'straws in the wind' which suggest that dementia — that hard core of the care of the elderly — may be becoming less common than previous studies have indicated. This, with a few other aspects of the epidemiology of the dementias, forms my next topic.

Are the dementias of old age becoming less common?

Until recently, despite variation in settings, in methodology and in case-

TABLE 2   Some recent surveys of 'marked' dementia

Study	Findings
Lundby (Hagnell et al 1983)	Fall in incidence over previous 25 years (all cases)
London (Gurland et al 1983)	2.3% prevalence, 65+ years (home cases)
Melton Mowbray (Clarke et al 1986)	4.5% prevalence, 75+ years (all cases); 3.7%, 80–84 years; 9.3%, 85+ years
Nottingham (Morgan et al 1987)	7.8% prevalence, 80+ years (home cases)
Compare e.g.: Newcastle, UK (Kay et al 1964)	5.6%, 65+ years; 22.0%, 80+ years (all cases)

finding criteria, there has been a relative consistency in the results of surveys of mental disorders in old people, suggesting a prevalence of something over 5% among persons aged 65 and above of dementias of 'moderate or severe' degree. (The prevalence of 'mild' dementias is another story, for here there is much greater variation; this group on follow-up is found to comprise people with transient cognitive impairments, and others with lifelong mental retardation, as well as those in the early stages of a dementing process.) Most studies have suggested that around one-fifth of all persons aged over 80 had 'moderate or severe' dementia. These studies have been conveniently summarized in a short booklet from WHO (World Health Organization 1986), and Ineichen (1987) has reviewed more recent studies; Table 2 refers to a few of these.

Incidence studies have been rare, but the first claim that there might be a fall in the incidence of dementia came from the total population study in Lundby, Sweden, where Hagnell et al (1983) found a decline in incidence over some 25 years of both Alzheimer and multi-infarct dementias.

More recently reports have begun to appear of prevalence studies which have found lower — sometimes strikingly lower — rates. Thus the US/UK studies of Gurland and Copeland (Gurland et al 1983) found not only low rates in old people living at home, but an as yet inadequately explained discrepancy between New York and London: the point prevalence of 'pervasive dementia' in subjects over 65 years, living at home, was 4.9% in New York compared with 2.3% in London. Differential mortality and institutionalization rates in this study suggest that any bias would be likely to be in the direction contrary to these findings, and the low rate found in London is without obvious explanation.

Perhaps most impressive of all in this respect is the study by our neighbours

TABLE 3   Prevalence (%) of cognitive impairment[a] in old people living at home in Nottingham

Age	Men	Women	Total
Total 65+[b]	1.6 (6)[c]	4.4 (21)	3.2 (27)
65–74	1.4 (3)	2.1 (6)	1.8 (9)
75–79	2.0 (2)	4.3 (7)	3.4 (9)
80+	2.9 (2)	9.7 (18)	7.8 (20)

[a] Defined by cut-off score of less than seven on the CAPE (Clifton Assessment Procedures for the Elderly) (Pattie & Gilleard 1979).
[b] Weighted total population over 65 years.
[c] Numbers in parentheses.

in Leicester University (Clarke et al 1986) of the total (home and institutional) population of persons aged 75 and over in the small town of Melton Mowbray in Leicestershire. They found a prevalence of 'marked cognitive impairment' of only 4.5% in those over 75 years. In contrast with a 22% prevalence in those over 80 in Newcastle, the figure for those aged 80–84 years in Melton Mowbray was only 3.7%; for those over 85, it was 9.3%.

We in Nottingham have made similar findings in old people living at home (Morgan et al 1987). We found a prevalence of cognitive impairment of 7.8% in people over 80 years, living at home (Table 3).

Although, as Clarke et al (1986) emphasize, rates in such studies are generally based on small numbers, and thus have wide confidence intervals, the figures gain some force from the relatively consistent changes between the findings of the earlier and later studies.

What is one to make of this? Possibly very little! Certainly one echoes the pleas, made in the WHO report already referred to, for the adoption of a common methodology in these studies so that results can better be interpreted and compared. But these reports probably do begin to have some cumulative significance. Do they mean that incidence is falling? We know that survival of the demented, particularly the very aged with dementia, seems to be increasing (Christie 1985), which would tend towards increased rather than lower prevalence rates. Epidemiological studies rarely differentiate reliably (even when they attempt to do so) between the Alzheimer dementias and those of vascular origin, and even if this apparent fall is real, we have little evidence of which type of dementia may be most affected; and of course there is variation in the mix of the dementias especially between, for instance, Japan and Western countries (Hasegawa et al 1985).

Gurland et al in New York (1983), Cooper in Mannheim (1984), and most recently Weissman and colleagues in New Haven (1985) have found a suggestion of an inverse relationship between socioeconomic status and the prevalence of dementia, and it may be that we are seeing also here some 'cohort effects' deriving from lifestyles (that is, the effects of different influences bearing on generations of people born at different times). If the factors involved can be clarified, this could suggest lines of prevention (Arie 1984). We know that various potentially preventable factors which may have altered between successive cohorts bear on the development of dementia: for instance, high blood pressure (both as a precursor of multi-infarct dementia and through the synergistic effects between vascular change and the Alzheimer process); or trauma (boxers' dementia is relevant); or diet; or cigarette or alcohol use. If there does prove to have been a fall in incidence, this may reflect such changes in life and behaviour.

Although the studies referred to here are interesting and suggestive, they are anything but conclusive — least of all do they suggest that the time is coming when we shall be able to dismantle our facilities for caring for the demented. Indeed, quite the opposite: in Melton Mowbray in the 1980s no less than half of all severely demented people were in institutions, whereas in Newcastle in the 1960s four-fifths of severe cases were at home. Here is another 'cohort' effect — the consequence of changes in the family, in the life horizons of women, and in general expectations that relief will be given from the direct burden of caring for the demented at home.

Broadening the therapeutic base

My last topic derives from our studies of the lives of 1042 randomly sampled old people living at home in Nottingham, half of them aged 65 to 74, half aged 75 and over. These studies are chiefly concerned with the relationship between activity levels, 'well-being', health, and the use of services. Of my colleagues in this Activity and Ageing project, chief in the present context is Dr Kevin Morgan. In what I report here, and in my reflections on the data, I may need to be even more tentative than in the previous section.

As old age psychiatry develops it is becoming increasingly concerned, as I have indicated, not only with the traditional problems of psychiatric morbidity in old age, but also with new problems, the recognition and management of which fall (or ought to fall) within its scope. Currently prominent among these, and deservedly so, is stress among carers of the elderly mentally infirm. Simply to acknowledge such issues is to broaden the therapeutic base of psychogeriatrics.

I have chosen here three other topics which represent the medical, social, and economic domains, respectively. Each is presented as an example rather than as a priority. My topics are mobility, loneliness, and poverty.

I shall look at some of our findings in relation to mood state and other relevant variables. Mood state (such as the presence of depression) may be either explicit (in the scores on our rating scales) or inferred (for example,

from antidepressant or anxiolytic drug use); but in our studies the categoriz-
ation of depression is based on a score of eight or more (the more conservative threshold from our Nottingham study) on the Symptoms of Anxiety and
Depression (SAD) scale described by Bedford et al (1976): in fact, a lower
cut-off point of six or more was suggested by Bedford as indicating psychiatric
illness. Also quoted are our own Social Engagement Score (Morgan et al
1987), which was designed to measure the degree to which the individual
participates in the social milieu, and a modified version (Wood et al 1969) of
the Life Satisfaction Index of Neugarten et al (1961). (In the remarks that
follow, 'more likely' or 'associated with . . .' indicates a significant chi-square
value at $P < 0.01$ or less; 'higher/lower levels' indicates a significant t value at
$P < 0.01$ or less.)

First, *mobility*. We defined as 'ambulant' those who can and do get out and
about independently, and as 'impaired' those who for whatever reason are
unable to do so, being either temporarily or permanently housebound. Just
over 90% (90.9%) of our sample were ambulant and just under 10% were
impaired. We found that impaired people were significantly more likely to be
very old (over 75); and they were more likely to be depressed. They showed
lower levels of life satisfaction than those who were ambulant and lower levels
of social engagement. They were more likely to have seen their family doctor
during the previous month. However, mobility showed no sex relationship,
and impaired people were no more likely than the ambulant to be receiving
psychotropic drugs.

What could this mean? Partly the findings are obvious and to that extent
tend to validate our measuring instruments. But we have identified unhappy
people, many of whom are clinically depressed. (We found, incidentally, that
depression in our total sample of old people was not related to age, the
prevalence of depression being approximately 10% for all age groups up to
the over-80s.) We do not know details of the help that these impaired subjects
are getting from the family doctors whom they see more often than other
subjects, but evidently they are not receiving more antidepressant or anxiolytic drugs. This may be good, in that they may be receiving other forms of
help which are deemed more appropriate than drugs; equally it may be bad,
in that symptoms which may be pharmacologically treatable are not always so
treated, perhaps in the light of the doctor's perception of such dysphoric
states as being 'no more than appropriate' to the impairment of the individual. Further detailed studies will be needed to elucidate this, but the
questions are important and familiar.

Next, *loneliness*. We defined as 'lonely' those who reported feeling lonely
'often'. Those who reported feeling lonely only 'sometimes' or 'never' we
defined as 'not lonely'. Just over 17% of our sample were lonely (17.4%). Not
surprisingly, the great majority (80%) of the lonely lived alone: but 20% did
not. The lonely were more likely to be very aged (over 75). They were, again,

more likely to be depressed and more likely to receive antidepressant medication; 11% of the lonely were taking antidepressants, compared with only 1.8% of the not lonely. They were more likely also to receive anxiolytics (10%) compared with the not lonely, of whom only 3.1% were receiving these drugs. They showed lower levels of life satisfaction and of social engagement, and they too were more likely to have seen their family doctor in the previous month.

Finally, *poverty*. We defined the poor as those receiving a State supplementary pension. They made up exactly 20% of our sample. Poor people were more likely to be very aged and to be women. They were more likely to be depressed than the non-poor — indeed, very nearly twice as likely to be depressed; and they showed lower levels of life satisfaction and of social engagement. Poor people were no more likely than the non-poor to be receiving antidepressant or anxiolytic drugs or to have seen their general practitioner in the previous month.

Such findings raise questions rather than settle them. They open or re-open areas of inquiry, such as the relationship between poverty and depression, and between various measures of life satisfaction and age. Not all studies by any means have reported the 'old old' as being less satisfied with their lives than the 'young old'. The studies of Mark Abrams (1978) reported higher levels of dissatisfaction in the 'young old', suggesting perhaps a 'cohort effect' of increased expectations being carried into old age. Questions arise too concerning the extent to which medical and other care services are directed to those most at risk and most in need, and concerning the possibility of differential responses by health professionals according to the socioeconomic condition of patients — questions such as have been the subject of study since (and even before) the famous work of Hollingshead & Redlich (1958) in America. Finally, the findings remind us of the links between poverty and mental disorders, which in this world of high unemployment have tended to be studied more in younger people than in the aged. It is too early at this stage of our studies to draw firm conclusions from these findings, but they obviously suggest hypotheses which we shall be exploring in greater detail.

What I am saying, in short, is that geriatric psychiatry, although it is inevitably aware of the mass of gross 'traditional' morbidity, for which manpower and resources are now beginning to be made available, must not forget its obligation to explore the well-being of old people in a broader sense — an activity which also offers scope for the better understanding of the social roots and associations of the psychosyndromes of old age, and which surely must ultimately yield further possibilities of prevention. It is encouraging that an apparatus of manpower, resources and training designed specifically to respond to the psychological disturbances of old age, such as I discussed in the opening part of this paper, is now beginning to be available in both the US and the UK. These developments in services and in education are surely as important as the exciting growth in biological knowledge, with which it must and will go hand in hand.

Acknowledgements

The Activity and Ageing project is supported by the Grand Charity. I am grateful to Dr John Wattis for allowing me to quote recent unpublished data. An earlier version of part of this paper was given at the University of Granada, Spain, in October 1986.

References

Abrams M 1978 Beyond three-score years and ten. Age Concern, Mitcham, Surrey

Arie T 1970 The first year of the Goodmayes psychiatric service for old people. Lancet 2:1179–1182

Arie T 1984 Prevention of mental disorders of old age. J Am Geriatr Soc 32:460–465

Arie T 1985 Education in the care of the elderly. Bull NY Acad Med 61(6):492–500

Arie T 1987 Caring for the elderly. In: Angell D, Snell P (eds) Medicine and management. Nuffield Provincial Hospitals Trust for Trent Regional Health Authority, Sheffield

Arie T, Jolley DJ 1982 Making services work: organisation and style of psychogeriatric services. In: Post F, Levy R (eds) The psychiatry of late life. Blackwell Publications, Oxford

Arie T, Jones RG, Smith CW 1985 The educational potential of old age psychiatry services. In: Arie T (ed) Recent advances in psychogeriatrics. Churchill Livingstone, Edinburgh

Bedford A, Foulds GA, Sheffield BF 1976 A new personal disturbance scale. Br J Soc Clin Psychol 15:387–394

Birren JE, Sloane RB 1977 Manpower and training needs in mental illness of the aging. Ethel Percy Andrus Gerontology Center, Los Angeles

Christie AB 1985 Survival in dementia: a review. In: Arie T (ed) Recent advances in psychogeriatrics. Churchill Livingstone, Edinburgh

Clarke M, Lowry R, Clarke S 1986 Cognitive impairment in the elderly. Age & Ageing 15:278–284

Cooper B 1984 Home and away: the disposition of mentally ill old people in an urban population. Social Psychiatry 19:187–196

Gilleard CJ 1985 Living with dementia. Croom Helm, London

Gurland B, Copeland JRM, Kelleher MJ, Kuriansky J, Sharpe L, Dean L 1983 The mind and mood of ageing. Croom Helm, London

Hagnell O, Lanke J, Rorsman B, Öhman R, Öjesjö L 1983 Current trends in the incidence of senile and multi-infarct dementia. Arch Psychiatry Neurol Sci 233:423–438

Hasegawa K, Homma A, Imai Y 1985 An epidemiological study of age-related dementia in the community. Int J Geriatr Psychiatry 1:45–55

Hawks D 1975 Community care: an analysis of assumptions. Br J Psychiatry 127:276–285

Hollingshead AB, Redlich FC 1958 Social class and mental illness. Wiley, New York

Ineichen B 1987 Measuring 'The Rising Tide'. Br J Psychiatry 150:193–200

Kay DWK, Beamish P, Roth M 1964 Old age mental disorders in Newcastle Upon Tyne. Part I: A study of prevalence. Br J Psychiatry 110:146–158

Lewis AJ 1946 Ageing and senility: a major problem of psychiatry. J Ment Sci 92:150–170.

Morgan K, Dallosso H, Arie T, Byrne EJ, Jones R, Waite RJ 1987 Mental health and psychological wellbeing among the old and the very old living at home. Br J Psychiatry 150:801–807

National Health Service Health Advisory Service 1982 The Rising Tide. Developing services for mental illness in old age. Sutton, Surrey

Neugarten B, Havighurst RJ, Tobin SS 1961 The measurement of life satisfaction. J Gerontol 16:134–143

Norman A 1987 Severe dementia: the provision of long stay care. Centre for Policy on Ageing, London

Pattie AH, Gilleard CJ 1979 Manual of the Clifton Assessment Procedures for the Elderly (CAPE). Hodder & Stoughton, Sevenoaks, Kent

Wattis J, Arie T 1984 Further developments in psychogeriatrics in Britain. Br Med J 289:778

Wattis J, Wattis L, Arie T 1981 Psychogeriatrics: a national survey of a new branch of psychiatry. Br Med J 282:1529–1533

Weissman MM, Myers JK, Tischler GL 1985 Psychiatric disorders (DSM-111) and cognitive impairment among the elderly in a US urban community. Acta Psychiatr Scand 71:366–379

Wood V, Wylie M, Sheafar B 1969 An analysis of a short self-report measure of life satisfaction: correlation with rater judgements. J Gerontol 24:465–469

World Health Organization 1986 Dementia in later life: research and action. Report of a WHO Scientific Group. WHO, Geneva

Zarit SH, Todd PA, Zarit JM 1986 Subjective burden of husbands and wives as caregivers: a longitudinal study. Gerontologist 3:260–266

DISCUSSION

A. Williams: I am particularly interested in evaluative studies showing the differential impact of the way health services are deployed. There is an enormous gap between the basic research and how it is translated into action in services for ageing populations. There are very tenuous links between the two. There is the problem that, however good the fundamental research, and however well therapeutic activities are conducted in the setting of teaching hospitals or well-resourced communities, if such research is to make any impact on a broad population it must have a major impact at a much lower level of service provision, in the hands of much less skilled people.

Some studies in Britain have shown that a major obstacle is the way that different professional groups see their role and their scope for action. On the whole, they take too narrow a view of their role. As we know, the medical conditions affecting old people are often multifactorial, and the responsibility for dealing with them is multiprofessional. That is a recipe for disaster as regards therapeutic effectiveness at a practical level. We therefore need to devise ways in which services could be organized and incentives generated at the lower levels of provision, for people to deploy services more effectively.

Some projects have been set up in Britain on this: for example, in the Kent Community Care project, where old people had been referred for residential care, their social workers were given notional budgets amounting to two-thirds of the cost of that care, to see how long they could keep such a person living at home. The social workers in this scheme were given much more freedom of manoeuvre than is usual, including the possibility of paying neighbours to keep an eye on the old people, or to prepare their meals, or to help them get up in the morning and get back to bed at night.

My point here is the importance of setting such studies up as randomized controlled trials. What scope is there for such trials in the evaluation of services, at this level? That is the way forward, methodologically speaking.

Arie: Our service in Nottingham is totally unselective: people over about 65 years (and especially the very aged) in Nottingham, simply by living there, regardless of the nature of their disorder, are *our* responsibility if they wish to use our services. In no way is it an elite service, and we impress this non-selectivity on our students. The service is also intensely 'multidisciplinary'—our team of nurses, remedial therapists, and psychologists, physicians and psychiatrists work together, and there is much overlap of role and function. The aim is that users of the service should get what, after assessment, they need—regardless of which section of our service they have made contact with.

You mention the project in Kent where social workers were given cash to use to enable elderly people to remain in their homes (Challis & Davies 1986). I am always puzzled that local projects of that kind, which seem to work in one locality, so rarely spread to others. Some had argued that the service that I set up in London was not transportable—that it was a service for that type of hospital in that type of place. They held that you cannot transpose a service working in that style (multidisciplinary, preventive as far as possible, rapidly interventive, very supportive, being centred on people's homes) into a university teaching setting. People did not believe that this could be done, yet it is working well. That is another piece of hypothesis testing, and thus, in a sense, of evaluation.

Macfadyen: One can test the hypothesis that psychogeriatrics make no difference, for example. This has been tested with controlled trials of psychogeriatric assessment (Bergmann 1981) and of psychogeriatric day care (Washburn & Vannicelli 1976). In recent trials the investigators have been interested in the results of the care, not only for the patients, but for the family members (Gilleard 1986) and the staff (Bond 1984). So people are beginning to grapple with the methodology of randomized controlled trials in psychogeriatrics, and some aspects of psychogeriatric care have shown up well in the results of these trials.

Arie: I think so too, and I am much encouraged. I am glad that you mention the third group—the staff. Where staff in this field are enjoying their work and have a glint in their eyes, the work is usually being done well. It must be worthwhile; it must be reinforcing. I can see all sorts of pitfalls to that hypothesis, but it has stood me in good stead.

Solomons: Where do the people with marked senile dementia go to die, in the UK?

Arie: We have a rather different system in Britain from the USA, but it is changing. Demented patients who need institutional care go to a variety of settings, depending chiefly on the nature of their disability. The placement of such people who have been referred to our service and, if they are severely impaired, their actual care, is our responsibility (including that of our university service), and we will see them through until the end. If they are very disturbed behaviourally and very infirm, such patients tend to receive long-stay care in a hospital-controlled unit (not necessarily in the main hospital), as part of the National Health Service. I have fifty such beds that I am responsible for, with a colleague. These are long-stay nursing beds. Alternative placements are in the privately run nursing homes which have begun to spring up in Britain, and in residential care units run by local social services. The latter take people who are not very infirm or behaviourally disturbed. The private sector is still finding its way. It sometimes operates a selection against the most disabled demented people, but not always; some private nursing homes take very disabled people. The private sector has been a small part of our care system, but this is no longer so.

T.F. Williams: The USA inherited from Great Britain the county system of 'port of last responsibility': the counties have to provide care in the last analysis. So we have a common historical thread, although we may have met the needs in different ways.

Fries: I am not yet happy with the evidence that some old-age mental disorders are becoming less prevalent. Much as I would like to, I don't find the evidence for this trend that has been presented so far to be convincing. Internationally there is relatively little information, and your data, Dr Arie, emphasize that. Definitions of diseases change, studies done in different locations are being compared with each other and, above all, the 'Gompertz' phenomenon which governs the prevalence of these conditions means that you cannot compare people over 75 in one study with those over 80 in another. It looks to me as though those differences alone explained much of the prevalence, because with the Gompertz phenomenon of logarithmic increase in incidence with time one expects almost a doubling of incidence rates in each five-year cohort (Fries 1984).

Arie: I was comparing like with like in Table 2, but giving different instances from different studies, because the data were presented differently. But the data are there for comparing the different age groups. Taken together, the studies, which I quoted, suggest a lower prevalence.

T.F. Williams: Let me raise a more general methodological issue. We have already heard about problems of assessing cognitive status, including the difficulties encountered in different cultures; we are told that that is surmount-able. We also see rather striking differences in results from different popula-tions. The study in Melton Mowbray is impressive. The over-75s were showing a prevalence of 'marked cognitive impairment' of only 4.5%, in a very careful study of the whole population. That is strikingly different from other people's figures. The difference may be partly due to differences in methodology, but perhaps we ought to think about where further research is needed. It seems to me that a big challenge is methodological.

Arie: Obviously methodology is crucial, but the Melton Mowbray figure for those aged 80 to 84 was 3.7%: for those aged 85+, it was 9.3%. These are very low prevalence figures (Clarke et al 1986).

White: In your study, cognitive impairment was defined operationally using a cut-off value of seven on the CAPE. Obviously, many factors in addition to cognitive impairment determine performance in a single test. An interesting point is that the usual error is to over-estimate the prevalence of impairment. Neuropsychologists have usually assumed that in evaluating a person's state of mental health, you should pick out his or her best level of performance after several tests, since there are many factors determining levels of performance on a test beyond cognitive impairment and dementia.

Mor: The possibility of a cohort effect has to be considered. It probably has no basic biological implications, but rather one related to the interaction between education and life experience, and performance on a standardized test. Our own studies have shown an extraordinarily strong relationship be-tween educational level and performance on mental status tests.

Wenger: I wonder if your results are better than those of others, Dr Arie, because your staff are skilled in dealing with an elderly population and are likely to take problems with vision and hearing impairment into account? We have seen visual and auditory limitations cause difficulty in scores of standar-dized questionnaires when those were not items of concern. Perhaps one should also factor in medications, and the fact that your elderly population was not over-medicated—a feature that has often caused problems.

Secondly, how how much are you or your staff, because of these skills, called upon to evaluate, in an acute medical-care setting, for example, whether an individual elderly patient has the cognitive or emotional stability to be a candidate for extensive invasive procedures, such as cardiac surgery? Are you asked to help decide whether that person's emotional and mental status will constitute a barrier to planned complex treatments?

Arie: We are often, but not always, called upon to do this. We are well placed to be available; our department must be one of the few places in the world where internists and psychiatrists actually live together! We are totally avail-able to help each other's patients, both in our weekly formal joint rounds, and informally. So we are often consulted for that sort of decision, and also when decisions are needed about competence, legal capacity and so on.

Andrews: On the assessment of dementia, it seems to me that we are using a fairly rough clinical screening test as an epidemiological tool, which is akin to doing a study of blood pressure in the community just by taking erratic measures, using a cuff, and reading the pulse. It is not surprising that one ends up with difficulty in comparing the results of different studies. We ought now to draw on the skills available from our neuropsychological colleagues to develop a better approach to assessing dementia, rather than just trying to improve our current mental status measures (rather like trying to improve the situation by having a better cuff).

Katzman: Dr Arie's results are dramatically different from our experience. We studied a group which was not a complete population, so the people followed longitudinally may have been unrepresentative initially. Nevertheless, over five years, the number of new people with a diagnosis of dementia is about the same each year. The *incidence* is running in these 80-year-old people at about 3% a year, and you are talking about a *prevalence* of 4% a year. That is a dramatic difference. Our patients are diagnosed on a mental status test and a four-hour neuropsychological examination by a psychiatrist and neurologist: we repeat this annually, to see if there is progression. So our figures should be conservative: yet we are so different from you that there seems to be a real difference between these cohorts.

Arie: There does seem to be a difference between the USA and the UK, at least between London and New York (Gurland et al 1983). On Gary Andrews' point, the methodology he describes may be crude, and the limitations of simply doing a cuff blood pressure measurement are obvious. But if people have been doing that for decades, and they suddenly start to get different readings, with the same primitive cuff, with no obvious bias, it suggests that something real may be going on.

Andrews: You suggest that there is a consistent trend, but my impression from the literature is that it is a bit all over the place—as exemplified by what we have just heard about the findings in the UK and the USA.

Solomons: In epidemiology, factors in the selection of the study population are often more responsible for the error in the results than the precision or accuracy of the measuring instrument. If there is a systematic bias in the instrument—for example, if a person can't see and is given a visual test, or can't hear and is given an auditory test—which is a systematic bias in one direction, that will produce an error with the instrument. But, in general, the instrument may have a crudeness or imprecision about it, yet it is used constantly and reproducibly.

Going back to problems of cross-cultural comparisons, perhaps we should cross over the investigators? We could exchange research teams between UK and USA, to do the same tests as we usually do, to see whether the same numbers come out with the same instruments and the same investigators.

White: We have done a set of health surveys called the EPESE, an acronym for Established Populations for Epidemiologic Studies of the Elderly. These were done in two counties in Iowa, in East Boston, and in the city of New Haven. Later we shall have data from a fourth site in the Durham (North Carolina) area. As part of the survey we administered the short portable mental status questionnaire developed by Pfeiffer (1975), in turn based on the mental status questionnaire developed by Kahn et al (1960). At each of the three sites we found the expected shift with advancing age towards poorer MSQ performance. When we compared the three communities, studied under standardized conditions, we found that the extent of that shift and the actual levels of performance varied dramatically between these three US populations. They varied to the extent that we could choose a cut-off point of five or more errors, and would find that at age 75, say, in East Boston, 60% of people were failing that test, whereas in Iowa only 8–9% were failing it; New Haven was somewhere in the middle (White et al 1986).

We first wondered if these cross-community MSQ performance differentials could be explained by differences in the distribution of education among the three communities. Some, but not all, was explainable that way. We then began looking for other explanations, not wishing to accept the proposition that something causing cognitive decline in the elderly is occurring in epidemic proportions in East Boston while sparing the elderly of Iowa. The most plausible explanation involves differential pre-selection for residence in the community; that is, individuals who experienced declining cognitive capacities may remain in the community longer in East Boston than in Iowa.

In East Boston the population consists largely of blue collar (working class) Italian families, Catholic, and with many children. They live in a very tight community where older people are cared for by the family at home. In addition, the excellent health services of the East Boston Neighborhood Health Center include nurses who make home visits. In Iowa the population is different. It is far more affluent and there are fewer children per family. The older person is often more conveniently cared for in a nursing home than in the community. The lesson is that when we make this sort of 'ecological' comparison, we need to remember that there are many reasons for inter-community differences besides the possibility that something biological is changing.

Fries: There are three additional reasons why I distrust cross-national comparisons. One has to do with the differences in investigators. We were involved in X-ray studies of ankylosing spondylitis in which workers from Perth in Australia found a 1% prevalence among HLA-B27-positive subjects, and people from the USA found 20%. When everybody met in Hawaii with the X-rays it turned out to be 11%. Both groups could agree when they were in the same room reading the same X-rays but, had that not been done, there would have been thought to be a vastly different prevalence and incidence of ankylosing spondylitis in Australia and in the USA.

Second, there are changes in the cohorts themselves which affect responses.

In the Health Interview Survey in the USA, the investigators have tried to ask the same question every five years but have failed to note that the questions have a different meaning each time. For example, when people are asked how healthy they are compared with a hundred other people, or how healthy they feel they should be, the responses are conditional on the expectations of the cohort. Changing expectations alter the way people respond, independent of their actual state of health. Perhaps there are cohort effects as well in examiners; study-examiners who classify patients as demented or not demented are conditioned by normative expectations of what people at a particular age should be like, and that is unlikely to be constant over time.

A third possible partial explanation for Dr Arie's findings is that in general, in clinical medicine, population-based groups or community-based groups tend to have a more benign prognosis than groups enrolled through medical providers. So the fact that your population is relatively unselected in comparison with other studies might also contribute to the apparently falling prevalence of marked dementia.

T.F. Williams: There has been interest in the USA in the possible therapeutic value of tetrahydroaminoacridine (THA) in dementia of Alzheimer type. This is a blocker of cholinesterase and should lead to a better preservation of acetylcholine levels in the brain. The Institute on Aging expects to begin a randomized clinical trial of this compound in about 17 centres in the USA, with the hope of having more definitive evidence about efficacy within about a year.

Katzman: THA is relatively straightforward—it will either improve cognition and function or it will not. With drugs such as nerve growth factor, and other trophic factors that might be introduced—drugs designed to prevent the progression of the illness—initial calculations indicate that the number of individuals in a study will need to be very large. Unless a drug reverses the condition, it will not be easy to know when something is effective.

Arie: Something else bothers me about the 'anti-dementia drugs', namely that we have a ceiling effect with the very demented, where effects on people who rate at the limit of our rating scales may still be significant but will not show up in ratings if the subjects remain beyond the 'worst' point on the scale. We need scales that discriminate within the range beyond what is conventionally the end of a scale. This applies especially to the very severely disabled people in long-term care. This raises another question—for which patients should we be trying these drugs? Assuming there are the late (type I) and early (type II) forms of Alzheimer's disease (Bondareff 1983), should we be trying the drugs on the late-onset patients, who have smaller transmitter deficits than the early-onset Alzheimer's patients, and so one might consider that there is only a small amount of deficit needing to be made good by the drug? Or should we try them on the early-onset patients with big mental impairments and big transmitter deficits, where one could argue that the deficits are so great that, like a gross vitamin deficiency, a little bit of replacement should go a long way?

Katzman: The measuring tools here are not good enough to discriminate between patients who are severely impaired; therefore, to see whether the drug works, you must try it on people with mild to moderate dementia.

Coleman: When one is dealing with a very advanced case of Alzheimer's disease, that person has lost many neurons. To try a treatment designed to enhance transmitter levels in somebody whose neurons aren't there is like putting gasoline in a car with no engine. But in cortex, for example, the loss is not so immense so there should be some potential left there. I agree that one should try the drugs on patients at earlier phases of the disease rather than the advanced ones.

Solomons: One problem with clinical trials of drugs in Alzheimer's disease is the irregular, non-uniform natural progression of the disease from one patient to the next. One needs a way of 'staging' the clinical expression of Alzheimer's such that drug therapy would be aimed at comparable phases of the disease in all patients in a trial. If that cannot be done, we are left with a hotch potch of clinical description, with all the problems of subjective assessment. Alzheimer's is—unfortunately—a very 'pathological' disease where we have a series of non-universal clinical measures: against that, we plan to throw some minimal-effect drugs. If I were in this field, I would not be particularly enthusiastic about the prospect of success for drug therapy.

Arie: Nevertheless, I think we are entitled to end this discussion on an optimistic note. For years research on the dementias was almost stagnant; now it is moving fast and fruitfully. For years it was widely held that clinical work with mentally ill old people was dull and professionally unrewarding; had that proved to be so, it would have been a disaster in relation to the prominence of these disorders among the demands on health services. Happily it is clear that this is fascinating work and that it is being widely taken up by gifted and effective people.

References

Bergmann K 1981 Geronto-psychiatric prevention. In: Magnusson K et al (eds) Epidemiology and prevention of mental illness in old age. Proc Nordic Geronto-Psychiatric Symp, Silkeborg

Bond J 1984 Evaluation of long-stay accommodation for elderly people. In: Bromley DB (ed) Gerontology: social and behavioural perspectives. Croom Helm, Beckenham

Bondareff W 1983 Age and Alzheimer disease. Lancet 1:1447

Challis D, Davies B 1986 Case management in community care. Gower, Aldershot

Clarke M, Lowry R, Clarke S 1986 Cognitive impairment in the elderly. Age & Ageing 15:278–284

Fries JF 1984 The compression of morbidity, Benjamin Gompertz, the two types of chronic disease, and health policy. In: Forum Proceedings; exploring new frontiers of US health policy. UMDNJ–Rutgers Medical School, New Jersey

Gilleard GJ 1986 Predicting the outcome of psychogeriatric day care. Gerontologist 25:280–285

Gurland B, Copeland JRM, Kelleher MJ, Kuriansky J, Sharpe L, Dean L 1983 The mind and mood of ageing. Croom Helm, London

Kahn RL, Goldfarb AI, Pollack M, Peck A 1960 Brief objective measures for the determination of mental status in the aged. Am J Psychiatr 117:326–328

Pfeiffer E 1975 A short portable mental status questionnaire for the assessment of organic brain deficit in elderly patients. J Am Geriatr Soc 23:433–441

Washburn S, Vannicelli M 1976 A controlled comparison of psychiatric day treatment and inpatient hospitalisation. J Consult Clin Psychol 44:665–675

White LR, Kohout F, Evans DA, Cornoni-Huntley J, Ostfeld A 1986 Related health problems. In: Cornoni-Huntley J et al (eds) Established populations for epidemiologic studies of the elderly. National Institute on Aging. US Dept HHS, Public Health Service. NIH Publication No. 86-2443

Cardiovascular disease in the elderly

Nanette K. Wenger

Department of Medicine (Cardiology), Emory University School of Medicine, 69 Butler Street, S.E., Atlanta, Georgia 30303, USA

Abstract. Cardiovascular disease is the major cause of death and disability in the elderly. Atherosclerotic coronary heart disease is the most prevalent problem, followed by hypertensive cardiovascular disease. Calcific aortic stenosis is the most common haemodynamically important valvular lesion; surgical correction significantly improves the prognosis. Pulmonary embolism occurs frequently, related to immobilization and co-morbidity. Congestive heart failure is both under-diagnosed and over-diagnosed. Complete heart block and sick sinus syndrome increase with age; appropriate pacemaker therapy can improve the length and quality of life. Clinical evaluation of elderly patients is often hampered by multiple co-existing diseases involving other organ systems, problems in reporting symptoms, and associated functional and structural changes of ageing that may mimic or mask cardiovascular disease. Presentations of cardiac illness often differ from those in a younger population. Most of the available data on therapy and prognosis do not apply to contemporary practice, so that clinical decisions are often extrapolated from information acquired in younger patients. Elderly patients are at high risk of complications of most diagnostic and therapeutic procedures, more related to co-morbidity than to age; they have more frequent and serious adverse drug reactions, due both to co-morbidity and to multiple medications. Age as such should not constitute a barrier to cardiac care; in the USA at least one-third of all cardiovascular procedures are performed in elderly patients. The goals of therapy are improvement in function and postponement of debilitating illness, enabling an extended active independent lifestyle.

1988 Research and the ageing population. Wiley, Chichester (Ciba Foundation Symposium 134) p 106–128

Cardiovascular disease is the major cause of death and disability in the elderly. Despite this fact, most contemporary clinical practice, in regard both to diagnosis and to therapy, is based on information extrapolated from studies conducted primarily in younger populations (Wenger et al 1987). Because of this, uncertainties remain as to what constitutes quality care for elderly patients with cardiovascular disease. Further, the use of health services by elderly cardiac patients does not necessarily reflect their need for these services; the availability and accessibility of health services, rather than patient needs, are the bases for most statistical data (Heller et al 1984), hence the needs of elderly patients for cardiac care are not precisely known.

Recognition of specific cardiovascular problems in the elderly is hampered by the varying alterations in cardiovascular structure and function with age (Weisfelt 1980), including increased vascular stiffness, adaptive increases in left ventricular wall thickness, decreased myocardial compliance with diminution of ventricular early diastolic filling, decreased maximal heart rate and catecholamine responsiveness, and decreased maximal oxygen uptake. The lessened functional reserve capacity of the aged heart may potentiate disease-related cardiovascular impairments.

On physical examination, the arterial pulsations are characteristically brisk and the pulse pressure widened, owing to diminished arterial elasticity with ageing (Messerli et al 1983). An S4 is characteristic, reflecting decreased ventricular compliance, and basal systolic murmurs are common even in the absence of significant valvular disease (Kotler et al 1981). Orthostatic hypotension is frequent, due to attenuated baroreceptor responsiveness (Caird et al 1973), and may constitute a barrier to therapy for hypertension, congestive heart failure, and the like. In addition to these cardiovascular changes of ageing that may obscure or mimic findings of specific cardiovascular illnesses, many non-invasive diagnostic procedures, such as perfusion lung scanning, radionuclide ventriculography, and so on, have less predictive accuracy in an older population. Changes in the function of many organ systems and — at times — activity restriction and malnutrition, as well as the effects of multiple medications, may further complicate the presentation. The accurate evaluation of cardiovascular disease may be further hindered by the frequent concomitant non-cardiac illnesses present in this age group, as well as by the mental problems related to ageing, illness, and drug therapy that may limit the validity of the clinical history.

Coronary atherosclerotic heart disease

The occurrence of clinical manifestations of coronary atherosclerotic heart disease and its complications increases dramatically with age. Co-morbidity rather than age *per se* appears to determine the excess of complications. In most industrialized nations the anatomical alterations of coronary atherosclerosis are so ubiquitous as to suggest that it may be more important to identify the precipitating features of the appearance of clinical symptoms than the presence of anatomical coronary obstruction as such (Wenger et al 1986). Further, it remains speculative whether the rate of progression of the severity of coronary atherosclerosis varies with age, a feature important in assessing preventive and therapeutic interventions.

The clinical presentations of coronary disease vary significantly from those in a younger population (Hill et al 1985). Both angina and myocardial infarction are less likely to be effort-related, in part owing to the habitual sedentary lifestyle of many elderly patients. Indeed, associated medical problems characterized by hypotension, hypoxaemia, blood loss and the like are often the precipitants of both angina and myocardial infarction. Further, the predominance of clinical coronary disease among men disappears after age 70 years (Latting & Silverman 1980).

Exercise testing, using a low-level treadmill or bicycle protocol (or arm ergometry when musculoskeletal problems or claudication limit leg testing), is feasible in many elderly patients; evidence of early ischaemia at exercise testing identifies patients with an unfavourable prognosis who may warrant more invasive interventions. An unmet need is a test with which to challenge the oxygen transport system in patients unable to perform conventional exercise tests. Therapy for low-risk older patients with stable angina is as for younger persons.

Painless myocardial infarction, although not necessarily asymptomatic infarction, is more common with increased age. It is not known whether this represents a lesser sensitivity to pain with ageing or the relationship to the concomitant diabetes mellitus and systemic arterial hypertension that are also associated with painless infarction. Atypical presentations, including pulmonary oedema, cerebrovascular accident, syncope, acute confusion, altered mental status and peripheral arterial embolism, are frequent (Svanborg et al 1982). The diagnosis is further hampered in that the total creatine kinase (CK) level may not be increased, despite elevation of its MB fraction (Heller et al 1983). Indeed, normal levels for total CK in an elderly population are not known. The electrocardiographic diagnosis of infarction may also be more difficult because of preexisting abnormalities due to infarction and conduction disorders; further, non-Q wave infarction occurs more often. The prognosis of unrecognized myocardial infarction is comparable to that with the classical presentation. However, since the clinical, enzymic and ECG components for the diagnosis of myocardial infarction differ from those in younger populations, difficulty can be anticipated in delineating criteria for inclusion in clinical trials involving patients with myocardial infarction over a broad age range, including the elderly.

The increased incidence of multivessel coronary disease in the elderly, as well as the frequent co-morbidity, explains the characteristically more complicated course of acute myocardial infarction that determines the significantly higher in-hospital mortality and longer hospital stay than in a younger population (Williams et al 1976, Marchionni et al 1981, Akman 1983). Atrial fibrillation and flutter as well as other atrial arrhythmias, conduction defects, and heart block are increased in frequency; the proportion of these problems present before infarction, and the proportion due to infarction, have yet to be delineated; congestive heart failure and cardiogenic shock are far more likely to occur, as is subsequent left ventricular aneurysm; and there is an increased incidence of cardiac rupture that may involve the papillary muscle, ventricular septum, or left ventricular free wall.

Ventricular fibrillation is less likely to occur, even in the presence of ventricular ectopic complexes; this, coupled with the increased risk of central nervous system complications of lidocaine therapy, suggests that the prophylactic use of lidocaine may not be warranted and that therapeutic use of the drug should involve a decrease in dosage (Wenger et al 1987). The lesser risk of ventricular ectopic activity may relate to its presence at baseline, rather than as a reflection of infarction; frequent ventricular ectopic complexes and short bursts of ventricular tachycardia are encountered on ambulatory ECGs in elderly persons even in the absence of cardiovascular disease (Fleg & Kennedy 1982, Kantelip et al 1986).

There is a marked increase in adverse drug responses in elderly patients in general and in elderly patients with acute cardiac illnesses in particular. Lower doses of narcotic analgesics are appropriate. Therapy with vasodilator drugs carries an increased risk of postural hypotension; there is a greater likelihood of impaired atrioventricular conduction and depression of myocardial function with verapamil and diltiazem; ventricular dysfunction, symptomatic bradycardia, and abnormalities of atrioventricular conduction are more likely to occur with beta blockade; and digitalis is more likely to engender toxic tachy- and bradyarrhythmias. Typically, elderly patients have been excluded from or under-represented in clinical trials of these drug therapies for myocardial infarction. Further, thrombolytic therapy in the acute stage of myocardial infarction has not been demonstrated to be of benefit in an elderly population (GISSI 1986) in whom the risk of bleeding complications is increased; other approaches designed to avert infarction or limit infarction size have not been tested in elderly populations.

Age should not constitute a bar to admission to a coronary care unit, as elderly patients derive equal benefit from intensive care and defibrillation when appropriate (Berman 1979). Pulmonary artery catheter-derived data are often needed to guide management of the increasingly frequent congestive heart failure in this age group. Also, elderly patients appear to gain equal benefit, in terms of survival, as younger persons from the use of beta-blocking drugs after infarction (Gundersen et al 1982). Nevertheless, elderly patients with uncomplicated infarction and a normal predischarge exercise test response have an excellent prognosis for recovery and rehabilitation (Wenger 1984). Early ambulation and multifaceted education and counselling, including the modification of coronary risk factors, are appropriate (Kannel & Gordon 1978, Mellström et al 1982, Jajich et al 1984), as is exercise rehabilitation after leaving hospital and a return to the preillness lifestyle (Peach & Pathy 1979). Contrary to the practice of earlier years, when patients aged 60 years and older were systematically excluded from exercise rehabilitation programmes, a progressive walking programme is excellent exercise rehabilitation for an elderly population, because walking entails a significant percentage of the age-related decreased physical work capacity. Elderly patients require longer periods of warm-up and cool-down activities and longer intervals at low-level activity, because of the increased time needed for their exercise heart rate to return to normal (Montoye et al 1968, Williams et al 1985).

Elderly patients also show an increase in late deaths after infarction and greater residual disability. Despite the slightly higher incidence of complications of coronary arteriography, it is tolerated well by elderly patients (Gersh et al 1982). Further, although there is a higher operative risk of coronary bypass surgery beyond age 70, the relief of angina and long-term survival after successful myocardial revascularization are excellent in appropriately selected patients (Elayda et al 1984, Gersh et al 1983). Cerebrovascular and peripheral vascular complications, neuropsychiatric problems, and the need for postoperative intracardiac pacing and intra-aortic balloon support are the major contributors to perioperative morbidity (Knapp et al 1981). Thus surgery (or coronary angioplasty) should be considered for those elderly patients with severe or unstable angina or with life-threatening coronary obstructive lesions who do not have contraindications to operation. Although the increased risk of angioplasty in elderly patients was described in the initial years of the procedure, the success rate and complication rate of percutaneous transluminal coronary angioplasty (PTCA) in the elderly are now comparable to those of a younger population (Mock et al 1982). It is not yet known whether re-stenosis rates differ in the elderly. Also, favourable responses to surgical correction have been described in elderly patients with cardiogenic shock related to surgically remediable complications of myocardial infarction (Weintraub et al 1986).

Systemic arterial hypertension

The prevalence of hypertension increases with age and, in many populations, hypertension is present in more than half of elderly persons. It constitutes a major risk factor not only for atherosclerotic coronary heart disease and stroke, but for congestive cardiac failure, renal failure, aortic dissection, and claudication as well (Amery et al 1981). The higher the blood pressure, both systolic and diastolic, the greater the risk of complications; isolated systolic hypertension in the elderly is also associated with increased cardiovascular morbidity and mortality (Rowe 1983).

The prevalence and seriousness of hypertension in the elderly population mandates careful evaluation for its presence and serial surveillance for the adequacy of the control of blood pressure. Control of hypertension has markedly reduced the occurrence of fatal stroke and of fatal myocardial infarction, by almost half in many populations (Amery et al 1985). However, most clinical trials that serve as a data base for recommending pharmacotherapy for hypertension have not included patients above 70 years of age (Hypertension 1979).

The current recommendations of the US Working Group on Hypertension in the Elderly (Statement 1986) are that therapy is warranted for elderly patients with a systolic blood pressure in excess of 150 mmHg and a diastolic pressure greater than 90 mmHg. Non-pharmacological measures, including restriction of dietary sodium intake, weight control, low-level exercise, and moderation in alcohol consumption, are initially recommended for patients with diastolic blood pressures between 90 and 94 mmHg (Amery et al 1980), since they entail little risk, expense or inconvenience; at higher levels of blood pressure, these measures must often be supplemented by pharmacological management. The goal of pharmacological therapy is to reduce diastolic blood pressure below 90 mmHg and systolic blood pressure below 140–160 mmHg. Because complications of antihypertensive therapy are more common in the elderly (Wood & Feely 1981), the initial drug dosage should be low, with small incremental increases, and there should be regular ascertainment of potential complicating orthostatic hypotension by checking blood pressures in both the sitting and standing positions. Although beta-blocking drugs, diuretics, angiotensin-converting enzyme inhibitors, or calcium-blocking drugs may be used as initial therapy, only beta-blocking drugs, converting enzyme inhibitors and methyldopa seem to limit or reverse left ventricular hypertrophy, an adverse prognostic feature. This does not seem to occur with arteriolar vasodilator therapy. Potential complications of beta-blocking drugs include the exacerbation of conduction system disease or ventricular dysfunction; however, orthostatic hypotension is rarely seen. Treatment with thiazide diuretics may engender hypovolaemia with orthostatic complications and hypokalaemia, and may aggravate pre-existing glucose intolerance. Vasodilator drugs often cause palpitations and headache, and reserpine, methyldopa and beta-blocking drugs may potentiate depression. Calcium-blocking drugs require surveillance to avoid hypovolaemic hypotension, and conduction disturbances and ventricular dysfunction are described; converting enzyme inhibitors appear to favourably affect preload and afterload. However, the comparative testing of antihypertensive drugs to define their risk–benefit characteristics in an elderly population has yet to be initiated.

Although definitive information is not available on the benefit of controlling isolated systolic hypertension, many physicians currently treat elderly patients with isolated systolic hypertension in excess of 150 mmHg; in the pilot phase of the Systolic Hypertension in the Elderly Program (SHEP), drug and placebo therapy produced comparable adverse effects (Hulley et al 1985).

Secondary hypertension is unusual in the elderly, but generally can be managed medically; consideration should be given to angioplasty or surgery if renovascular hypertension is present (Delin et al 1982).

Common complications of cardiovascular diseases: congestive heart failure and arrhythmias

The prevalence of heart failure also increases with increasing age (McKee et al 1971); the major aetiologies underlying its occurrence in the elderly are coronary atherosclerotic heart disease and hypertensive cardiovascular disease. Calcific aortic valve disease must also be considered as aetiological, and unrecognized thyrotoxicosis may cause high-output cardiac failure (Kennedy 1975). As is the case with symptomatic myocardial ischaemia, the onset of congestive cardiac failure in elderly patients is also commonly related to specific precipitating events. These include ischaemic episodes, brady- or tachyarrhythmias, fever, blood loss, infection, excessive dietary sodium intake, the use of pharmacological agents that depress myocardial function (such as beta-blocking drugs, calcium channel-blocking drugs and some anti-arrhythmic agents), or poor compliance with the medical regimen. These events challenge the diminished cardiovascular reserve capacity of ageing.

Congestive cardiac failure is both under- and over-diagnosed in an elderly population; the features complicating its recognition include the frequent sedentary lifestyle, easy fatiguability that may be attributable to other diseases, confusion with symptoms of the frequent concomitant respiratory disorders, and the increased likelihood of diastolic dysfunction as a cause of heart failure. Heart failure may at times present as disordered mental function, restlessness or agitation, profound fatigue, anorexia, or insomnia, with resultant problems in recognition and in the initiation of therapy. The presence of a normal-sized heart is often erroneously considered to rule out congestive cardiac failure. The use of echocardiography has provided an important advance in the recognition of congestive cardiac failure, since cardiac chamber size, wall thickness, cardiac valve characteristics, and systolic and diastolic ventricular function can be determined.

Therapy does not differ from that in younger patients save for the need to limit excessive immobilization, to use diuretic therapy with caution so as to avoid hypovolaemia and hypotension, and to avoid digitalis toxicity. The latter is increasingly likely when the manifestations of respiratory disease are misdiagnosed as heart failure and digitalis glycosides administered. Whether the improved survival seen in younger populations with heart failure (Cohn et al 1986) when vasodilator therapy was added to digitalis and diuretics will occur as well in elderly patients is not known. Recent data suggest that exercise rehabilitation can improve the functional capacity of elderly patients with compensated congestive cardiac failure.

Brady- and tachyarrhythmias commonly complicate the course of coronary and hypertensive cardiovascular diseases. Both the sick sinus syndrome and trifascicular block due to primary conduction system disease are far more common in the geriatric population than in younger age groups (Fleg & Kennedy 1982, Kantelip et al 1986, Martin et al 1984). Ventricular ectopic activity is frequent in an elderly population, even in the absence of cardiac disease, and asymptomatic ventricular ectopic activity generally should not be treated. The same is the case with asymptomatic sick sinus syndrome without haemodynamic consequences. Ambulatory electrocardiography is the best procedure by which to identify arrhythmias and to correlate their occurrence with symptoms such as lightheadedness, dizziness, palpitations, unexplained falls or syncope.

Anti-arrhythmic drug therapy carries an increased risk in elderly people because of their altered handling of drugs, the frequently associated conduction system disease and ventricular dysfunction, and the problem of drug interactions; only highly symptomatic or life-threatening ventricular arrhythmias should be treated and decreased doses of antiarrhythmic drugs should be used. Similarly, pacemaker therapy is warranted only for symptomatic brady-arrhythmias or to permit the drug therapy of tachyarrhythmias in patients with the sick sinus syndrome (Report 1984); at all ages, appropriate pacemaker implantation can improve survival and life quality. Pacemakers that permit the atrial contribution to ventricular filling or are rate-responsive may enable improved function in active, ambulatory elderly patients.

Of concern is the need for anticoagulation in elderly patients with atrial fibrillation, a common complication of mitral valve disease, coronary and hypertensive cardiovascular diseases, and other causes of ventricular dysfunction. Despite the increased risk of anticoagulant-related haemorrhage in the elderly, patients with prior embolic phenomena, those with mitral valve disease, particularly mitral stenosis, and those with heart failure appear at greatest risk of embolic complications and probably warrant anticoagulation.

Syncope occurs frequently in aged patients. As is the case with heart failure, a cardiovascular aetiology for syncope and for other manifestations of arrhythmia may be both under- and over-diagnosed in the elderly. Tachyarrhythmias and bradyarrhythmias may both produce syncope, and a specific aetiology should be defined for treatment to be instituted. The occurrence of arrhythmias secondary to excessive drug therapy poses a further problem in diagnosis. Often a single syncopal episode in an elderly patient has no definable explanation.

Valvular heart disease

Degeneration of collagen with secondary calcification is common in the aortic and mitral valves of elderly patients (Sugiura et al 1982). Although the determinants of calcification are not known, an understanding of the mechanism(s) might suggest preventive approaches to limit the calcification. Haemodynamically significant calcific aortic stenosis is the most common valvular lesion that requires surgical intervention in the elderly population. Recognition is often difficult, in that the vascular changes of ageing may mask the usual slow-rising small volume carotid pulse contour, hypertension may be present even with severe aortic stenosis, the murmur may become soft or almost disappear as the cardiac output decreases, and the frequent concomitant heart failure and coronary disease complicate the presentation. At times, the high frequency components of the basal systolic murmur are heard throughout most of systole along the lower left sternal border and toward the cardiac apex, mimicking the murmur of mitral regurgitation. A basal systolic thrill radiating into the neck, and evidence of left ventricular hypertrophy on clinical examination or at electrocardiography, suggest important aortic valvular obstruction. The occurrence of angina, heart failure, or effort syncope suggest haemodynamically significant aortic stenosis; however, all these symptoms may be due to other problems in an elderly patient with a basal systolic murmur without haemodynamic consequences. Further, the sedentary lifestyle of many elderly patients precludes activity-related symptoms. The onset of atrial fibrillation may precipitate heart failure.

The absence of aortic valvular calcification on the chest film and at echocardiography virtually excludes significant aortic valve obstruction, a feature suggesting that preventing calcification may have beneficial effects. Exercise testing is inappropriate if significant aortic stenosis is suspected, because of the excessive risk of exercise-precipitated sudden death. Doppler echocardiography has provided a major advance in the non-invasive recognition of potentially severe aortic valvular obstruction, enabling the selection of patients for cardiac catheterization who are likely to benefit from surgical therapy. The correlation of Doppler echocardiographic with cardiac catheterization data remains controversial in elderly patients with calcific aortic stenosis; also, coronary arteriography is required to evaluate for associated severe coronary atherosclerotic obstruction, which has been concomitantly successfully corrected (Smith et al 1976). Despite increased age, and indeed often despite significant left ventricular dysfunction and heart failure, surgery entails an acceptably low risk (5–10%), even in Class III and IV patients. The symptomatic and functional improvement after valve replacement in patients with critical aortic stenosis (Logeais et al 1984) is pronounced and has been maintained to 10 years; 10-year survival is enhanced by surgical intervention as well (Murphy et al 1981). Few elderly patients survive more than three years once angina, heart failure or syncope occur, and sudden death is common. Factors that limit the potential benefits of surgery because they increase operative mortality include inoperable coronary disease, severe chronic obstructive pulmonary disease, renal failure, peripheral vascular disease, malnutrition, and the like. The role of balloon valvuloplasty remains uncertain, although this investigational technique may offer promise (Cribier et al 1986).

Aortic regurgitation of varied aetiology is best managed medically in elderly patients, using diuretics, vasodilator drugs and digitalis to control the cardiac failure. Massive acute aortic regurgitation due to trauma or infective endocarditis often requires valve replacement; because the presentation is typically that of acute pulmonary oedema and the diastolic murmur is soft or inaudible, an incorrect diagnosis of myocardial infarction may be made.

Mitral valvular disease in the elderly is typically mitral regurgitation due to rheumatic heart disease, papillary muscle dysfunction, myxomatous mitral valvular degeneration or calcification of the mitral annulus; the latter predominates in women. Mitral stenosis is rarely diagnosed initially in the elderly. However, the onset of atrial fibrillation may cause haemodynamic deterioration in an elderly patient with mitral regurgitation (Clancy et al 1985), or cause peripheral arterial embolism or cardiac decompensation when mitral stenosis is present. Mitral valvular disease can usually be managed medically, save for the severe acute mitral regurgitation related to chordal or papillary muscle rupture, as occurs with infective endocarditis or myocardial ischaemia. Emergency mitral valve replacement may be necessary, with intra-aortic balloon support during cardiac catheterization and preoperatively. The results of mitral valve replacement are less satisfactory than with aortic valve replacement; surgical mortality is 10–14% with mitral valve replacement, in part related to the concomitant ventricular dysfunction or emergency surgery (Hochberg et al 1979). The results of surgery for aortic regurgitation are less favourable than for aortic stenosis.

It remains controversial whether mechanical or bioprosthetic valves are preferable in elderly patients. Bioprostheses may avert the risk of anti-coagulation (Wintzen et al 1982), but valvular degeneration may necessitate reoperation at an older age. It is not known whether the rate of degeneration of bioprostheses differs in the elderly, nor if the currently recommended lower-dosage anticoagulation therapy will significantly decrease the excess bleeding risks of an elderly population.

Atrial septal defect is the most common congenital cardiac lesion in the elderly; supraventricular tachyarrhythmias may produce symptoms and require treatment.

Infective endocarditis is frequent in elderly patients with both acquired valvular and congenital heart disease, operated and unoperated (Thell et al 1975), with aortic valve endocarditis most common. An increased occurrence of *Streptococcus bovis* endocarditis is thought to be due to gastrointestinal problems and of enterococcal endocarditis to genitourinary procedures in elderly men. The high mortality described in this age group may reflect the frequent atypical presentation, with the patient often being afebrile; late diagnosis; and thus delayed initiation of therapy. Recommendations for prophylaxis against infective endocarditis are as for younger patients (Committee 1984).

Cardiomyopathy

Hypertrophic cardiomyopathy is not uncommon in elderly patients and appears to have a good prognosis; the risk of serious arrhythmias appears to be less than among younger patients. The presenting complaints may include chest pain, dyspnoea, palpitations, or syncope (Krasnow & Stein 1978). Its recognition is often difficult, as there are many other causes for a systolic murmur and a prominent fourth heart sound, and the electrocardiogram may mimic myocardial infarction. The detection of a bisferiens carotid pulse or a double apex impulse provides a clue to the diagnosis; the systolic murmur decreases with squatting and is accentuated with a Valsalva manoeuvre; echocardiography is confirmatory. Patients with hypertrophic cardio-myopathy are particularly sensitive to volume depletion, as may occur often in elderly patients in the setting of surgery or other associated medical problems; and treatment with digitalis, diuretics and nitrate drugs that may be given as therapy when an incorrect diagnosis is made may exacerbate the outflow obstruction and worsen the clinical status; beta-blocking drugs are indicated for symptomatic patients (Hamby & Aintablian 1976).

Dilated cardiomyopathy is less frequent than in a younger population, although it may at times be erroneously misdiagnosed as ischaemic heart disease in the elderly. Alcohol excess may precipitate or exacerbate cardiac decompensation. Therapy is as for heart failure due to ventricular systolic dysfunction. Rarely, cardiac amyloidosis or haemochromatosis may produce a restrictive cardiomyopathy in elderly patients.

Cardiopulmonary disease

The two major cardiopulmonary problems in elderly people are pulmonary embolism and chronic obstructive pulmonary disease; both may be accentu-ated by the decline in pulmonary function with ageing.

Pulmonary embolism is particularly common in the elderly because of multiple problems leading to prolonged immobilization and the frequent occurrence of congestive cardiac failure and arrhythmias. The diagnosis may be difficult because of concomitant cardiac and pulmonary diseases; the major non-invasive test — perfusion lung scanning — has far less specificity than in a younger population, because areas of decreased perfusion are present in the absence of pulmonary embolism. Pulmonary embolism is often misdiagnosed as pneumonia or heart failure. Anticoagulation, despite the increased risk of bleeding, remains the therapy of choice (Wintzen et al 1982); when anticoagulation is contraindicated, a transvenously inserted vena caval obstructing device is the preferred management.

Chronic obstructive pulmonary disease is the most common cause of right-sided cardiac failure in an elderly population. As in younger patients, those with a resting pO_2 lowered below 55 torr benefit from continuous oxygen therapy, if respiratory depression does not occur with oxygen administration; this treatment improves both clinical status and survival. The therapy of associated supraventricular tachyarrhythmias remains controversial, in that digitalis toxicity is common in elderly patients with chronic lung disease, and treatment with verapamil may depress myocardial contractility. Exercise rehabilitation is often also appropriate once cardiac failure has been controlled, and can further improve functional status.

Summary

The increasing percentage of elderly persons in most developed countries and the anticipated increased longevity of this elderly population mean that we require more information specific to their cardiovascular problems and the delineation of an appropriate approach to care. The highly heterogeneous character of the elderly population requires that determinants other than chronological age guide decisions about therapy: prominent among these determinants are physiological status, mental status, and associated diseases, because chronological age poorly predicts functional capabilities (Wenger et al 1987). As life expectancy continues to increase, there will be an increased need to assess the vocational and leisure/recreational capabilities of elderly patients with cardiovascular disease whose functional status has been reasonably well maintained.

Preventive approaches to the care of elderly patients should be designed to delay debilitating cardiovascular illnesses and the resulting dependency. Control of blood pressure facilitates the management of angina pectoris and congestive heart failure; control of obesity decreases cardiac work. Physical activity of reasonably modest intensity can improve the functional capacity of many elderly patients with cardiovascular disease, particularly previously sedentary individuals (Hodgson & Buskirk 1977). Elderly patients typically are interested in preserving their health and are able and willing to adhere to medical care recommendations. The goal of therapies for cardiovascular disease in elderly patients should be an improvement in functional status, limitation of morbidity, and maintenance of the functional capacity to enable self-sufficiency and an independent lifestyle, rather than simply a prolongation of life regardless of its quality.

Drug therapy in elderly patients entails an increased risk of adverse reactions because of age-related pharmacokinetic and pharmacodynamic changes (Greenblatt et al 1982, Lowenthal & Affrime 1981, Ouslander 1981); multiple medications increasing the likelihood of drug interactions; and hearing, visual and memory impairments that may engender errors in the taking of medication. Major adverse drug effects in elderly patients are described with digitalis, diuretics, antihypertensive drugs, antiarrhythmic agents and anticoagulants (Lavarenne et al 1983).

Adequate attention has not been paid to the psychosocial complications of cardiac illness in elderly patients that may limit recovery and the resumption of the previous lifestyle (Pathy & Peach 1980). Social isolation and inadequate social support may adversely affect survival (World Health Organization 1987) and inadequate expectations of the outcomes of cardiovascular illness may limit the demands for care by elderly persons.

Appropriate management requires an appreciation of the characteristics of cardiovascular illness unique to the elderly, including disease mechanisms, rate of progression of severity, and prognosis, coupled with the selection of those clinical approaches to recognition and therapy that may increase the likelihood of a favourable outcome (Coodley 1985, Messerli 1984).

References

Akman D 1983 Treatment of acute myocardial infarction in the elderly. Geriatrics 38:46

Amery A, Bulpitt C, Fagard R et al 1980 Does diet matter in hypertension? Eur Heart J 1:299

Amery A, Hansson L, Andren L et al 1981 Hypertension in the elderly. Hypertension seminars at Ostra Hospital, Göteborg, Sweden. Acta Med Scand 210:221

Amery A, Birkenhager G, Brisko P et al 1985 Mortality and morbidity results from the European Working Party on High Blood Pressure in the Elderly Trial. Lancet 1:1349

Berman ND 1979 The elderly patient in the coronary care unit. I. Acute myocardial infarction. J Am Geriatr Soc 27:145

Caird FI, Andrews GR, Kennedy RD 1983 Effect of posture on blood pressure in the elderly. Br Heart J 35:527

Clancy KF, Iskandrian AS, Hakki A-H et al 1985 Age-related changes in cardiovascular performance in mitral regurgitation: analysis of 61 patients. Am Heart J 109:442

Cohn JN, Archibald DG, Ziesche S et al 1986 Effect of vasodilator therapy on mortality in chronic congestive heart failure. Results of a Veterans Administration cooperative study. N Engl J Med 314:1547

Committee on Rheumatic Fever and Infective Endocarditis of the Council on Cardiovascular Disease in the Young 1984 Prevention of bacterial endocarditis. Circulation 70:1123A

Coodley EL (ed) 1985 Geriatric heart disease. PSG Publishing Co, Littleton, Massachusetts

Cribier A, Saoudi N, Berland J et al 1986 Percutaneous transluminal valvuloplasty of acquired aortic stenosis in elderly patients: an alternative to valve replacement? Lancet 1:63

Delin K, Aurell M, Granerus G et al 1982 Surgical treatment of renovascular hypertension in the elderly patient. Acta Med Scand 211:169

Elayda MA, Hall RJ, Gray AG et al 1984 Coronary revascularization in the elderly patient. J Am Coll Cardiol 3:1398

Fleg JL, Kennedy HL 1982 Cardiac arrhythmias in a healthy elderly population: detection by 24-hour ambulatory electrocardiography. Chest 81:302

Gersh BJ, Kronmal RA, Frye RL et al 1982 Coronary arteriography and coronary artery bypass surgery: morbidity and mortality in patients ages 65 years or older. Circulation 67:483

Gersh BJ, Kronmal RA, Schaff HV et al 1983 Comparison of coronary artery surgery and medical therapy in patients 65 years of age or older. A nonrandomized study from CASS registry. N Engl J Med 313:217

GISSI 1986 Study of streptokinase in acute myocardial infarction. Lancet 1:397

Greenblatt DJ, Sellers EM, Shader RI 1982 Drug therapy: drug disposition in old age. N Engl J Med 306:1081–1088

Gundersen T, Abrahamsen AM, Kjekshus J et al 1982 Timolol-related reduction in mortality and reinfarction in patients ages 65–75 years surviving acute myocardial infarction. Circulation 66:1179

Hamby RI, Aintablian A 1976 Hypertrophic subaortic stenosis is not rare in the eighth decade. Geriatrics 31:71

Heller GV, Blaustein AS, Wei JY 1983 Implications of increased myocardial isoenzyme level in the presence of normal serum creatine kinase activity. Am J Cardiol 51:24

Heller TA, Larson EB, LoGerfo JP 1984 Quality of ambulatory care of the elderly: an analysis of five conditions. J Am Geriatr Soc 32:782

Hill RD, Glazer MD, Wenger NK 1985 Myocardial infarction in the elderly. In: Hurst JW (ed) Clinical essays on the heart, vol 5. McGraw-Hill, New York, p 293

Hochberg MS, Derkac WM, Conkle DM et al 1979 Mitral valve replacement in elderly patients: encouraging postoperative clinical and hemodynamic results. J Thorac Cardiovasc Surg 77:422

Hodgson JL, Buskirk ER 1977 Physical fitness and age, with emphasis on cardiovascular function in the elderly. J Am Geriatr Soc 25:385

Hulley SB, Furberg CD, Gurland B et al 1985 Systolic Hypertension in the Elderly Program (SHEP): antihypertensive officacy of chlorthalidone. Am J Cardiol 56:913–920

Hypertension Detection and Follow-up Program Cooperative Group 1979 Five-year findings of the Hypertension Detection and Follow-Up Program. II. Mortality by race, sex, and age. JAMA (J Am Med Assoc) 242:2572

Jajich CL, Ostfeld AM, Freeman DH Jr 1984 Smoking and coronary heart disease mortality in the elderly. JAMA (J Am Med Assoc) 252:2831

Kannel W, Gordon T 1978 Evaluation of cardiovascular risk in the elderly: the Framingham Study. Bull NY Acad Med 54:573

Kantelip JP, Sage E, Duchene-Marulla ZP 1986 Findings on ambulatory electrocardiographic monitoring in subjects older than 80 years. Am J Cardiol 57:398

Kennedy RD 1975 Drug therapy for cardiovascular disease in the aged. J Am Geriatr Soc 23:113

Knapp WS, Douglas JS Jr, Craver JM et al 1981 Efficacy of coronary artery bypass grafting in elderly patients with coronary artery disease. Am J Cardiol 47:923

Kotler MN, Mintz GS, Parry WR et al 1981 Bedside diagnosis of organic murmurs in the elderly. Geriatrics 36:107

Krasnow N, Stein RA 1978 Hypertrophic cardiomyopathy in the aged. Am Heart J 96:326

Latting CA, Silverman ME 1980 Acute myocardial infarction in hospitalized patients over age 70. Am Heart J 100:311

Lavarenne J, Dumas R, Cayrol C 1983 Effets indésirables des médicaments chez les personnes âgées. Bilan des observations recueillies pendant un an par l'Association Française des Centres de Pharmacovigilance. Therapie (Paris) 36:485

Logeais Y, Luguerrier A, Rioux C et al 1984 Surgery of calcified aortic stenosis in patients age 70 and over: immediate results: apropos of the series of 229 cases. Ann Cardiol Angeiol 33:385

Lowenthal DT, Affrime MB 1981 Cardiovascular drugs for the geriatric patient. Geriatrics 36:65

McKee PA, Castelli WP, McNamara PM et al 1971 The natural history of congestive heart failure: the Framingham Study. N Engl J Med 285:1441

Marchionni N, Pini R, Vannucci A et al 1981 Intensive care for the elderly with acute myocardial infarction. J Clin Exp Gerontol 3:46

Martin A, Bembo LJ, Butrous GS et al 1984 Five-year follow-up of 101 elderly subjects by means of long-term ambulatory cardiac monitoring. Eur Heart J 5:592

Mellström D, Rundgren Å, Jagenburg R et al 1982 Tobacco smoking, ageing and health among the elderly: a longitudinal population study of 70-year-old men and an age cohort comparison. Age & Ageing 11:45

Messerli FH (ed) 1984 Cardiovascular disease in the elderly. Martinus Nijhoff, The Netherlands

Messerli FH, Ventura HO, Glade LB et al 1983 Essential hypertension in the elderly: haemodynamics, intravascular volume, plasma renin activity, and circulating catecholamine levels. Lancet 2:983

Mock M, Holmes D Jr, Vlietstra R et al 1982 Percutaneous transluminal coronary angioplasty (PTCA) in patients > 60 years of age registered in the NHLBI Registry. Circulation 66 (suppl II):II-329 (abstr)

Montoye HJ, Willis PW, Cunningham DA 1968 Heart rate response to submaximal exercise: relation to age and sex. J Gerontol 23:127

Murphy ES, Lawson RM, Starr A et al 1981 Severe aortic stenosis in patients 60 years of age and older: left ventricular function and 10-year survival after valve replacement. Circulation 64 (suppl II):II–184

Ouslander JG 1981 Drug therapy in the elderly. Ann Intern Med 95:711

Pathy MS, Peach H 1980 Disability among the elderly after myocardial infarction: a 3-year follow-up. J R Coll Physicians Lond 14:221

Peach H, Pathy J 1979 Disability in the elderly after myocardial infarction. J R Coll Physicians Lond 13:154

Report of the Joint American College of Cardiology/American Heart Association Task Force on Assessment of Cardiovascular Procedures (Subcommittee on Pacemaker Implantation) 1984 Guidelines for permanent cardiac pacemaker implantation, May 1984. J Am Coll Cardiol 4:434

Rowe JW 1983 Systolic hypertension in the elderly. N Engl J Med 309:1246

Smith JM, Lindsay WG, Lillehei RG et al 1976 Cardiac surgery in geriatric patients. Surgery (St Louis) 80:443

Statement on hypertension in the elderly 1986 The Working Group on Hypertension in the Elderly. JAMA (J Am Med Assoc) 256:70

Sugiura M, Matsushita S, Ueda K et al 1982 A clinicopathological study of valvular diseases in 3,000 consecutive autopsies of the aged. Jpn Circ J 46:337

Svanborg A, Bergström G, Mellström D 1982 Epidemiological studies on social and medical conditions of the elderly. European Reports and Studies 62. WHO Regional Office for Europe, Copenhagen

Thell R, Martin FH, Edwards JE 1975 Bacterial endocarditis in subjects 60 years of age and older. Circulation 51:174

Weintraub RM, Wei JY, Thurer RL 1986 Surgical repair of remediable post-infarction cardiogenic shock in the elderly: early and long-term results. J Am Geriatr Soc 34:389

Weisfelt ML (ed) 1980 The aging heart: its function and response to stress. Raven Press, New York

Wenger NK 1984 The elderly coronary patient. In: Wenger NK, Hellerstein HK (eds) Rehabilitation of the coronary patient, 2nd edn. John Wiley, New York, p 397

Wenger NK, Furberg CD, Pitt E (eds) 1986 Coronary heart disease in the elderly. Working Conference on the Recognition and Management of Coronary Heart Disease in the Elderly, held September 4–6, 1985, at the National Institutes of Health, Bethesda, MD, USA. Elsevier, New York

Wenger NK, Marcus FM, O'Rourke RW (eds) 1987 Bethesda Conference #18: Cardiovascular disease in the elderly. J Am Coll Cardiol 10:suppl A

Williams BO, Begg TB, Semple T et al 1976 The elderly in a coronary unit. Br Med J 2:451

Williams MA, Maresh CM, Esterbrooks DJ et al 1985 Early exercise training in patients older than age 65 years compared with that in younger patients after acute myocardial infarction or coronary artery bypass grafting. Am J Cardiol 55:263

Wintzen AR, Tijssen JGP, deVries WA et al 1982 Risk of long-term oral anticoagulant therapy in elderly patients after myocardial infarction. Second report of the sixty plus Reinfarction Study Research Group. Lancet 1:64

Wood AJJ, Feely J 1981 Management of hypertension in the elderly. South Med J 74:1503

World Health Organization 1987 Report of a Scientific Group on the Epidemiology of Aging 1983. Geneva, Technical Report Series, in preparation

DISCUSSION

Grimley Evans: I am interested in your view of the nature of the relationship between blood pressure and morbid outcomes in the elderly. In the South Wales study (Miall & Brennan 1981) the relationship (in people over 65) appeared to be J-shaped: in other words, very low blood pressures were worse in terms of mortality than slightly higher blood pressures, for both sexes. We found the same for men in our Tyneside study (Evans 1987). (There was no relationship between blood pressure and either stroke or mortality, in women.) Cruickshank et al (1987) have recently suggested that this up-turn of mortality at the lower end of the blood pressure distribution is due to people who have coronary artery disease and need a higher blood pressure, to maintain life. Some years ago, Anderson (1978) re-examined some of the Framingham data, which have always shown a steady monotonic relationship, and suggested that the Framingham mode of analysis distorted the relationship of blood pressure to morbidity at the bottom end of the distribution. I am interested in whether the American data show this J-shaped curve, to see whether or not there is an environmental difference between elderly people in the two countries, and whether there is increased mortality at the lowest end of the blood pressure distribution in the USA.

Wenger: This may be the same issue as in patients whose Q wave disappears or persists after myocardial infarction; one critical variable is the presence or absence of an intercurrent event. In a patient documented previously to have hypertension, who now has an extensive myocardial infarction, resulting ventricular dysfunction, and cannot maintain a reasonable cardiac output, the blood pressure will fall. We know that the ventricular dysfunction *per se* is the major determinant of mortality in that population. Are we, therefore, looking at mortality due to the ventricular dysfunction that is the cause of the lowered blood pressure? Again, to return to the myocardial infarction example, if the patient sustains a contralateral infarction and this causes the Q wave to disappear, the outcome will be far less favourable than if the patient had no intercurrent cardiac event. The latter scenario is compatible with a small infarction that has healed with formation of a small, firm and fibrous scar, rendering the prognosis better. So we must determine intercurrent cardiovascular events and resultant changes in ventricular function; this is not easy to study, except prospectively. Most blood pressure studies have documented intercurrent events, but did not look for resultant ventricular dysfunction as the basis for whether the elevated blood pressure fell after a hospitalization for an intercurrent event. So the lowered blood pressure may actually reflect another variable, added to the constellation of problems the patient has.

Svanborg: I wonder to what extent the up-turn of the lower part of the curve of blood pressure against age, mentioned by Grimley Evans, is due to the higher occurrence of smoking. We know that tobacco smokers have significantly lower blood pressure than non-smokers (Mellström et al 1982). At the same time they have a higher risk of cardiovascular disease (Mellström & Svanborg 1987). At the age of 70, male smokers weighed on an average 4.5 kg less and at the age of 75, 7 kg less than non-smokers. It has long been known that there is a relationship between body mass and blood pressure.

Let me also comment on the occurrence of coronary heart disease in the elderly. Anginal pain in elderly individuals is roughly as common in men as in women, and this similarity between the sexes in the prevalence of anginal pain seems to persists at least up to the age of 80. The risk of myocardial infarction, on the other hand, in elderly women is much lower than in men.

You mentioned some other electrocardiographic changes in the elderly, Dr Wenger. One problem is that 'clinical reference values' for possible physiological changes in the electrocardiographic picture of the elderly are not really known. The difficulty when we use the Minnesota coding system might be that this is not adapted to taking into consideration ECG changes that might be physiological in the elderly.

Wenger: The electrocardiograms that were used in the formulation of criteria for the Minnesota code did not include ECGs of significant numbers of elderly patients. We know that conduction abnormalities are seen in the elderly, in the absence of 'obvious' coronary disease; but this absence of 'obvious disease' is the problem, because autopsy studies of an apparently well elderly population, even including some elderly individuals tested by various non-invasive means who did not show clinical evidence of disease, often revealed significant coronary atherosclerosis at post-mortem examination.

Svanborg: And, of course, this might also be the case in younger populations.

Wenger: But much more so in older populations, and with more extensive and more multivessel coronary disease. Often the individual arterial obstruction is not a critical one, but multivessel coronary disease seems to be more typical of the older population. I am not sure that we can, using the intensity of exercise testing we typically impose, readily reach the activity threshold where that extent of coronary disease may become clinically manifest. This is one of our unmet needs—a physiological test to challenge the oxygen transport system that can be safely performed by a reasonable number of elderly individuals. The role of studies using dipyridamole must be assessed in older persons. Basically, an exercise test is designed to precipitate myocardial ischaemia; this may pose an excessive risk in an older population, who may not be able to tolerate even transient ischaemia without complications.

T.F. Williams: The work of Lakatta and his colleagues in older people free of demonstrable coronary heart disease indicates that the heart maintains a remarkable function into the later years (Rodeheffer et al 1984); so, as you were emphasizing, it appears to be the co-morbid features that lead to cardiac problems. These co-morbid problems are very common, and we are therefore interested in them from a preventive or long-range point of view. This is one perspective.

When it comes to addressing these problems, once the patient has cardiovascular disease, an important point that you made is that we know so little about responses in older people, particularly to drugs, especially in people who may also need other drugs for other disease conditions. The Food and Drug Administration in the USA believes that we should expect or require drug testing to be done in older people for drugs that will be commonly used in such people, although guidelines and a formal requirement have yet to be set. This presents a challenge, again especially because a new drug would need to be tested in people who already have many other medical problems—besides heart disease they may also have diabetes, chronic pulmonary disease, and so on. Thus testing becomes an even larger issue. We need to see where the priorities lie.

Wenger: Some features of the clinical presentation of myocardial infarction or of angina pectoris suggest that it may not be feasible to combine populations of younger and older patients for study, because the criteria for entrance into a study may limit the accession of either the younger or the older subgroups. We may have arbitrarily to choose an age range within which to look at the disease, and to determine whether it differs from subsets of people in an advanced age range. We are uncertain whether age 65–70 is categorically different from age 80–85 in many of the features of the clinical presentation of coronary disease. In an elderly population, the variance of any variable is greater than at younger ages, and chronological age is not a good marker, except very grossly, by which to differentiate between the very frail and the less frail elderly. Their degree of co-morbidity may be far more important.

In this regard, clinical trials typically have enrolled patients with as few concurrent diseases as possible, to facilitate the interpretation of the results. We shall be less likely to see isolated coronary disease in studies of elderly patients. The majority of US patients over 65 have at least one chronic illness. The elderly constitute the largest population using medically prescribed drugs, and yet most drugs have not been tested specifically in the elderly. We shall have to examine drug benefits and risks both in individuals with apparently isolated disease (and therefore less likely to be receiving other drugs) as well as in elderly patients who are very prone to drug interactions because of their multiplicity of diseases and therapies.

Arie: The situation is even worse than simply that drugs are insufficiently tested on elderly people. Claims are made for their safety and efficacy in elderly people on the basis of inappropriate evidence. We in the UK have also been trying to press the regulatory bodies to adopt a protocol for testing drugs, namely that old people (and particularly the very old) should be represented in the test samples in at least the proportions they form of the general population or, better, the proportions they are likely to form of potential users. We reviewed six major journals over a year and found 96 articles purporting to report effects of drugs in old people (Smith et al 1983). We found that claims concerning effects on old people, or safety in old people, often depended on the inclusion of perhaps only a couple of people in their early sixties; alternatively, no data were given on the age distribution of subjects, so valid inferences could not be drawn. Where unwanted effects were reported, these were commonly not related to age in the published material. There is a lot of tidying up to be done here, and we should all be pressing the regulatory bodies in our countries to get this right.

Wenger: Once we recommend this, we must be aware of the problems to be faced in including elderly patients in any clinical trial, in terms of recruitment, conduct of the study, format, venue, follow-up and so on. These may have to be conducted in different ways from the usual clinical trials. In the US Systolic Hypertension in the Elderly trial, the pilot phase (Hulley et al 1985) provided a number of surprises, and considerable information and suggestions as to a reasonable way (at least in the USA) to include the elderly population in a research study. The surprises related to the general opinion that systolic hypertension in the elderly would be very difficult to control; many of us thought that the choice of drugs was unwise, in that these elderly individuals would respond extremely poorly to diuretic therapy. But, at least as can be judged from the pilot study, we were quite wrong; elevated systolic blood pressure was reasonably easy to control, and the reported side-effects were trivial. Armchair reasoning is obviously not the way to recommend drug therapy in an elderly population.

Arie: The point we have to keep emphasizing is the *very* elderly, because that is where problems and unwanted effects commonly arise.

Wenger: We have also not addressed the non-pharmacological management of hypertension in an elderly population; that component may be extremely important. Sodium restriction in the diet will limit the problem of hypokalaemia related to diuretic use, and lessened sodium intake may even limit the drug dosage needed to control blood pressure. Other features of non-pharmacological management may be important, including physical activity, weight control, avoidance of excessive alcohol intake, smoking cessation, and the like, and we have not yet addressed them, either.

Katzman: You mentioned that operations are freely done nowadays on patients over 70 or even 75 years of age, Dr Wenger. How far do you go? Is the morbidity or mortality after such operations the same in people over 80, or even over 90 or 95? Is there an age-determined limit?

Wenger: Once you consider the oldest old (those over age 85), there is very stringent selection for operation. Chronological age and physiological age may differ considerably, often related to co-morbidity. For instance, we performed coronary by-pass graft surgery on a 92-year-old gentleman who wanted to continue to play golf, but could not do so because of incapacitating angina. Within a few weeks of the operation he was back on the golf course. That person was 92 years old chronologically, but 65 or 70 physiologically. The problem is that the patients who undergo cardiac surgery in their late 80s and early 90s are so carefully and specifically selected that I am not sure we can say much about age *per se* and relative risk. The individual who is well, has no other major illness, is alert and has an active lifestyle may be physiologically very different from others of the same age without these characteristics; we need different markers of ageing for that group.

Solomons: Frank Williams suggested that we should look at some of the information presented here in terms of its relation to the delivery of health care. You, Dr Wenger, have been involved in a number of population studies, rigorously designed. But when you project your experience and interest to facing the elderly population, you may have run up against the limits to which conventional experimental designs can be applied in studies of the aged. You have emphasized the presence of heterogeneity; as age advances, the co-morbidities combine; you have a flaring of possible presentations, almost to infinity, such that each patient in the end may represent a unique and individual phenomenon—almost an epiphenomenon. Generally, science tries basically to deal with nature by grouping and selecting and describing relatively homogeneous sets. Dr Williams' Institute is responsible for allocating research funds for ageing research. When we do this research, will we be doing only phenomenology and ethology when we look at this potentially infinite number of combinations of variables? And have we not, in fact, reached the limits of the conventional research approach in trying to draw conclusions from a myriad of such heterogeneous combinations?

T.F. Williams: This is a major challenge for much of what we do in research in older people; it is very specifically a challenge when we talk about drugs. This may call for a new approach to strategies, and I don't minimize the problems.

Fries: We always make an agonized plea for more data, because the questions are arising faster than they are being answered, and the number of questions is huge. You used 'co-morbidity' as a singular term, Dr Wenger, but 'co-morbidity' is itself infinitely divisible into different types. Such heterogeneity cannot, I maintain, be studied by traditional reductionist science in the human situation—that is, by isolating a single variable and doing a randomized controlled trial with 100 or 200 people in each group in order to answer one question—because you in fact haven't answered even that question for the next patient who comes along, who is in another subgroup. So you cannot get there from here, in a heterogeneous world. The only approach that I know to the study of these complexities is the longitudinal, observational, non-intrusive tracking of large numbers of patients, and the use of multivariate statistics to analyse the data, rather than the univariate statistics which are appropriate for a reductionist type of experiment (Fries & McShane 1986).

Wenger: This approach is feasible, even for drugs that are already licensed for clinical use; it is termed in the USA 'post-marketing surveillance'. The FDA could specifically mandate detailed surveillance of this type in selected subgroups of elderly individuals and develop some guidelines for the collection and analysis of data. The problem is that we typically look at major unwanted or unusual affects, rather than the typical multiplicity of mild complications of therapy that compromise well-being that are seen so frequently in the elderly and are attributed to 'old age'. There is a way of getting this information, but we have not yet tried to do so.

A. Williams: I want to pursue this matter further and go beyond the point where Nanette Wenger's paper finished, which was with the objectives of treatment of cardiovascular disease. I am wondering how frequently evaluative trials are pursued to the stage where data are generated on variables such as the general quality of life and the functional capacity of the person. More specifically, may I ask what, on the basis of your present knowledge, you would do if you were put in the position of having a prespecified budget for expanding the provision of cardiological services for the elderly? Where would you put your money to do the most good possible, in terms of increases in life expectancy and quality of life? This ties in with the question of the selection of potential patients by age or condition or treatment.

Wenger: I would certainly like to see the delineation of high-risk elderly patients as one objective. The high-risk elderly coronary patient uses the greatest amount of high technology expensive care when a recurrent infarction recurs, with all the complications. This reinfarction is often one from which hospital survival is unlikely but from which patients die very slowly. This is one of the major problems in caring for this high risk subset, but some of the complications of recurrent infarction may be potentially avertible by earlier intervention.

Mor: In designing such studies I agree that one needs to follow large numbers of patients prospectively, but the population one chooses and the care systems to which they are exposed are very important in selecting the cohort to be followed. Additionally, more could be learned with the application of multivariate hypothesis testing using existing clinical-trial data, which is generally not done. The problem of further examining the effect of age on treatment outcome is that often there are insufficient numbers of aged patients in the chosen population. That is because most clinical trials have excluded the aged.

Andrews: Over the past 10–15 years or so in many developed countries there has been, for middle-and old-age populations, a significant increase in life expectancy, out of proportion to anything that occurred for many decades previously. This has been accounted for in Australia and the USA almost totally by a reduction in mortality from coronary heart disease, a phenomenon not observed in the UK. I wonder whether we have learned anything from this astounding natural experiment, and whether we have any clues to the factors that contributed to this reduction. Clearly, they don't fall into the category of any major medical intervention.

Wenger: Those of us who believe in the value of coronary prevention will say that the preventive measures adopted in recent years have been responsible for the decrease in coronary mortality. If you talk to the cardiovascular surgeons, they will no doubt say that surgery is an important factor. The pharmacological therapy has expanded amazingly; a further major feature, I think, is that our bases for diagnosis have changed. In recent decades we have increasingly used enzyme-based diagnosis of myocardial infarction, which means that we probably identify less extensive infarctions, the non-Q wave infarctions. However, we are beginning to learn that non-Q wave infarction (previously termed subendocardial infarction) tends to be a stuttering infarct—it will recur repeatedly until it finally does its major damage. If we become skilful in detecting when the first 'bite' at the myocardium occurs, and we can intervene in those patients who are at high risk for repeated infarction, this intervention may be life-saving; it may also be one of the most cost-effective interventions we can undertake. The problem is that we lack a test that can be applied widely to an elderly population to identify with reasonable certainty the subset of people who are at excessive risk and for whom intervention may be feasible.

References

Anderson TW 1978 Re-examination of some of the Framingham blood-pressure data. Lancet 2:1139–1141

Cruickshank JM, Thorp JM, Zacharias FJ 1987 Benefits and potential harm of lowering high blood pressure. Lancet 1:581–584

Evans JG 1987 Blood pressure and stroke in an elderly English population. J Epidemiol Community Health, in press

Fries JF, McShane DJ 1986 ARAMIS (The American Rheumatism Assoc Medical Information System): a prototypical national chronic disease data bank. West J Med 145:798–804

Hulley SB, Furberg CD, Gurland B et al 1985 Systolic Hypertension in the Elderly Program (SHEP): antihypertensive efficacy of chlorthalidone. Am J Cardiol 56:913–920

Mellström D, Svanborg A 1987 Tobacco smoking—a major cause of sex differences in health. Compr Gerontol 1:34–39

Mellström D, Rundgren Å, Jagenburg R, Steen B, Svanborg A 1982 Tobacco smoking, ageing and health among the elderly. A longitudinal study of 70-year-old men and an age cohort comparison. Age & Ageing 11:45–58

Miall WE, Brennan PJ 1981 Hypertension in the elderly. In: Onesti G, Kimm KE (eds) Hypertension in the young and old. Grune & Stratton, New York, p 277–283

Rodeheffer RJ, Gerstenblith G, Becker LC, Fleg JL, Weisfeldt ML, Lakatta EG 1984 Exercise cardiac output is well maintained with advancing age in healthy human subjects: cardiac dilatation and increased stroke volume compensate for a diminished heart rate. Circulation 69:203–213

Smith C, Ebrahim S, Arie T 1983 Drug trials, the 'elderly', and the very aged. Lancet 2:1139

Osteoporosis and age-related fracture syndromes

B. L. Riggs and L. J. Melton III

Endocrine Research Unit, Division of Endocrinology, Metabolism, and Internal Medicine, and Department of Medical Statistics and Epidemiology, Mayo Clinic and Mayo Foundation, Rochester, Minnesota 55905, USA

Abstract. Osteoporosis is one of the most important age-related diseases. Each year in the United States it causes at least 1.2 million fractures and costs 7 to 10 billion dollars. The main cause of the fractures is increased bone fragility due to low bone density, although in the elderly an increase in the frequency of falls and in the trauma produced by the falls also contributes to fractures. Low bone density in osteoporosis has multiple causes which can be grouped into the categories of low initial bone mass and bone loss due to ageing, menopause, and sporadic factors. Given the magnitude of the problem, prevention is the only cost-effective approach. Enough is known about causes of bone loss leading to osteoporosis that an effective programme of prevention can be designed. Its implementation in the population should substantially reduce the incidence of this major public health problem.

1988 Research and the ageing population. Wiley, Chichester (Ciba Foundation Symposium 134) p 129–142

The problem of osteoporosis

Osteoporosis has aptly been called the silent epidemic. Bone loss occurs gradually over many years and, often, over several decades without clinical manifestations. As bone mass falls more and more below the fracture threshold (the level required to maintain skeletal integrity during the activities of everyday life), fractures begin to occur after minimal trauma. Fractures due to osteoporosis have their onset in middle life, and they become progressively more frequent with ageing. At least 1.2 million fractures in the United States each year are attributable to osteoporosis (Riggs & Melton 1986, and Table 1).

The pattern of fracture incidence with ageing depends on the content of trabecular and cortical bone at the site of fracture (Riggs & Melton 1986). The patterns of the three most common fractures — the vertebrae, proximal femur, and distal forearm (Colles' fracture) — are given in Fig. 1. The vertebrae and ultradistal radius contain large amounts of trabecular bone,

TABLE 1 Estimated fractures attributable to osteoporosis in the United States each year

Site	No. of cases
Vertebrae	538 000
Hip	227 000
Distal forearm	172 000
Other limb sites	283 000

and the incidence of fractures at these sites increases soon after menopause. For Colles' fractures, the incidence continues to increase with age until age 65 when it plateaus, whereas for vertebral fractures the incidence continues to rise well into advanced life. Hip fractures, by contrast, increase slowly with ageing until late in life, when an exponential increase leads to very high rates of fracture. Fractures of the proximal humerus, proximal tibia and pelvis follow a similar pattern. The sites of all these late-occurring fractures contain substantial amounts of both cortical and trabecular bone. Fractures of the shafts of the limb bones (predominantly cortical bone) do not increase with age and are mainly related to trauma.

One-third of women over 65 will have vertebral fractures. By extreme old age, one of every three women and one of every six men will have had a hip fracture. This catastrophic fracture leads to death in 12 to 20% of cases. One-quarter of the survivors require long-term nursing-home care and one-half of them are unable to walk without assistance. The direct and indirect costs of osteoporosis are estimated to be 7 to 10 billion dollars annually in the United States (Culliton 1987). As more and more of the population survive

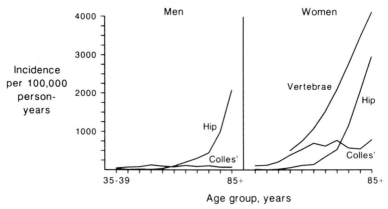

FIG. 1.   Incidence rates for the three common osteoporotic fractures (Colles', hip, and vertebral) in men and women, plotted as a function of age at the time of fracture. (By permission of the *New England Journal of Medicine*.)

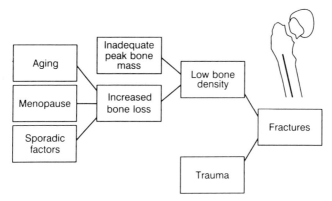

FIG. 2.   Model for the development of fractures due to osteoporosis. See text for details. (From Riggs 1987 by permission of W.B. Saunders Company.)

into advanced age, these already enormous costs will increase further unless the incidence of osteoporosis is reduced by the institution of preventive measures.

Pathogenesis of osteoporosis

Osteoporosis is a complex disorder with multiple causes. These can be grouped mechanistically into several categories, as shown in the model (Fig. 2). The main cause of age-related fractures is a low bone density. Bone density, at any age, depends upon two main variables — the amount of bone made during growth and its subsequent rate of loss. Thus, a greater peak bone mass is protective against osteoporosis whereas a lesser one increases risk. Over their lifetimes, women lose about 50% of their trabecular bone and about 35% of their cortical bone; men lose two-thirds of these amounts. The causes of this bone loss can be grouped into three categories. The first category represents the sum of all age-related endogenous factors that occur universally in the general population and include decreased osteoblast function, impaired calcium absorption, and other abnormalities that impair the response of bone to direct and indirect stresses. This term accounts for the slow bone loss that occurs over life in both sexes. It begins in both sexes around age 35 and increases in magnitude as age increases. This process accounts for the loss of 20 to 25% of cortical bone and 30 to 35% of trabecular bone in both women and men. The second category is sex steroid deficiency. The menopause produces an accelerated phase of bone loss that lasts up to 10 years. The accelerated bone loss attributable to the menopause may be 10 to 15% for cortical bone and 15 to 20% for trabecular bone. In men, this accelerated phase does not occur except in a small number in whom hypogonadism develops. The third category of bone loss includes a number of sporadic factors affecting some, but not other, members of the population. When present, these conditions increase the rate of bone loss. Finally, the propensity of the elderly to fall is an independent risk factor for fractures.

Initial bone mass

It is becoming more and more clear that insufficient accumulation of skeletal mass by young adulthood predisposes to fracture later in life as age-related bone loss ensues. The effects of heredity, race and sex on the incidence of osteoporosis can apparently be explained, in part, by their influence on peak bone mass. White women have the lightest skeletons and black men have the heaviest; white men and black women have skeletons of intermediate density. This rank order corresponds to the rank order for the occurrence of fractures. Peak bone mass has a strong genetic component and may explain the tendency of osteoporosis to run in families (Smith et al 1973). Finally, an epidemiological study in Yugoslavia (Matkovic et al 1979) showed that residents of a high calcium intake district had greater metacarpal bone density in young adult life than did compatriots who lived in a low calcium district. In the same two districts, those with a high calcium intake also had fewer hip fractures. The difference in bone density was apparent in young adulthood and did not diverge further with ageing, suggesting that the main effect of calcium was on peak bone mass.

Age-related factors

The two major age-related factors that have been thus far demonstrated are decreased bone formation (at the cellular level) due to impaired osteoblast function and decreased calcium absorption.

Impaired osteoblast function.   As assessed by the measurement of mean wall thickness of trabecular packets in biopsy samples (Lips et al 1978), from age 30 onward less bone is formed than is resorbed at individual bone remodelling units, and this abnormality becomes more pronounced with ageing. Although this defect could be caused by osteoblast senescence, the observation that fracture healing in the elderly is not impaired suggests that the osteoblasts are capable of responding to appropriate stimuli. It is possible that there is impaired regulation of osteoblast function by one or more of the various bone-derived growth factors that have been recently shown to be made by bone cells (Centrella & Canalis 1985).

Impaired calcium absorption.   Calcium absorption decreases in both sexes with ageing, especially after age 65 years. There is increasing evidence that this abnormality is associated with increased parathyroid function with ageing

(Insogna et al 1981). Serum levels of 1,25-dihydroxyvitamin D (1,25($OH)_2$D), the physiologically active vitamin D metabolite, have been shown by several, but not all, studies to decrease with ageing and are a possible cause of the decreased calcium absorption (Tsai et al 1984). A primary impairment in 25-hydroxyvitamin D_3 (25-OH-D) 1α-hydroxylase, the renal enzyme responsible for the conversion of 25-OH-D to 1,25($OH)_2$D, has been found in kidney slices from ageing rats. An analogous effect in elderly humans has been found by demonstrating that the rise in serum 1,25($OH)_2$D during the infusion of parathyroid hormone is blunted (Tsai et al 1984). Also, there is some evidence to suggest that a primary defect in intestinal calcium transport may contribute to the defect in calcium absorption. The increased parathyroid function causes an increase in bone turnover (there is increased activation of new bone remodelling units) but because bone formation is decreased at the cellular level at each bone remodelling unit, an increase in bone turnover leads to increased bone loss.

Other age-related hormonal factors. Serum concentrations of both growth hormone and the growth hormone-dependent insulin-like growth factor I (IGF-I) decrease by about 50% with ageing (Rudman et al 1981). IGF-I is the major factor stimulating the growth of bone and cartilage cells. Serum calcitonin, a major antiresorptive hormone, does not decrease with ageing but, at any age, is consistently lower in women than in men (Body & Heath 1983).

Menopause

Women who have had an oophorectomy in young adult life have lower bone density values in later life than age-matched control women (Richelson et al 1984). Administration of oestrogen at the menopause prevents the accelerated phase (Lindsay et al 1980), but not the slow phase, of bone loss. Nonetheless, case–control and cohort studies have found that the postmenopausal administration of oestrogen reduces the occurrence of fractures of the vertebrae, hip and distal radius by about one-half (Ettinger et al 1985). This is consistent with the estimate that one-third to one-half of overall bone loss in women is caused by the menopause.

Sporadic factors

Nutrition. The dietary requirement for calcium is relatively high because there are obligatory fecal and urinary losses of about 150 to 250 mg/day. When the calcium absorbed from the diet is insufficient to offset these losses, calcium must be withdrawn from the bone which contains 99% of all the body reserves. The recommended daily allowance — the level of nutrient intake that will protect 95% of the population from deficiency — has not been rigorously established for calcium. Currently, it is set at 800 mg/day. A recent survey by the United States Public Health Service showed that, although American men have an average dietary intake that approximates this level, middle-aged and elderly women have an intake of only 550 mg/day.

Attempts to determine the level of intake required to prevent negative calcium balance using metabolic balance techniques have given conflicting results. Heaney et al (1978) found that 1000 mg/day was required for pre-menopausal women whereas 1500 mg/day was required for postmenopausal women. But Nordin et al (1979) found that only 550 mg/day of calcium intake was required. Population studies have in general not demonstrated a strong relationship between calcium intake and bone density. Three of six controlled trials found significant short-term slowing of bone loss from the appendicular skeleton with increased calcium intake, but the reduction in bone loss was less than that achieved with oestrogen therapy. Two recent studies showed that 1500 mg/day of calcium administered to women shortly after the menopause could not substitute for oestrogen in preventing bone loss from the vertebrae (Ettinger et al 1987, Riis et al 1987). Thus, the evidence defining the role of calcium intake in modulating bone loss is conflicting and more studies are needed.

Other nutritional factors seem to be less important. A high protein intake increases the urinary excretion of calcium and, possibly, increases calcium requirements. Serum levels of 25-OH-D decline moderately with ageing and may be even lower in some patients with recent hip fracture (Meller et al 1985). Nonetheless, because of the fortification of food, nutritional deficiency of vitamin D probably is not a major risk factor for osteoporosis in the United States, except in certain elderly housebound persons with inadequate dietary intake.

Behavioural factors. Various behavioural risk factors for bone loss include decreased physical activity, a high alcohol consumption, and smoking. The stresses of weight bearing stimulate osteoblast function, whereas immobiliz-ation causes bone loss. Muscle mass and bone mass are directly related, and a recent study (Pocock et al 1986) showed that there was a positive correlation between physical fitness (as assessed by measurement of oxygen consump-tion) and the bone density of the vertebrae and proximal femur. Active intervention with exercise programmes in postmenopausal women has been shown to slow the rate of bone loss as compared with a control group. Both smoking and a high alcohol intake each increase the risk of osteoporosis two-fold, and when both factors are present, the risk is increased four-fold (Seeman et al 1983). These agents appear to have direct toxic effects on bone cells. Obesity protects against bone loss (Seeman et al 1983), both because of increased loading stress to the spine and, in postmenopausal women, because of increased conversion of adrenal androgens to oestrogen by fat cells.

Medical conditions and drug use.   Certain diseases, surgical procedures, and medications may also be associated with the development of osteoporosis. The most common conditions are early oophorectomy (in women), hypogonadism (in men), subtotal gastrectomy, thyroid hormone excess, hemiplegia, chronic obstructive lung disease, and the use of glucocorticoid and anticonvulsant drugs. Thiazide diuretics may protect against bone loss by causing renal retention of calcium.

Trauma

Risk of fracture is related both to the nature of the force applied to bone and to the ability of the bone to withstand that force. The risk of fracture increases as the amount of force that is applied increases, and the risk also increases as bone fragility increases as a consequence of bone loss. The elderly fall frequently because of failing vision, neurological diseases and their sequelae, arthritis of the lower limb joints, and the use of sedatives and other drugs; their falls entail increased trauma because impaired coordination and slowed reflexes reduce their ability to break the impact of a fall (Melton & Riggs 1985). Nonetheless, most falls do not result in fractures in the elderly. In a nursing-home study, only 1.4% of falls resulted in major injuries (Rodstein 1964). Thus, the interaction between low bone density and trauma in producing fractures in the elderly is not well understood, and other factors may contribute to the susceptibility to fracture. For example, it is possible that changes in the quality of bone in the elderly contribute, such as reduced microfracture repair, altered physical properties of elderly bone, structural changes in trabecular pattern resulting from bone loss, and subclinical osteomalacia (Melton & Riggs 1985). The more likely explanation, however, is that biomechanical factors associated with unique characteristics of the individual fall determine whether the fall results in skeletal fracture.

Prevention of osteoporosis

Given the magnitude of the problem, prevention is the only cost-effective approach. There are several measures that, if adopted widely in the population at risk, would substantially reduce the incidence of fractures due to osteoporosis. First, an attempt should be made to reduce or eliminate remediable causes of falls in the elderly. This can be accomplished by an intensive education campaign targeted to the elderly population and to health-care professionals providing domiciliary care for the elderly. Common causes of

TABLE 2   General measures to reduce bone loss

---

1. Treat women with premature menopause with oestrogen until age 50
2. Increase physical activity
3. Eliminate tobacco usage
4. Use alcohol in moderation
5. Increase calcium intake to 1500 mg/day in adolescence and 1000 mg/day in adults. Higher intake recommended for individuals with risk factors for osteoporosis
6. Ensure adequate vitamin D intake in elderly

---

falls in the elderly include slipping on highly waxed floors or loose throw rugs, instability caused by wearing shoes with high, narrow heels, and the use of drugs that impair coordination. A night-light should be provided in the bathroom. Great care should be exercised in walking on ice and other slippery surfaces. Elderly women with an unsteady gait should use a cane or a walker. Second, an attempt should be made to remove risk factors for bone loss in the general population, as listed in Table 2. Brody et al (1984) estimated that if bone loss could be retarded by only 5.5 years, the incidence of hip fracture — the major cause of morbidity in osteoporosis — would be reduced by one-half. Third, women who have bone density values in the lower part of the normal range at the time of menopause should be considered for long-term oestrogen replacement therapy.

In addition, it should become possible in the future to identify subjects who are at risk for fracture because of low bone density and to treat them with regimens that will increase bone density. This is not yet possible, because we do not have sufficient information to accurately forecast the risk of fracture from the bone density of the vertebrae or hip, and because effective and safe programmes for stimulating bone formation are not available. Nonetheless, these deficiencies should be resolved in the foreseeable future. Progress is already being made in defining fracture risk. It has been demonstrated that fractures do not occur in the absence of severe trauma until bone density falls below the fracture threshold of about 1.0 g/cm^2 for both vertebrae and femur (Riggs et al 1982). Moreover, with further decreases in bone density below the fracture threshold, the incidence of hip fractures and the prevalence of vertebral fractures increase (Fig. 3). A further refinement of this approach may allow definition of the lifetime fracture risks associated with specific levels of bone density. Also, progress is being made on developing regimens that stimulate bone formation and, thus, have the theoretical potential of increasing bone mass substantially and reducing the risk of new fractures. Of the several regimens currently being investigated, however, only therapy with sodium fluoride has been widely evaluated (Riggs 1984). This drug stimulates osteoblasts directly and in many instances can result in a doubling of trabecular bone mass in the axial skeleton. Sodium fluoride is relatively toxic,

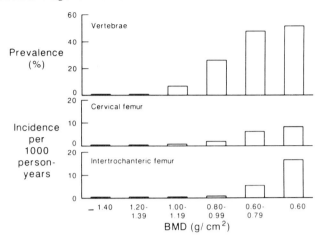

FIG. 3. Occurrence of vertebral and proximal femoral fractures at various levels of vertebral and proximal femur bone mineral density (BMD). Data are from random samples of women in Rochester, Minnesota, and from a sample of patients from the same population with hip fractures or vertebral fractures. (By permission of the *New England Journal of Medicine*.)

however, and it has not been unequivocally demonstrated that fluoridic bone is as strong as an equivalent amount of normal bone. A more promising approach is treatment with physiological growth factors. A concerted effort is in progress to isolate and characterize the various local skeletal growth factors (Centrella & Canalis 1985). Stimulating bone formation in osteoporotic patients physiologically by using growth factors produced by recombinant DNA technology is an exciting prospect.

Enormous scientific strides have been made in recent years in understanding how osteoporosis develops, how bone-cell activity is regulated physiologically, and how it can be manipulated pharmacologically. Further progress is expected in the immediate future. Thus, there is reason to be optimistic that osteoporosis can be brought under control within the coming decade.

References

Body J-J, Heath H III 1983 Estimates of circulating monomeric calcitonin: physiological studies in normal and thyroidectomized man. J Clin Endocrinol Metab 57:897–903

Brody JA, Farmer ME, White LR 1984 Absence of menopausal effect on hip fracture occurrence in white females. Am J Public Health 74:1397–1398

Centrella M, Canalis E 1985 Local regulators of skeletal growth: a perspective. Endocrinol Rev 6:544–551

Culliton BJ 1987 Osteoporosis re-examined: complexity of bone biology is a challenge. Science (Wash DC) 235:833–834

Ettinger B, Genant HK, Cann CE 1985 Long-term estrogen replacement therapy prevents bone loss and fractures. Ann Intern Med 102:319–324

Ettinger B, Genant HK, Cann CE 1987 Postmenopausal bone loss is prevented by treatment with low-dosage estrogen with calcium. Ann Intern Med 106:40–45

Heaney RP, Recker RR, Saville PD 1978 Menopausal changes in calcium balance performance. J Lab Clin Med 92:953–963

Insogna KL, Lewis AM, Lipinski BA, Bryant C, Baran DT 1981 Effect of age on serum immunoreactive parathyroid hormone and its biological effects. J Clin Endocrinol Metab 53:1072–1075

Lindsay R, Hart DM, Forrest C, Baird C 1980 Prevention of spinal osteoporosis in oophorectomised women. Lancet 2:1151–1153

Lips P, Courpron P, Meunier PJ 1978 Mean wall thickness of trabecular bone packets in human iliac crest: changes with age. Calcif Tissue Res 26:13–17

Matkovic V, Kostial K, Simonovic I, Buzina R, Brodarec A, Nordin BEC 1979 Bone status and fracture rates in two regions of Yugoslavia. Am J Clin Nutr 32:540–549

Meller Y, Kestenbaum RS, Shany S et al 1985 Parathormone, calcitonin, and vitamin D metabolites during normal fracture healing in geriatric patients. Clin Orthop 199:272–279

Melton LJ, Riggs BL 1985 Risk factors for injury after a fall. Symposium on falls in the elderly: biological and behavioral aspects. Clin Geriatr Med 1:1–15

Nordin BEC, Horsman A, Marshall DH, Simpson M, Waterhouse GM 1979 Calcium requirement and calcium therapy. Clin Orthop 140:216–239

Pocock NA, Eisman JA, Yeates MG, Sambrook PN, Eberl S 1986 Physical fitness is a major determinant of femoral neck and lumbar spine bone mineral density. J Clin Invest 78:618–621

Richelson LS, Wahner HW, Melton LJ III, Riggs BL 1984 Relative contributions of aging and estrogen deficiency to postmenopausal bone loss. N Engl J Med 311:1273–1275

Riggs BL 1984 Treatment of osteoporosis with sodium fluoride: an appraisal. In: Peck WA (ed) Bone and mineral research. Annual 2: a yearly survey of developments in the field of bone and mineral. Elsevier, New York, p 366–393

Riggs BL 1987 Osteoporosis. In Wyngaarden JB, Smith LH (eds) Cecil textbook of medicine, 18th edn. Saunders, Philadelphia

Riggs BL, Melton LJ III 1986 Involutional osteoporosis. N Engl J Med 314:1676–1686

Riggs BL, Wahner HW, Seeman E et al 1982 Changes in bone mineral density of the proximal femur and spine with aging: differences between the postmenopausal and senile osteoporosis syndromes. J Clin Invest 70:716–723

Riis B, Thomsen K, Christiansen C 1987 Does calcium supplementation prevent postmenopausal bone loss? A double-blind, controlled clinical study. N Engl J Med 316:173–177

Rodstein M 1964 Accidents among the aged: incidence, causes and prevention. J Chronic Dis 17:515–526

Rudman D, Kutner MH, Rogers CM, Lubin MF, Fleming GA, Bain RP 1981 Impaired growth hormone secretion in the adult population: relation to age and adiposity. J Clin Invest 67:1361–1369

Seeman E, Melton LJ III, O'Fallon WM, Riggs BL 1983 Risk factors for spinal osteoporosis in men. Am J Med 75:977–983

Smith DM, Nance WE, Kang KW, Christian JC, Johnston CC Jr 1973 Genetic factors in determining bone mass. J Clin Invest 52:2800–2808

Tsai K-S, Heath H III, Kumar R, Riggs BL 1984 Impaired vitamin D metabolism with aging in women: possible role in pathogenesis of senile osteoporosis. J Clin Invest 73:1668–1672

DISCUSSION

Fries: My worry about most current views on osteoporosis relates to the lack of longitudinal data—that is, following an individual's bone density through life. A question that concerns me is whether someone who is deprived of calcium in adolescence and subsequently has adequate calcium intake, adequate weight-bearing exercise, and so forth, ever gets back to the level of bone density that he or she should be at.

We are doing a study of runners and non-runners, looking longitudinally at bone density changes. We find changes in bone density which suggest that control subjects who begin exercising (and running) make as much as a 10% gain in a year in their bone mineral; people who *have* been running (including postmenopausal women who have maintained bone density by exercise) and who stop may lose 10–20% of their bone mineral in a year, as though they were trying to get where they would have been on the curve based on cross-sectional data. These studies are giving us a much more dynamic feel for calcium balance than one gets from cross-sectional studies (Lane et al 1986).

Riggs: Longitudinal data are certainly needed, and cross-sectional data can be misleading. The main problem with longitudinal data on bone density is the large number of measurements that must be obtained to compute a statistically significant individual slope. This is because we are assessing small changes in bone density, of only a few per cent, using methods with a precision of 3–5%. So a long period of observation is needed to establish each person's rate of bone loss. Also, it is becoming increasingly difficult to do longitudinal studies, because the general population is well informed on the need to prevent osteoporotic fractures, and people are taking supplementary calcium, and are becoming more physically active. More and more postmenopausal women are taking oestrogens. This makes it difficult to assess the natural rate of bone loss, yet it is the only way to resolve certain important issues.

Wise: An increasing number of postmenopausal women are being given oestrogen and progesterone sequentially, because this regime suppresses the negative effects of oestrogen on several tissues and physiological systems. Do you have sufficient data to know whether the oestrogen/progesterone treatment is as effective in maintaining bone mass as is oestrogen alone?

Riggs: The combination of oestrogen and progesterone seems to offer considerable protection against the complication of endometrial carcinoma and to be as effective as oestrogen alone in preventing bone loss. The problem is whether the progestin has an adverse effect on the development of atherosclerosis. The 19-nor progestins probably do have such an effect, because they are androgen derivatives, whereas the 17-acetyl group, such as Provera (medroxyprogesterone acetate) have little or no effect.

Svanborg: We have data to show that if nothing preventive is done in Göteborg, by the year 2000 we shall have approximately twice as many hip fractures as can be explained by the ageing of the population. Similar data have been reported from Malmö and Stockholm in Sweden, from Oslo in Norway and from Dundee in Scotland. Our colleague, Dr Siv Mannius, has recently also shown that in a predominantly farming area in the south of Sweden there has been no significant increase over the last decade in the occurrence of hip fractures, contrary to the experience in the city of Göteborg. Unfortunately, we have not been able to measure bone density in this rural area. Are there any known regional differences in the incidence of hip fractures in the USA?

Riggs: I don't know any data in the United States on this, but perhaps the best epidemiological study was that of Matkovic & coworkers (1979), which I mentioned. They compared two districts in Yugoslavia which differed substantially in calcium intake. There was a marked difference in the number of hip fractures between the two districts. There was also a difference in bone density, but only in the earliest age group, of those in their twenties, suggesting that the higher calcium intake was exerting its effect during growth and had little effect after that. There are no good epidemiological studies on the level of physical activity. But the big problem with osteoporosis, as with the other areas discussed at this symposium, is that so many interacting factors are operating that it is difficult to control the independent variables.

Svånborg: You mentioned fluoride as a possible preventive measure. We know that it increases bone density; do we really know whether this increases skeletal strength?

Riggs: I would agree that we do not know whether the increase in bone mass with increased fluoride intake decreases the fracture rate. This is the main purpose of our ongoing double-blind clinical trial. Earlier retrospective studies, by ourselves and by others, however, suggest that it does. Therefore even if fluoridic bone is less strong than normal bone, a substantial increase in bone mass may result in a net increase in strength. Fluoride has not been approved for treatment by the US Food and Drug Administration, however, because it is relatively toxic. I consider it only an interim approach to the problem of treating osteoporosis.

Svanborg: Has the 1500 mg calcium daily requirement for postmenopausal women been accepted by the FDA?

T.F. Williams: They don't take a stand on that.

Kirkwood: I am interested in possible pleiotropic effects of calcium intake and calcium metabolism. George Williams (1957), in advancing a theory on the evolution of ageing based on pleiotropic gene effects, suggested as an example of pleiotropy that a gene which promoted a high rate of calcification of bone would be an advantage early in development but could be disadvantageous if it contributed to cardiovascular disease later in life. Is there any evidence of deleterious effects of calcium supplementation? And, in relation to the same point, you have very clear evidence of race differences in bone density. Do these differences correlate with differences between races in the primary causes of age-related morbidity, and could that be evidence of some kind of balancing under natural selection of one age-related deterioration against another?

Riggs: Calcium supplementation appears to be quite safe. It has not been carefully investigated for subtle adverse effects, such as calcification of the aortic valve, but provided the individual does not already have kidney stones, hypercalcuria or hypercalcaemia, it is safe to take up to a level of two grams per day.

There is interesting recent work by Norman Bell in South Carolina showing that black people, who appear to be well protected against osteoporosis, are also protected against the bone-resorptive effects of agents such as parathyroid hormone and 1,25-dihydroxyvitamin D.

Hollander: There are indications that jogging and running in women upset the menstrual cycle and induce an 'artificial menopause'—that is, an increased risk of osteoporosis. Is that true or not?

Riggs: Amenorrhoea certainly occurs, but mainly in women running over 50 miles a week. It is interesting that an increase in bone density occurs in women runners who are menstruating and in those in whom amenorrhoea has been induced, although those who are not menstruating have less bone. It seems that when a certain level of running is reached, you turn off the hypothalamic regulating centres and stop menstruating, and that is deleterious to bone mass. Until that point, running appears to be beneficial, in terms of its effect on the skeletal mass.

Fries: The general feeling is that when a women falls below 7% body fat and stops menstruating, at that point she may be doing a variety of harmful things. But the concept of moderation in the amount of physical activity still allows plenty of room for exercise before that point is reached; it appears to require running more than 2000 miles a year.

White: We are currently looking at data on hip fracture, primarily using the Epidemiologic Follow-up of the first National Health and Nutrition Examination Survey (NHANES I). It appears that systolic hypertension itself may be an independent risk factor. The more potent risk factors, however, are measures of skinfold thickness, which serves as an indication of the amount of fat in the body, and the calculated arm muscle area, which reflects muscle mass. These are striking associations. You mentioned, Dr Riggs, that excessive leanness may be a risk factor. In fact, we saw the relationship throughout the range of muscle mass and skinfold thickness. A high lean body mass was protective. A high skinfold thickness was also protective. When we looked simply at body weight and relative weight, high values were also quite protective. However, absolute and relative weight were (1) no longer protective after the effects of arm muscle area and skinfold thickness were taken into account, and (2) not as predictive as the combined effect of arm muscle area and skinfold thickness. So, to what extent is weight just reflecting a correlation between bone strength and body size? The factors making a bone strong include the forces placed on it, in terms of how much you stand on it (weight bearing), how much muscle force is put on it (exercise), and what the osteoblasts are allowed to do by virtue of their endocrine and calcium milieu.

These influences may well mediate some of the known race and sex differences. Perhaps much of the difference between men and women can be explained simply by the fact that men are, on average, bigger. Again, the differences between black and white people may be largely explained by differences in body size and composition. We may not need to look for major genetic factors beyond those which produce anthropometric differences. In our analyses of hip fracture we found no differences between black and white men, but a two-fold increase in risk of white women compared with black women (Farmer et al 1984). Body weight and relative weight in late life are similar for black and for white men. In contrast, black women at age 65–75 are slightly taller, but about 20lb heavier than white women (White et al 1986).

References

Farmer ME, White LR, Brody J, Bailey KR 1984 Race and sex differences in hip fracture incidence. Am J Public Health 74:1347–1380
Lane NE, Bloch DA, Hones HH, Fries JF 1986 Long-distance running, bone density, and osteoarthritis. JAMA (J Am Med Assoc) 255:1147–1151
Matkovic V, Kostial K, Simonovic I, Buzina R, Brodarec A, Nordin BEC 1979 Bone status and fracture rates in two regions of Yugoslavia. Am J Clin Nutr 32:540–549
White LR, Kohout F, Evans DA, Cornoni-Huntley J, Ostfield A 1986 Related health problems. In: Cornoni-Huntley J et al (eds) Established populations for epidemiologic studies of the elderly. National Institute on Aging. US Dept HHS, Public Health Service. NIH Publication No. 86-2443
Williams GC 1957 Pleiotropy, natural selection, and the evolution of senescence. Evolution 11:398–411

Ageing and infection

J. P. Phair, C. S. Hsu and Y. L. Hsu

Section of Infectious Disease, Department of Medicine, Northwestern University School of Medicine and Cooperative Studies Program Coordinating Center, Hines Veterans Administration Hospital, Chicago, Illinois 60611, USA

Abstract. An increased morbidity and mortality due to infectious disease has been noted in the ageing. Two alternative explanations may account for this. Changes in the immune system and inflammatory responses with age or an increase in age-related diseases may underlie the increased susceptibility. A review of studies of healthy older individuals demonstrates changes in the immune system with ageing but minimal change in the inflammatory response. Investigations of severe infection in older nursing-home patients requiring hospitalization indicate that infection as a cause of admission and death is significantly more common in individuals who are bedridden because of serious cardiovascular or neurological disease and require urinary catheterization. The evidence indicates that underlying disease, not the senescence of host resistance, leads to severe infection in the ageing.

1988 Research and the ageing population. Wiley, Chichester (Ciba Foundation Symposium 134) p 143–154

It is accepted clinically that infections in the elderly occur with increased frequency, present obscurely, and are a common cause of high morbidity and mortality (Gardener 1980). Two potential explanations for this poor response to infection have been offered: (a) deterioration of the inflammatory and immune responses with age, and (b) the age-associated diseases which enhance susceptibility to infection. Investigations attempting to define the impact of age upon host responses to microbial infection independent of age-associated diseases have been impeded by the lack of an accepted marker of senescence. Therefore, most investigations have used chronological age to define the population to be studied. This can result in a survey of survivors, a potentially physiologically younger group of individuals.

Examples of infections associated with increased mortality and morbidity in the elderly include bacteraemic pneumonia (Austrian & Gold 1964), staphylococcal endocarditis, and nosocomial (hospital-acquired) infections which are frequently bacteraemic and lethal in this population (Haley et al 1981, Watanakunakorn 1973). In addition there are suggestions that specific infections occur more frequently in aged individuals. Tuberculosis, during the past 50 years predominantly a disease of persons over 60 years (Stead 1981), and recurrent herpes zoster (shingles), are two often-cited examples. Tuberculosis in older patients usually represents reactivation infection, implying that a waning of immunity with age underlies the recrudescence of infection due to this intracellular pathogen. An alternative explanation is available for the association of tuberculosis and ageing. Individuals over 60 are the major population in industrial countries who have been exposed to tuberculosis and therefore the group most capable of developing reactivation disease. Thus, the localization of this infection to this age group may be the result of public health measures and availability of treatment which have effectively reduced the number of younger individuals at risk for reactivation tuberculosis, and not a result of an alteration in the resistance of older people.

There can be no doubt of the association of herpes zoster and the waning of virus-specific immunity (Miller 1980). However, it is also apparent that shingles is not exclusively a disease of older people and is often seen in younger individuals.

A review of our knowledge about alterations of host defences in older individuals indicates that important changes do occur in immunity and, to a lesser extent, in the inflammatory response. The ability to control microbial invasion is based on a complex set of cellular interactions which are relatively specific for particular organisms. Cell-mediated immunity depends on the ability of macrophages to ingest and kill certain fungi and intracellular bacteria and on the cytotoxic effect of lymphocytes on virus-infected cells. Cell-mediated immunity involves the processing of microbial antigen by macrophages and the production of monokines, which trigger the sensitization of thymic-dependent lymphocytes. The lymphocytes in turn produce lymphokines, which enhance the microbicidal activity of the macrophage. Included in the progeny of the stimulated lymphocytes are cytotoxic cells capable of killing virus-infected cells. The regulatory cell of this cellular interaction is the thymic or T helper/inducer (CD4) lymphocyte (McDevitt 1984).

The production of antibody results from the interaction of the antigen-processing macrophage, CD4 cells, and the B lymphocytes which are the precursors of the immunoglobulin-producing plasma cells. In contrast to defects in cell-mediated immunity, which are associated with infection by intracellular pathogens, deficits in antibody production are marked by recurrent infections produced by encapsulated pyogenic microorganisms, such as *Streptococcus pneumoniae* (Levitt & Cooper 1984).

Infections due to *Staphylococcus aureus*, aerobic Gram-negative bacilli and certain fungi are seen with increased frequency in persons with defects in the non-specific inflammatory response. Patients with reduced numbers of polymorphonuclear leucocytes (neutrophils) in the circulation are the example most often cited. The inflammatory system involves the interaction of neutrophils, components of the complement system, and (to a lesser extent) specific antibody. Deficiencies of particular components of the complement cascade, notably C_3, result in infection by the same organisms that cause disease in neutropenic individuals (Armstrong 1980).

Studies of healthy people aged 65 years and over demonstrate alterations in cellular immunity. Anergy is more prevalent in older subjects and is associated with alterations in thymic lymphocyte (T cell) function. The number of circulating T lymphocytes, including both helper/inducer and suppressor/cytotoxic cells, is normal, but the proportions of the two kinds appear to be altered in some studies (Nagel et al 1981). The number of cells that respond to antigens or mitogens *in vitro* is decreased and the response is altered. The cell cycle, which results in the division, proliferation and clonal expansion of the responsive cells, is prolonged (Inkeles et al 1977, Tice et al 1979). There is increased activity of suppressor T cells, and recent evidence indicates that the production of interleukin 2, the lymphokine required for macrophage activation and natural killer cell activity, is decreased (Giles et al 1981). These changes may underlie the increased frequency of reactivation infections in the elderly. This perturbation of cell-mediated immunity, however, is subtle and does not represent the aged equivalent of the acquired immune deficiency syndrome (AIDS).

The elderly often demonstrate a polyclonal increase in the amounts of immunoglobulins IgG and IgA, although in a subgroup decreases in IgG have been noted (Buckley et al 1974). *In vitro* studies, and some *in vivo* studies, indicate that the response to immunization is depressed in the elderly (Phair 1978a). There are advocates of altered immunization schedules for the vaccination of older persons or the use of more immunogenic vaccines in this age group, especially in those with chronic disease. It is worthy of note that individuals over age 55 who are free of serious illness have an 'excellent' response to pneumococcal vaccine antigens (Simberkoff et al 1986).

A major infectious disease problem for the elderly is the augmented risk of nosocomial infections due to aerobic Gram-negative bacilli and *S. aureus* (Haley et al 1981). This suggests a defect in the inflammatory responses involving neutrophils or serum opsonins such as complement. However, complement function (as measured by the function of the classical antibody dependent pathway and the alternate pathway) is normal in healthy individuals of 65 years and older and, in general, serum opsonic function for *Escherichia coli* and *S. aureus* is normal (Phair 1978b).

Normal numbers of neutrophils are produced and released by the bone marrow of aged individuals. The ability of the cells to adhere (the first morphologically recognizable manifestation of the inflammatory response) is also normal (Corberand et al 1981). Neutrophils of older healthy persons are capable of movement but there are conflicting reports about the responses of these cells to chemotactic stimuli (Phair et al 1978b, Corberand et al 1981). Bacteria are ingested normally by neutrophils from older subjects but some investigators have noted a reduced reduction of the dye, nitroblue tetrazolium, indicating changes in oxidative metabolism, which is usually stimulated by phagocytosis (Corberand et al 1981). Although killing of *S. aureus* is normal (Phair et al 1978b) there are studies showing decreased fungicidal activity. In summary, cross-sectional studies of healthy older individuals have failed to demonstrate a major defect in the inflammatory response to explain the increased prevalence of nosocomial infection in this population.

The adherence of bacteria to mucosal surfaces is implicated in the pathogenesis of bacterial pneumonia and urinary tract infections, two common infections of older persons. The question of whether ageing alters the interaction of bacteria and host cells, thereby increasing colonization and the resultant infection, remains unanswered. The process of adherence has been summarized by Beachey (1981). It involves the interaction of adhesins on the surface of microorganisms with receptors on host cell surfaces. The availability of host cell receptors may be modulated by proteins which block linkage with bacterial adhesins; an alteration in the concentration of such 'blocking factors' with age could increase the susceptibility of the older patient to bacterial colonization and infection. Fibronectin, a protein present on the surface of upper respiratory tract epithelial cells, prevents bacteria from binding to receptors. Enhanced proteolytic activity of respiratory tract secretions is associated with a blocking of receptor sites by fibronectin (Woods et al 1981). The effect of stress in the aged person on the proteolytic activity of respiratory secretions remains undefined, however. Increased proteolytic activity might be derived from inflammatory or other cells or, alternatively, from the decreased release of normally present proteases. The relationship of altered humoral or cellular immunity to bacterial adherence has not been delineated, although secretory IgA is known to inhibit adherence of bacteria to mucosal surfaces.

Bacterial colonization plays a significant role in the pathogenesis of urinary tract infections. It again is not clear whether age affects the interaction of bacteria and cells which leads to adherence, a necessary precondition of colonization. In younger populations, urinary tract infections occur predominantly in women and recurrences are associated with the persistence of vaginal (Fowler & Stamey 1977) and periurethral colonization (Kallenius & Winberg 1978). There is no evidence that the increase in urinary tract infection in older men and women is associated with changes which increase local colonization. Mechanical factors, such as pelvic floor relaxation and hypertrophy of the prostate, leading to pooling of urine, undoubtedly contribute greatly to the increased risk of bacteriuria in the elderly.

In contrast to the paucity of information derived from the investigation of healthy elderly people that is available to explain increases in infection, there is much relevant data on the association of chronic disease and infection in the over-60 age group. Much of this information is the result of investigations into infection in nursing-home patients (Garibaldi et al 1981, Cohen et al 1979). In

TABLE 1   Risk factors for the occurrence of infection in nursing-home patients

Infection	Risk factor	Odds ratio	Probability (P value)	95% confidence limits
All	Immobility	3.03	<0.001	1.72–5.34
	Urinary catheter	4.69	<0.001	2.55–8.64
Pneumonia	Medical device	4.92	<0.001	2.42–9.97
	Age 27–68	1		—
	69–78	1.48		1.03–2.15
	79–85	1.82		1.04–3.25
	86–102	2.39	0.039	1.06–5.53
Septicaemia	Immobility	5.10	0.04	1.06–24.6
	Medical device	7.99	<0.001	2.40–26.5

our studies, infection was the primary reason for hospitalization in more than 50% of 326 admissions to the hospital of patients in nursing homes, and was a frequent secondary diagnosis. The mean age of the nursing-home population studied was 75.4 years ± 14 (standard deviation) and ranged from 27 to 102. Only 30 patients were under 60 years, and all had neurological or psychiatric disease. Infection accounted for only 27.8% of the hospital admissions in those under 60.

The two findings most commonly associated with infection were immobility, usually due to cardiovascular or cerebrovascular disease, and the chronic use of a urinary catheter (Table 1). Soft tissue infections were also prevalent in elderly diabetics. Pneumonia was a more frequent diagnosis with each increase in the age quartile of the population and was associated with use of a gastric or jejuneostomy tube for feeding.

The impact of the consequences of severe disease associated with immobility, or the use of a urinary catheter or intravenous cannula, on the frequency of infection is clearly demonstrable in older patients. It remains to be shown that age-associated alterations in the host response alone contribute significantly to the problem of infection in the elderly.

Acknowledgements

This work is supported in part by the Samuel J. Sackett Endowment and the Northwestern Memorial Foundation.

References

Armstrong D 1980 Infections in patients with neoplastic disease. In: Verhost J et al (eds) Infections in the immunocompromised host. Pathogenesis, prevention and therapy. Elsevier, North-Holland Biomedical Press, Amsterdam, p 129–158
Austrian R, Gold J 1964 Pneumococcal bacteremia with especial reference to bacteremic pneumococcal pneumonia. Ann Intern Med 60:759–776

Beachey SH 1981 Bacterial adherence: adhesion–receptor interactions mediating the attachment of bacteria to mucosal surfaces. J Infect Dis 143:325–345

Buckley CE, Buckley EG, Dorsey FC 1974 Longitudinal changes in serum immunoglobulins in older humans. Fed Proc 33:2036–2039

Cohen ED, Hierholzer WJ, Schilling GR et al 1979 Nosocomial infections in skilled nursing facilities: a preliminary survey. Public Health Rep 94:162–165

Corberand J, Ngyen F, Laharrague P et al 1981 Polymorphonuclear functions and aging in humans. J Am Geriatr Soc 29:391–397

Fowler JE, Stamey TA 1977 Studies of introital colonization in women with recurrent urinary infections. VII. The role of bacterial adherence. J Urol 117:472–476

Gardener ID 1980 The effect of aging on susceptibility to infection. Rev Infect Dis 2:801–810

Garibaldi RA, Brodine S, Matsumiya S 1981 Infections among patients in nursing homes. N Engl J Med 305:731–735

Giles S, Kosak R, Durante M, Weksler M 1981 Immunological studies of aging. Decreased production of and response to T-cell growth factor by lymphocytes from aged humans. J Clin Immunol 67:937–942

Haley RW, Hooton TM, Culver DH et al 1981 Nosocomial infection in U.S. hospitals, 1975–1976. Estimated frequency by selected characteristics of patients. Am J Med 70:947–959

Inkeles B, Innes J, Kuntz MM et al 1977 Immunologic studies of aging. III. Cytokinetic basis for the impaired response of lymphocytes from aged humans to plant lectins. J Exp Med 145:1176–1187

Kallenius G, Winberg J 1978 Bacterial adherence to periurethral epithelial cells in girls prone to urinary tract infections. Lancet 2:540–543

Levitt D, Cooper MD 1984 B-cells. In: Stites DP et al (eds) Basic and clinical immunology. Lange Medical Publications, Los Altos, California, p 76–86

Miller AE 1980 Selective decline in cellular immune response to varicella zoster in the elderly. Neurology 30:582–587

McDevitt HO 1984 Cellular interaction in the immune system. In: Fortner JG, Rhoads JE (eds) Accomplishments in cancer research. Lippincott, Philadelphia, p 151–156

Nagel JE, Chrest FJ, Adler WH 1981 Enumeration of T lymphocyte subsets by monoclonal antibodies in young and aged humans. J Immunol 127:2086–2088

Phair JP, Kauffman CA, Bjornson A, Adams L, Linnemann C Jr 1987a Failure to respond to influenza vaccine in the aged: correlation with B-cell number and function. J Lab Clin Med 92:822–828

Phair JP, Kauffman CA, Bjornson A, Gallagher J, Adams L, Hess EV 1978b Host defenses in the aged: evaluation of components of the inflammatory and immune responses. J Infect Dis 138:67–73

Simberkoff MS, Cross AP, Al-Ibrahim M et al 1986 Efficacy of pneumococcal vaccine in high risk patients: results of a Veterans Administration Cooperative Study. N Engl J Med 315:1318–1327

Stead WW 1981 Tuberculosis among elderly persons: an outbreak in a nursing home. Ann Intern Med 94:606–610

Tice RR, Schneider EL, Kram D et al 1979 Cytokinetic analysis of the impaired proliferative response of peripheral lymphocytes from aged humans to phytohemagglutinin. J Exp Med 149:1029–1041

Watanakunakorn C, Tan J, Phair JP 1973 Some salient features of *S. aureus* endocarditis. Am J Med 54:473–481

Woods DE, Straus DC, Johanson WG et al 1981 Role of salivary protease activity in adherence of gram-negative bacilli to mammalian buccal epithelial cells in vivo. J Clin Invest 68:1435–1440

DISCUSSION

*T.F. Williams:*Gregory Siskind (1987) has raised the philosophical question of whether we should view the decreased activity in the immunological system with age as good rather than bad. He points out that we have had adequate exposure in early life to most of the organisms with which our immune system helps us to deal, and we maintain our responsiveness to these as long as we live, so we are prepared for most infections. If we kept up a too vigorous immune system it might turn round and destroy, by an autoimmune reaction, rather than help. As a specific point in relation to that, what is the older person's response to vaccines and therefore the role of immunization against various viral and bacterial infections?

Phair: Weksler's (1983) concept of the increase in suppressive activity being protective is an interesting one. It raises the question of whether strategies that are effective for the immunization of young people can be used in older people. Derek Hobson in Liverpool has suggested that in influenza vaccine program-mes in older people we should increase the immunogenic dose, and instead of giving one booster we should give two, two weeks apart, with the killed vaccines (Hobson et al 1973). We may be able to overcome that problem with the live attenuated vaccines. However, for pneumococcal vaccines, Simber-koff's most recent paper reports that the pneumococcal vaccine does not prevent pneumonia in the population where we most want it to be effective, in older people (Simberkoff et al 1986). It works in African goldminers or in army recruits, but not in the ageing population. The question of whether it prevents bacteraemic pneumonia, and therefore increased mortality, has not been answered. None of the studies has included enough bacteraemic patients to answer that question.

Wenger: With some of the infectious illnesses, one problem in older patients may be the delay in diagnosis. Particularly in the elderly cardiac patient with infective endocarditis, who often doesn't manifest a febrile response, the disease may be advanced before it is recognized. The increased mortality is due in part to the delayed diagnosis and treatment. We also often see the elderly patient with pneumonia or urinary tract infection that is not detected until the patient stops eating or shows an alteration in mental status, simply because the febrile response, which is the usual trigger for the recognition of an infection, does not occur.

Phair: That is absolute right. The recognition of an infectious disease in an older person requires thinking about; the usual clues are obscure. Why that is so should be a good area for research. Carol Kauffman has shown that *in vitro* monocytes from older humans and older rats will produce the lymphokine, interleukin 1, equally as well as monocytes from younger individuals (Jones et al 1984). This is the trigger for the febrile response, so the trigger is not the problem. It is not clear whether the problem is in the hypothalamus or in the effector arm of the hypothalamic response to the prostaglandin-mediated stimulus for temperature elevation. There is a delay in the recognition of infection. Cholecystitis or acute appendicitis can be missed because they do not present in the usual way.

Coleman: There is a growing body of literature on the innervation of the organs of the immune system. We have found a tremendous reduction in the catecholaminergic innervation of the spleen in ageing rodents (Capocelli et al 1985). Felten and his co-workers found the same thing, and extended it to other organs of the immune system (Felten et al 1987). However, there is not total agreement about the effects that this innervation has on the functioning of the immune system.

Phair: Lymphocytes have the same receptors for certain of the enkephalins as are present on cells in the central nervous system. It would be presumptuous to think that the immune system doesn't work in a parallel way to many other body systems. The evidence for neurological input into the immune system is increasing all the time. It is very difficult, however, with present technology, to translate that input into changes in function. One of the most widely quoted studies in man is the study of spouses after the death of their partners. A period of alteration in function of the immune system has been documented (Bartrop et al 1977) but it is difficult to translate these changes into clinical illness. Furthermore, the intervening mechanisms are still unclear.

Fries: Dr Phair, you concluded that a role for the host was less important than the role of co-morbidity, in predisposing to infection. In light of our earlier discussion on 'disease' and 'ageing' and the appropriateness or otherwise of the terms, I would like to define 'host' more broadly and suggest that co-morbidity is part of the 'host'. Co-morbidity includes senescent processes that are probably quite important in predisposing to infection in the elderly, including, for example, hip fractures, diabetes and congestive heart failure. I feel reasonably sure that host factors must be dominant because anything that follows the Gompertz function (i.e. increases exponentially with age) must be related to the host, because that is what the Gompertz function seems to reveal (Fries & Crapo 1981).

An interesting though slightly tangential aspect of 'Gompertz data' with regard to infection is as follows. If you take the USA data and plot all-cause mortality as a Gompertzian curve, you see a perfectly straight line all the way to age 85, above which the data are not available. If you separate out specific causes of death, most of the major causes are remarkably parallel to the overall lines, and are roughly Gompertzian in form. However, there are two causes of death that, above age 75 or 80, become super-Gompertzian: in other words, they begin rising more exponentially than before. These are infection and cardiovascular disease. (Cancer, to 'compensate', becomes sub-Gompertzian at that level.) The explanation is almost certainly that death certificate-reporting practices are inaccurate because the death of an older person is often attributed to bronchopneumonia or heart failure, because that is the easiest thing to do; such deaths are never attributed to 'cancer', even though the actual cause isn't known and the host factors are all-important (Fries 1984).

Phair: In people over 70, the terminal phase of most illnesses is an infection—iatrogenic in many cases. My only message was that, given our present technological abilities, it is hard to define senescence of the lymphocyte–macrophage system, and the polymorphonuclear/opsonic system, independently of other disease states. That is not to say that the fact that patients develop pneumonia is not due to some change in the mucociliary elevator, which is age related, or that the skin of an older person is not the same as the skin of a younger person. These are important host defence mechanisms; but, if the discussion is limited to what we think of as classical host defence against microorganisms, we lack the data to show that there is a significant age-related deadline which could explain the observed increase in infection.

Fries: What seems to decrease linearly in most organs is maximum function—the reserve function of the organism; whereas body temperature, say, and pH tend to remain constant through life. What is lost is the ability to return from abnormal to normal by the homeostatic mechanism of a particular organ. The ability to mobilize polymorphonuclear leucocytes and lymphocytes is also part of the reserve function—the ability to mount the response rapidly and promptly, not measuring a white count in its steady state (Fries & Crapo 1981).

Phair: Unfortunately, we don't know how to measure the reserve function of polymorphonuclear leucocytes. In my studies and those of others we have looked at 75- or 80-year-olds who are feeling well (Phair et al 1978); the physician, however, faces a patient who may have been institutionalized for the first time in his or her life, not always because of medical illness but just because of societal problems; or may have had a hip fracture. The polymorph in that person might be totally different from that of a younger person who has a fracture.

Mor: I spend time with clinicians who comment constantly on the influence of depression during hospitalization on patients' health. When this is properly treated with antidepressants, the patients respond physiologically to their disease state better. In connection with the reduction in the immune response after bereavement, there is much evidence to suggest that the surviving spouse is also depressed, independent of any kind of physical disease. So the influence of psychological state on suppressed immune function may represent a common theme.

Phair: That would tie in with Dr Coleman's point about the neural input to the immune system.

Coleman: These are the kinds of evidence usually cited in support of the notion of a functional role for the innervation of the organs of the immune system. On the other hand, an attempt was made to alter the mental status and the mood of advanced cancer patients. That study found no effect on the progression of the cancer, but it has been criticized on the grounds that the disease was so far advanced that any successful intervention was very improbable.

Phair: We have done similar studies to try to assess the impact of the emotional state of patients with human immunodeficiency virus (HIV) infections. We cannot show any effect of depression. Subtle changes, possibly due to emotional effects, are lost because of the dominant effect of HIV infection.

Wenger: It may be, too, that depression is associated with an unfavourable alteration in nutrition, and in mobility and activity; so, is it the depression alone, with its neurological and neurophysiological consequences, or is it all the other features that accompany depression?

Phair: That is relevant, because when you think about these systems in older people, one of the first things to look at is nutrition. The difficulties in assessing the nutritional status of individuals have been a barrier to attacking that problem. Most studies of defence mechanisms in older individuals have been done in upper middle class white Americans who volunteer to be studied, which means that one is missing a whole segment of the population who may have a very different nutritional state.

Solomons: We know from very young people (infants and toddlers, at the lower end of the spectrum of the lifespan), that malnutrition increases the duration, severity and lethality of infections without increasing the incidence (Black et al 1984). We have no specific information on this issue at the far end of the age spectrum; but, as you say, most people who die do so from an infection; and most people die in a state of malnutrition. There are markers of the fact that they are about to die, such as low serum albumin and transferrin levels. This was first found in studies of intravenous nutrition (Koretz 1984): but when an attempt was made to reverse these markers, specifically by giving albumin and raising lymphocyte counts, the patients also died, because their deaths were not being *mediated* by the state of nutrition—they were only being *marked* by their poor nutritional status. Bad nutrition is usually a marker, but not necessarily a mediator, of the events which it predicts (Koretz 1984).

Phair: That is very relevant, because people have tended to focus on ameliorating malnutrition, in order to improve the response to infection, not realizing that it has been established that infection *induces* malnutrition: one day of high fever can put you into negative nitrogen balance for a week.

Solomons: It has also now been suggested that the wasting of infection is mediated by a soluble cytotoxin called cachectin or tumour necrosis factor (Beutler & Cerami 1987), and that feeding a person who is making a lot of cachectin my be counterproductive; in fact, the anorexia of infection may be protective for the infected person.

Phair: The Murrays reported that starved people developed tuberculosis when they were re-fed, not during the period of malnutrition (Murray & Murray 1977).

T.F. Williams: Again, despite the best of feeding, until intercurrent infection has been eliminated (which may be a bladder infection or an infection elsewhere), the healing of pressure ulcers is not likely to progress.

Macfadyen: Professor R.K. Chandra has worked on the relationship between immunity and nutrition in children. He has also looked at this in elderly people in Canada, where he showed that simple interventions, like increasing caloric intake and giving twice the recommended daily allowance of nutrients and minerals, improved their immune response (Chandra 1985). In control comparisons he showed that old people developed fewer post-operative complications if they had been on a regimen of that type for two weeks before the operation.

T.F. Williams: That was a preventive step, though, rather than a treatment?

Solomons: No, the analysis of the literature by Koretz (1984) showed that you could predict who was going to die or to have complications very reliably by assessing nutritional indices before surgery; however, attempts to *alter* the outcome by pre-surgical nutritional intervention were not very successful. The previously malnourished patients still had excess complications. The absolute level of albumin in the circulation was not as important, in fact, as the liver's ability to synthesize it. In other words, having a low albumin is a predictor of post-operative complications; simply raising the circulating level by infusing albumin or plasma does not alter the predicted course.

References

Bartrop RW, Luckhurst E, Lazarus L, Kiloh LG, Penny R 1977 Depressed lymphocyte function after bereavement. Lancet 1:834–836

Beutler B, Cerami A 1987 The endogenous mediator of endotoxic shock. Clin Res 35:192–197

Black RE, Brown KH, Becker S 1984 Malnutrition is a determining factor in diarrheal duration, but not incidence, among young children in a longitudinal study in rural Bangladesh. Am J Clin Nutr 39:87–94

Capocelli A, Bellinger D, Felten D, Coleman PD 1985 Age-related decrease in the catecholaminergic innervation of the mouse spleen. Abstracts, 1985 Meeting of the Society for Neuroscience

Chandra RK (ed) 1985 Nutrition, immunity and illness in the elderly. Pergamon, New York

Felten SY, Bellinger D, Collier T, Coleman PD, Felten D 1987 Decreased sympathetic innervation of spleen in aged Fischer 344 rats. Neurobiol Aging 8:159–165

Fries JF 1984 The compression of morbidity, Benjamin Gompertz, the two types of chronic disease, and health policy. In: Forum Proceedings; exploring new frontiers of US health policy. UMDNJ–Rutgers Medical School, New Jersey

Fries JF, Crapo LM 1981 Vitality and aging. Freeman, New York

Hobson D, Baher FA, Curry RL 1973 Effect of influenza vaccines in stimulating antibody in volunteers with prior immunity. Lancet 2:155–156

Jones PG, Kauffman CA, Bergman AG, Hayes CM, Kluger MG, Cannon JG 1984 Fever in the elderly. Production of leukocytic pyrogen by monocytes from elderly persons. Gerontology 30:182–187

Koretz RL 1984 What supports nutritional support? Dig Dis Sci 29:577–588
Murray MJ, Murray AB 1977 Starvation suppression and refeeding activation of infec-
    tion: an ecological necessity? Lancet 1:123–125
Phair JP, Kauffman CA, Bjornson A, Gallagher J, Adams L, Hess EV 1978 Host
    defences in the aged: evaluation of components of the inflammatory and immune
    responses. J Infect Dis 138:67–73
Simberkoff MS, Cross AP, Al-Ibrahim M et al 1986 Efficacy of pneumococcal vaccine in
    high risk patients: results of a Veterans Administration Cooperative Study. N Engl J
    Med 315:1318–1327
Siskind GW 1987 The immune system. In: Warner HR et al (eds) Modern biological
    theories of aging. Raven Press, New York
Weksler ME 1983 The thymus gland and aging. Ann Int Med 98:105–107

General discussion

Functional reserve and its possible decline with age

T.F. Williams: The concept of reserve function has considerable appeal, but we need evidence for it. We talk about declining capabilities with increasing age in many areas and we imply that that is a characteristic of ageing. Even though, on average, untrained people (in cross-sectional investigations) show a slow decline in their maximum aerobic capacity with age, there are older athletes who choose to exercise vigorously, and their values are almost as high as those of the young athletes. One can hardly say that these persons have lost reserve function just because of age. Furthermore, studies by Holloszy and his colleagues (Seals et al 1984) show that ordinary, 60–70-year-old previously sedentary people (not athletes) can increase their aerobic capacity as much as young people; they also improve their blood lipid levels and their glucose tolerance. So I am not sure what evidence there is for an inevitable loss of reserve function with age.

Fries: I agree with you. There is a large difference between trained and untrained people in almost any activity, and the magnitude of that variation usually dwarfs the age-related change. For instance, the age-related change in marathon running may be two minutes slower each year, but the training effect may be half an hour or more. But there is an age effect. There are only two good longitudinal studies of 'masters' athletes: in one, Clarence De Mar ran the Boston Marathon for 50 consecutive years and won it several times in his youth. His times declined an average of two minutes a year. There are similar longitudinal data for the famous marathon runner, John Kelley. The effects of training were apparent, in that these men were running well quite late in life. When De Mar died at 68 of cancer he had very large-calibre coronary arteries, although with quite a bit of atherosclerosis. So there is inevitably some biological decline, however heavily an athlete trains. However, most of us are not at our optimal physical (or mental) performance level, so we can improve as we age, rather than declining (Fries & Crapo 1981).

Wenger: When we compare younger and older athletes, different mechanisms play a part in the maintenance of their high degree of physical performance. Most certainly in the older athletes, because of their decreased ventricular compliance, there is an increased dependence on the 'Starling' mechanism (i.e., ventricular dilatation as a means of maintaining stroke volume) than at a younger age. The aged athlete has a lesser potential for increasing the heart rate, as the maximal heart rate decreases with age. Thus very different responses to exercise occur in older and younger athletes.

T.F. Williams: What about other organ systems? Do we have evidence there about reserve, or loss of reserve? In the nervous system, I gather that even though there is some loss of nerve cells with age, the extent of that loss is less clear in recent studies than used to be claimed. But does it make any difference? In any system, what are our grounds for arguing that our reserves become a major factor in functioning? I grant that some loss of reserve occurs, but how much of it is an important loss, in any organ system, with age?

Hollander: In a perfect, 'normal' situation such loss might do no harm at all, but if there are other functions or systems that interact with that loss, to give another deleterious effect, it might become important.

Katzman: Much is now known from longitudinal studies about what happens to certain brain functions. It is clear that for capacities such as one's voculabulary, or store of information, one stays the same or even improves over the period from age 20 to age 80. In one classic study a group of young people, aged 19, took an intelligence test as freshmen at the University of Iowa in 1919. These people were located again in their late fifties and early sixties and were found to obtain the same or better scores on exactly the same tests. This has also been followed through at the National Institute of Mental Health in a group studied from 1957 to 1967, who were in their mid 70s in 1957 and in their mid 80s in 1967. WAIS vocabulary scores actually improved. On the other hand, any 'timed' test gets worse when age 65 is passed: in the NIMH study the rate at which addition could be done got worse as the subjects aged. Although it has not been well demonstrated in longitudinal studies, cross-sectional studies seem to show that one's episodic memory—the learning of unrelated facts, such as the names of people—decreases late in life, whereas 'semantic memory' (the learning of ideas) does not decrease at all.

On the neurobiological side, the latest information is that the number of nerve cells that Dr Robert Terry (1987) has counted in cerebral cortex from people known to be mentally normal during life shows no loss between age 20 and age 80. However, the weight of the brain decreases; there is atrophy. There might well be some loss of dendritic connections.

Coleman: All the work on the numbers of neurons in the *human* cerebral cortex records the density of neurons. If one finds a constant density, coupled with the kind of shrinkage of the cortical mantle that is often seen in the ageing brain but has never been well quantified, it suggests some loss of neurons, even in studies demonstrating a constant neuronal density. We also have evidence suggesting that when neurons in some regions of the human brain are lost, their surviving neighbours compensate for their death by spreading additional dendritic material (Buell & Coleman 1979, Flood et al 1985). We now have preliminary Golgi–electron microscopic evidence for the sprouting of axon terminals, to go along with this dendritic proliferation.

T.F. Williams: Dr Jay Luxemberg and his colleagues have done repeated computed tomography measures of the lateral ventricles, comparing healthy controls (age- and sex-matched) with a group of demented subjects. In the follow-up CT scans, two years after the initial ones, there was no change in lateral ventricular size in the healthy people, whereas in all the demented subjects (presumably the dementia was of the Alzheimer type) there was an increase in ventricular size. This may be a useful confirmatory test in cases of questionable diagnosis, if you want to do a follow-up study; but at least in this measure the ventricles weren't changing in size in normal subjects.

Wise: In addition to the controversy over changes in the density of neurons, an important point that we are just beginning to appreciate is the capacity for postsynaptic sites to compensate for changing neuronal function. Receptors have been shown to up-regulate or increase in density in the presence of decreasing neurotransmitter release. Whether this continues to occur during ageing is still unclear. In terms of the selective changes that Dr Katzman discussed in Alzheimer's disease being limited to certain neurotransmitters, it will be interesting to see whether there is compensation for changing neuro-transmitter function on the part of receptors during ageing.

Arie: I have been impressed by work such as that of Marion Diamond (1985) on the effect on the cortical thickness of aged rats of enhanced stimulation and an enrichment of their environment. There is also Dr Scheibel's work (1982) on the spontaneous waxing and waning of dendrites—the tendency of the dendri-tic richness to decrease with age, but often with a compensatory (if that's the right word) regrowth of dendrites, though possibly not functional ones. Dendrites can be made to sprout by certain 'neurotrophic' substances, gang-liosides for instance (Dal Toso et al 1986). I would be interested to hear the views of others on the relevance of this work. One has always taken it for granted that the way we treat people obviously has a capacity for changing their behaviour, but it is an exciting thought that this may also be capable of changing the structure of the brain, and even the aged brain. Whether there are ways of putting this to therapeutic use in people with impaired brains is a much more open question.

*Coleman:*One of Marion Diamond's collaborators did some studies in my laboratory measuring dendrites in adult rats. There was an increase in dendritic extent that seemed to be attributable to the enriched environment (Uylings et al 1978). There have been other studies, mostly from Marion Diamond's laboratory (e.g. Connor et al 1982) showing increased dendritic extent in rats in enriched environments.

A major criticism has been made of all these studies of enriched environ-ments. Essentially the studies include three groups of animals, one in a so-called enriched environment, one in a standard environment (a laboratory cage with a companion), and another group in what is called the 'deprived environ-ment', where the rat is isolated in a cage with solid metal sides. The question is whether studies that show dendritic increases in an enriched environment are really studies of that type of environment, or studies of a deprived environ-ment, showing that it can lead to neuronal regression.

Arie: Nevertheless, the results seem to show that the environment is capable of influencing the structure of a mature brain, and that is very interesting.

Coleman: I agree; and there is no question that environment can influence structure in the adult brain. With regard to Dr Scheibel's work, he and I have had a friendly dispute for some years! He has called the dendritic proliferation that he has seen 'lawless growth', and has concluded that it is generally non-functional; but he does now seem to feel that a neuron may either proliferate new dendritic material or regress, and we differ only on some fine points of emphasis.

Wise: Transplantation of fetal brain tissue into aged rats can restore the cyclic reproductive function in females. This suggests that the responsive neural cells must remain responsive for prolonged periods of time.

Arie: What are the prospects for therapeutic applications in humans?

Katzman: In terms of possible treatment of Alzheimer's disease, transplantation works in one rat model. About 20% of rats over 24 months of age have difficulty in learning a water maze (a submerged platform in a swimming pool that can't be seen through the water). Once young rats have experienced this, they immediately go to the platform on a second trial. About 20% of older rats will not learn; they find the platform only by chance. Those older rats can have that ability restored by transplantation of fetal septal neurons into the hippocampus. Even more surprisingly, it can also be restored by the intraventricular injection of nerve growth factor, which has a specific action on the cholinergic system that projects to the hipppocampus and to the cortex. That is something that can be tried in Alzheimer patients as soon as we have an adequate supply of human NGF. If NGF helps patients, perhaps other trophic molecules could be made to work in a similar fashion.

Fries: I would agree with Frank Williams' point of departure, that with some organs like the kidney one can't necessarily find the same linear rate of decline by looking, say, at the glomerular filtration rate (GFR) as you can in other areas like maximum cardiac output or nerve conduction velocity. We may need to look deeper there. The kidney, for example, is an excretory organ; it has filtration, secretion, and reabsorption, not just filtration, as its functions. I have seen many people die of renal disease which was not recognized as renal disease but as digitalis toxicity which didn't get cleared, or inability to handle a water load adequately in an elderly person, or to handle a salt load. The GFR may have been perfectly adequate, but the reserve function of the kidney was not. None of the declines in single organ system function by themselves really explain what we see in terms of the increased vulnerability of the whole organism; one needs to invoke combined models of multiple organs in which there are linear declines of perhaps a dozen separate organ-related functions, and the cumulative effect of these is to increase vulnerability exponentially with age (Fries & Crapo 1981).

Andrews: It used to be fashionable to refer to a subgroup of people whom some called 'gerontocrats', who did not appear to show the decrements expected with advanced age. It would be interesting to discover from our longitudinal data whether such a subgroup exists, or whether these people represent the odd outlier, or are they the 'masters' athletes, and do we have anything to learn from such a group, if it is identifiable.

References

Buell SJ, Coleman PD 1979 Dendritic growth in the aged human brain and failure of growth in senile dementia. Science (Wash DC) 206:854–856

Connor JR Jr, Beban SE, Hopper PA, Hansen B, Diamond MC 1982 A Golgi study of the superficial pyramidal cells in the somatosensory cortex of socially reared old adult rats. Exp Neurol 76:35–45

Dal Toso R, Cavicchioli L, Calzolari S, Leon A, Toffano G 1986 Are gangliosides a rational pharmacological treatment of chronic neurodegenerative disease? In: Crook T et al (eds) Treatment development strategies for Alzheimer's disease. Mark Powley Associates Inc, Madison, Connecticut, USA

Diamond M 1985 The potential of the ageing brain for structural regeneration. In: Arie T (ed) Recent advances in psychogeriatrics. Churchill Livingstone, Edinburgh

Flood DG, Buell SJ, DeFiore C, Horwitz G, Coleman PD 1985 Age-related dendritic growth in dentate gyrus of human brain is followed by regression in the 'oldest old'. Brain Res 345:366–368

Fries JF, Crapo LM 1981 Vitality and aging. Freeman, New York

Luxemberg JS, Haxby JV, Creasey H, Sundaram M, Rapoport SI 1987 Rate of ventricular enlargement in dementia of the Alzheimer type correlates with rate of neuropsychological deterioration. Neurology 37:1135–1140

Seals DR, Hagberg JM, Hurley BF, Ehsani AA, Holloszy JO 1984 Endurance training in older men and women. I. Cardiovascular responses to exercise. J Appl Physiol 57:1024–1029

Scheibel AB 1982 Some neural substrates of aging and senescence in the central nervous system. In: Isaacs B (ed) Recent advances in geriatrics 2. Churchill Livingstone, Edinburgh

Uylings HBM, Kuypers K, Diamond MC, Veltman WAM 1978 Effects of differential environments on plasticity of dendrites of cortical pyramidal neurons in adult rats. Exp Neurol 62:658–677

Malignant disease and the elderly

Vincent Mor

Centers for Long Term Care Gerontology and Health Care Research, Brown University, Providence, Rhode Island 02912, USA

Abstract. Most cancers are diseases of the ageing. Approximately 50% of all cancers occur among those over 65 and nearly 60% of all cancer deaths occur among the elderly. The cumulative risk of acquiring cancer among those aged 65–85 is 17% in females and 23% in males. Cancer incidence increases steadily as a function of age, reaching 23 per 1000 population among those aged 85 and older. Recent estimates of age-specific cancer prevalence rates for women over 70 were 106 per 1000 population and were 118 per 1000 population among men over 70. The rapidly shifting age distribution in most industrialized nations, including the growth of the 'old-old', means that the actual number of older people with cancer will increase at least in proportion to the ageing of the population. This trend will have an impact on the health-care system and may affect social norms regarding the treatment of elderly cancer patients. This paper reviews these trends and presents data from a series of research projects and the related literature to examine how older people respond to cancer symptoms and treatment and whether the treatment received by aged cancer patients differs from that given to younger patients. The relationship between age and stage of disease at presentation is explored, together with the manner in which older cancer patients' disease is identified, the 'aggressiveness' of treatment pursued, and patients' responses to those treatments.

1988 Research and the ageing population. Wiley, Chichester (Ciba Foundation Symposium 134) p 160–176

Cancers are predominantly diseases of the ageing. Approximately 50% of all cancers occur in the age group over 65, and close to 60% of all cancer deaths occur after 65 years of age. The enormity of the impact of cancer on the aged is evident in Figs. 1 and 2, which present the incidence, mortality and prevalence rates of cancer as a function of age. The risk of developing cancer increases rapidly with age. At ages 50–54, the incidence is 4.9 per 1000 persons; it more than doubles to 10.3 per 1000 between the ages of 60 and 64. The incidence rates double again in the over-85 age group. The death rate due to cancer also increases rapidly with age, from 0.5 per 1000 among those 35 to 44 years of age to 14.3 per 1000 among those over 85. Incidence and mortality rates do not fully reflect the impact of the disease on various age groups, particularly the aged. Cancer prevalence rates are calculated on the basis of the sum of persons diagnosed, less those who die. Using Connecticut Tumor Registry data, Feldman et al (1986) estimated that in 1982 the prevalence rate

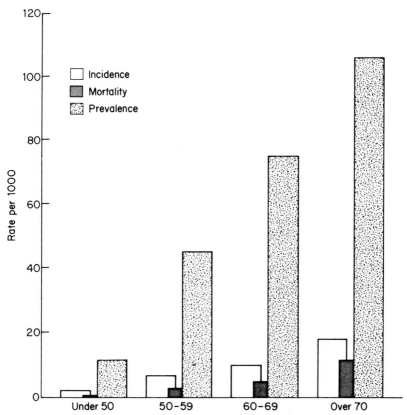

FIG. 1. Cancer rates in women per thousand, by age categories. Source: Connecticut SEERS (Surveillance Epidemiology and End Reporting System) data and Feldman et al (1986) Connecticut prevalence estimates.

of all cancers among those over 70 years of age was 118.1 per 1000. Among those aged 50–59, in contrast, the rate was 22.9 per 1000. The effect of cumulative incidence is apparent, since persons diagnosed and 'cured' in earlier years continue being counted as cancer 'cases' throughout their lives.

As the population ages, the number of cancer deaths will increase. The over-65 population currently constitutes just over 11% of the US population. However, by 2030 it will represent 18% of the population, or an estimated 55 million individuals (Yancik 1983). Since the death rate from heart disease has been dropping, even among those over 75, the numbers of older people who can be expected to survive to develop cancer is likely to increase even more rapidly than the size of the elderly population (National Center for Health Statistics 1986a). Janerich (1984) notes that increases in the effectiveness of cancer treatment in the form of a lengthened disease-free interval or a

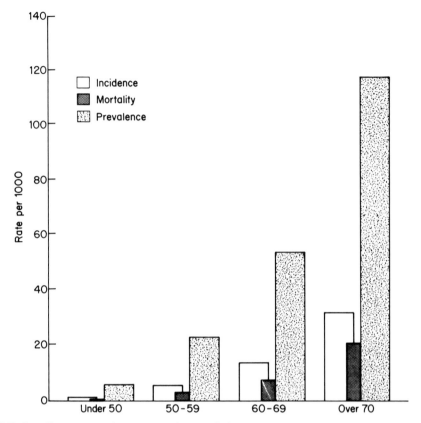

FIG. 2. Cancer rates in men per thousand, by age categories. Source: Connecticut SEERS data and Feldman et al (1986) Connecticut prevalence estimates.

lengthened 'clinical' period, as a result of early diagnosis, will also increase the prevalence of the disease and have substantial implications for the health-care system. The 'old-old' are the fastest growing segment of the ageing population; those between 75 and 84 will increase in number by 57% by the year 2000 and those over 85 by 91%. Applying Feldman's prevalence rates to the estimate of 55 million persons over 65 in the US in 2030 implies that there will be at least six million persons over 65 with cancer.

Past practice and recent evidence suggest that historically the elderly have not been treated as have younger persons with cancer. Whether that is attributable to the attitudes, knowledge and preconceptions of older people, or those of their families and health-care providers, is difficult to identify. Whatever the reason, if advances are made in cancer treatment and control they must be applied to the aged population in order to mitigate the substantial societal impact of the disease. The purpose of this paper is to summarize recent literature and an ongoing study that examines age differences in the recognition, diagnosis and treatment of cancer. Available data are intertwined with the discussion of each of these topics and the literature available about them.

Methods: Brown University Cancer and Aging Study

Newly diagnosed lung ($N = 399$), breast ($N = 499$) and colorectal ($N = 680$) cancer patients who were Rhode Island residents, between the ages of 45 and 90, and had a histologically confirmed diagnosis, were identified in nine Rhode Island Hospitals between July 1984 and February 1986. This represents approximately 75–80% of the population of patients diagnosed in the State. Patients were identified via pathology offices and their eligibility was confirmed by examining patients' charts. Those with *in situ* disease and those diagnosed at autopsy were excluded.

The purpose of this prospective study is to compare the pattern of diagnostic and treatment services received by older and younger cancer patients and to compare their psychosocial and physical response to the initial symptoms as well as subsequent medical interventions. Demographic and medical variables were obtained from medical records at the hospital of diagnosis for all patients. The referring physicians reported their post-diagnosis recommendations and the patients' performance status (their physical health, function, and capacity to carry out normal activities). All cancer-related surgical, medical and radiation oncology interventions received over the three years after diagnosis are documented and the patients' disease progress and condition is abstracted. A subsample of patients is interviewed periodically over the first year after diagnosis, and plans are under way to involve patients' family members in future interviews. Table 1 presents the demographic and medical characteristics of the sample by cancer type. The interview sample under-represents patients whose disease was most advanced at diagnosis, as well as older patients with other impairments, because these individuals were more likely to have died before interview contact, or to have refused to be interviewed, or their physicians chose not to allow us to contact them.

Knowledge of early detection

The key to the successful treatment of cancer is its early identification. Building on the knowledge that periodic use of mammography can increase survival among women of all ages with breast cancer, a concerted effort has been made to extend the notion of early detection to other cancers. However, to benefit from early detection programmes the population must know how to use them. Research has shown that those who make use of health promotion and prevention measures are more knowledgeable about health issues than

TABLE 1   Sample characteristics by cancer type in the Brown University Cancer and Aging Study

	Lung (N = 399)	Breast (N = 499)	Colorectal (N = 680)
Sex			
Female	32.3%	99.2%	48.2%
Age			
45–64	45.9%	44.7%	29.0%
65–74	36.3	28.7	34.9
75–90	17.8	26.7	36.2
Marital status			
Married	69.1%	48.2%	58.4%
Employed at diagnosis			
Yes	31.6%	27.1%	20.1%
Extent of disease			
Local	29.6%	57.9%	40.3%
Regional	35.3	34.3	43.7
Metastatic	35.1	7.8	16.1
Other chronic disease			
Yes	45.5%	32.5%	47.0%

those who do not. Furthermore, older persons are significantly less knowledgeable than are the young about the type of corrective actions that can be taken to reduce their risk of disease, particularly cancer.

Table 2 presents data from a random sample survey of men and women aged over 40 in Rhode Island that tested their knowledge about colorectal cancer (Masterson-Allen et al 1986). Respondents of 75 and over were less likely to know what colorectal cancer is (29.9%) than were those between 40 and 54 (14.1%) and were less likely to think that colorectal cancer was curable (61.5%) than were the youngest respondents (88.4%). The oldest respondents (75+) were significantly more likely to have reported that they didn't know how often they should be tested for colorectal cancer (18.1%) than were members of the youngest group (8.2%).

Advance data from the 1985 Health Interview Survey conducted by the National Center for Health Statistics reveals that only 39% of women 65 and older have had a breast examination within a year, as opposed to 52% of those aged 30–44. Women over 65 are twice as likely to report not knowing how to examine their own breasts as are women aged 45 to 64 (22% vs. 11% respectively). Even among those over 65 who report that they know how to examine their own breasts, older women are more likely to report never performing the procedure (National Center for Health Statistics 1986b).

TABLE 2   Knowledge of colorectal cancer in a random sample of Rhode Island residents over 40 by age

	Age categories			
	40–54 (N = 147)	55–64 (N = 115)	65–74 (N = 162)	75+ (N = 84)
Doesn't know what colorectal cancer is	14.1%	21.5%	24.0%	30.8%
Doesn't know whether colorectal cancer is curable	9.6%	9.7%	14.0%	29.5%
Doesn't know how often to be tested for colorectal cancer	8.2%	9.6%	12.7%	18.1%

Source: Masterson–Allen et al (1986).

Symptom recognition and delay

Without knowledge of the disease and its warning signals individuals are unlikely to know how to respond in the face of symptoms. Since the clinical stage of cancer at diagnosis is a principal determinant of survival, delay in the face of cancer-related symptoms can have a negative effect on survival. Wilkinson and his colleagues tested this hypothesis using Tumor Registry data for breast cancer cases. They found that those who delayed seeking medical care beyond two months after the onset of symptoms had significantly reduced survival over 60 months (Wilkinson et al 1979). As expected, delay was strongly associated with the stage of the disease at diagnosis. The authors summarize by noting that the disease stage has a direct effect on survival, while delay has an indirect effect on survival by tending to shift the stage to a more advanced level.

In the Brown Cancer and Aging Study we have found that older patients with colorectal cancer were less likely to have noticed their own symptoms than were younger patients (18.8% vs. 5.8%). Since patients over 75 were three or four times more likely to have heart disease or diabetes than younger patients, early detection in the oldest age group is likely to be attributable to more frequent visits to physicians for their other chronic diseases. Medical contact for unrelated purposes may have led to the identification of incipient cancer, despite these older people's lack of knowledge about the warning signs of cancer. Indeed, perhaps because of this fact, we did *not* find that older patients were more likely to delay seeking medical attention after having noticed a symptom that they attributed to cancer. Table 3 reveals that older patients with lung, breast or colorectal cancer were not more likely to have delayed seeking medical care more than three months after first noticing

TABLE 3   Percentage of cancer patients reporting that they delayed more than three months before seeking medical attention, by cancer type and age

Cancer type	Age categories		
	45–64	*65–74*	*75–90*
Lung cancer (N = 119)	20.8%	11.1%	12.6%
Breast cancer (N = 200)	14.9%	12.1%	18.2%
Colorectal cancer (N = 277)	34.0%	26.7%	15.9%

Source: Brown University Cancer and Aging Study (Mor et al 1986).

symptoms than were younger patients. In the case of colorectal cancer, older patients were half as likely as were younger patients to report delaying more than three months.

Age as a determinant of stage of disease at diagnosis

Since the stage of the disease at which cancer is diagnosed is such an important determinant of the prognosis, researchers have examined predictors of stage at diagnosis in order to develop better, more specific health education plans for the population. Results with respect to age have been mixed. Not only have the findings on the effect of age on the stage at diagnosis differed by type of cancer, but even within a cancer type they have not been terribly consistent (Mor et al 1986). Table 4 summarizes several of the population-based studies that examined the relationship between age and stage among breast cancer patients. In general, they do not reveal an effect of age. Studies showing an age effect tend to have been based on clinic populations or on data gathered in earlier decades. Studies of age and stage of disease at diagnosis among patients with colorectal cancer have consistently failed to reveal a difference. Studies of lung cancer patients either have failed to find a difference in stage due to age, or have found younger patients to have more advanced disease at diagnosis (Mor et al 1985). On the other hand, studies consistently reveal that older women with cervical or uterine cancers are identified later in the course of the disease (Holmes & Hearne 1981, Goodwin et al 1986).

The 'search for spread'

To ascertain cancer stage correctly requires many diagnostic procedures, some of which are invasive. Nonetheless, without them, plans for treatment for each patient may be inadequate because the tumour may have metastasized beyond the initial lesion, making conservative treatment inadequate.

TABLE 4   Percentage of breast cancer patients diagnosed with local disease, by study

Study	Age categories[a]			
	<54	55–64	65–74	75+
Brown University Cancer and Aging Study (Mor et al 1986)	60.8%	52.3%	63.2%	56.4%
Hawaii Tumor Registry (whites only) (Ward–Hinds et al 1982)	55.7%	55.4%		
Metropolitan Detroit Cancer Surveillance System (whites only) (Satariano et al 1986)	51.7%	48.3%	50.1%	52.3%
New Mexico Tumor Registry (Goodwin et al 1986)	55%	52%	57%	59%
Community Hospital Oncology Program (Chu et al 1987)	56%	57%	55%	63%
Duke Comprehensive Cancer Center (Allen et al 1986)	40.0%	43%	42%	40%

[a] Ten-year age categories, starting with <50.

Examining age differences in the 'search for spread' of the disease is important in its own right, for if we find that older patients are less likely to receive the comprehensive battery of diagnostic tests needed to determine disease stage conclusively, our finding of a general absence of differences in stage according to age may be incorrect.

Chu and his colleagues evaluated the Community Hospital Oncology Program and examined age differences in the types of diagnostic tests performed. Breast cancer patients diagnosed with local disease who were over 75 years of age were significantly less likely to have had lymph node dissection than were comparable patients between 45 and 74 (72% vs. 91%). Among patients with regional breast cancer, older women had fewer lymph nodes examined than did younger women ($P < 0.01$).

Our preliminary examinations of diagnostic tests performed in the Brown University Cancer and Aging Study revealed no consistent age bias within a given stage of disease (Mor et al 1986). For example, 10.2%, 18.7% and 25.7% of breast cancer patients with local, regional and distant metastatic disease were found to have had a liver scan to search for metastases to the liver. In no instance were older patients less likely to have had the test. The same was true for bone scans, bone marrow tests and brain computerized tomography (CT); although patients with metastatic disease were more likely to have had tests, within a particular disease stage there were no age differences. However, since age differences were examined within each disease stage, the results of diagnostic tests necessary for us to question or refute the stage classification of older patients could not be available.

When we examined the fit between the treatments given and the patients' clinical condition (histology, stage, node involvement, site of metastases, etc.) in the Cancer and Aging Study, we found certain anomalies. Patients 'staged' with local disease have been found *not* to have had surgery, but nevertheless to have died within several months of diagnosis. Obviously, the available records are incomplete. The diagnostic information given in pathology reports is only as complete as the tests clinically determined to be necessary. The physician's final notes synthesizing the clinical diagnosis of advanced disease may never be entered into the hospital file. The adequacy of the data has always been a challenge in epidemiology, and the validity of staging data is no exception.

Treatment recommendations

Considering and ultimately implementing cancer treatments is a complex process, spanning the physician recommending and the patient accepting treatment, and then the patient and family galvanizing the necessary resources and making arrangements to receive the recommended treatment. Historically, older patients were felt to be unable to sustain the debilitating effects of many types of surgical and medical cancer treatment (Patterson 1983). Until relatively recently, most Cooperative Groups in the US conducting clinical trials on chemotherapeutic agents excluded otherwise eligible individuals who were over 60 or 65 years of age.

Physicians' recommendations for treatment were examined in the Cancer and Aging Study. Since surgery is almost universally performed for breast cancer, we analysed only those who had had definitive surgery. We examined the probability of having been recommended for either radiation or chemotherapy. Of 128 local breast cancer patients, 23% were recommended to have one or the other form of treatment, presumably for adjuvant purposes, while 67% of the 82 patients with regional disease were recommended for one or other treatment. Age was unrelated to the recommendation for patients' treatment at either stage. The lack of consensus among the experts as to the proper treatment for breast cancer complicates our interpretation of these findings. A recent National Institutes of Health consensus conference did *not* recommend chemotherapy for stage II node-positive, oestrogen receptor-negative patients. Nonetheless, in a recent survey of 634 practising medical oncologists, over 76% said that they had recommended combination chemotherapy for their postmenopausal patients under 65 years of age, whereas 50% recommended it for those over 65 (Oncology News/Update 1987). Physicians' actual practice probably also deviates from their reported recommendations in response to family pressure, the perception of how well the patients can tolerate treatment-related toxicity, as well as other social and attitudinal factors.

We also found that 22% of the 220 patients with regional colorectal cancer were recommended for either chemotherapy or radiation therapy. Aged patients were significantly ($P < 0.01$) less likely to have had either of these treatments recommended for them than were younger patients, even after we controlled for whether patients had a pre-existing medical condition such as heart disease or diabetes, and the patients' judged ability to perform normal functions and activities. Since neither chemotherapy nor radiation therapy has been shown to have a measurable impact on survival, using standard therapies, in this instance older patients are not being deprived of treatments that could be beneficial.

Aggressiveness of treatment

Studies that have tried to compare types of treatment by age have generally focused on initial, surgical interventions. In the decades in which mastectomy, particularly radical mastectomy, was the treatment of choice for breast cancer, older patients were less likely to have the more radical procedures (Donegan 1983). A report of breast cancer patients from upstate New York diagnosed between 1955 and 1975 found that only 40.3% of women over 70 had a radical mastectomy, whereas 83.2% of women under 50 had that operation (Mueller et al 1978). Conversely, simple mastectomy was performed on 25.9% of women over 70 and on only 5.1% of women under 50. Since this study found no differences in the distribution of age by disease stage, differences in the intervention were *not* attributable to this factor.

More recently, Chu and his colleagues also examined differences in the pattern of treatment for breast cancer as a function of age (1987). They too found differences in treatment, with older patients being less likely to have had a modified radical mastectomy among women with local disease. Two-step surgery (biopsy and tumour excision performed separately) was less prevalent for older women with either local or regional disease. Radiation therapy was less likely to have been given to older women with local disease. This finding, in conjunction with the fact that older women were less likely to have mastectomy, suggests that if breast-conserving procedures were performed, they were not followed up with radiation therapy as is recommended. Finally, chemotherapy (not hormonal), which is fairly rare in local disease but more commonly recommended for patients with regional and distant metastases, was significantly less likely to be given to women over 65 or 75, regardless of the stage of their disease. For example, 78% of women with regional disease under 54 years were given chemotherapy while this was true for only 30% of similar women aged 75 and over. A similar pattern was found among breast cancer patients treated at Duke Medical Center between 1970 and 1984. Older women were less likely to have received any form of systemic therapy after having surgery (Allen et al 1986). Only a third of patients younger than 55 years received no systemic therapy at all, compared to 58% of those over 55.

It is often difficult to determine the appropriateness of the full treatment package that a patient has received after diagnosis. Using Tumor Registry data, Samet and his colleagues coded whether the combination of surgical, radiation or chemotherapeutic interventions given within the first few months after diagnosis was 'definitive' (Samet et al 1986). Different definitions were established for each major cancer type. In general, they found that older patients were less likely to have received 'definitive' treatment. Specifically, 96% of patients with local breast cancer under 55 were treated definitively, while that was true for only 69% of those aged 85 and over and for 84% of those 75–84 years of age. Differences were even greater for local lung cancer, where pneumonectomy was defined as treatment; 55% of those under 55, compared with none of those over 85 and only 13% of those between 75 and 84, had this treatment. The percentage of patients with local disease who received *no* treatment increased with age for all cancers combined and for many individual sites: 12% of breast cancer patients over 85 received no treatment; only 1% under 65 years of age received none.

Table 5 contrasts Samet's findings for breast cancer with the more recent data obtained in the Cancer and Aging Study. While the age effects are not as marked in the Rhode Island data, the trend is clearly in the same direction. When we examined these data for only those persons with pre-existing other chronic disease, such as heart disease and diabetes, we found the differences to be more striking. Among those with local breast cancer at diagnosis, 100% of those aged 45–65 had definitive treatment, as opposed to 83.3% of those aged 65–74 and 60% of those 75 and over ($P < 0.01$). This finding suggests that younger patients with similar presenting conditions are treated more aggressively even though local breast cancer is amenable to cure using appropriate therapies. Recently, Greenfield and his colleagues (1987) published similar results from their study of breast cancer patients identified at five hospitals. Using an expert defined algorithm they abstracted patients' charts to determine (1) whether they were treated appropriately, and (2) the severity of any other chronic diseases that the patients had at the time of cancer diagnosis. They found that among patients with local disease and only insignificant other chronic disease, those over 70 years of age were more than twice as likely to have had inappropriate treatment than were those under 70 (17% vs. 4.4%).

TABLE 5 Percentage of breast cancer patients with local and metastatic disease receiving 'definitive treatment', by age and study

Study	Age categories				
	45–54	55–64	65–74	75–84	85+
Brown University Cancer and Aging Study, Rhode Island 1984–1986					
Local disease	86.7%	88.5%	83.5%	70.5%	66.7%
Regional disease	96.2	96.4	93.2	83.7	—
	Age categories				
	≥54	55–64	65–74	75–84	85+
Samet et al 1986: New Mexico Tumor Registry, 1969–1982					
Local disease	96	96	95	84	69
Regional disease	95	93	93	83	81

Pursuit of treatment in the face of toxicity

Until relatively recently it was standard practice to exclude persons over 60 or 65 from clinical trials of chemotherapy or radiation therapy research protocols (Carbone et al 1983, Begg et al 1980). Indeed, initial studies of whether there were increased rates of treatment-related toxicity among the aged could barely be done, because so few patients over 65 or 70 were available for analysis. Carbone, and later Begg, did a series of analyses using data from the Eastern Cooperative Oncology Group to address this issue. Fewer than 10% of lung cancer and 15% of colorectal cancer patients studied were 70 or over. Although older patients had higher rates of haematological toxicity, particularly from treatments including methotrexate, this was to be expected in view of the known renal clearance of this drug and the diminished creatinine clearance among the elderly (Carbone et al 1983). Even for haematological reactions, the prevalence of life-threatening toxicity was no more common among the aged than in younger patients. In other respects, chemotherapy-related toxicity was no greater among patients over 70 than among younger persons (Begg et al 1980).

Nerenz and his colleagues (1986) recently reported similar results for patients receiving oncological care from a Veterans Administration hospital. While older patients were somewhat less likely to receive the full chemotherapeutic dose of methotrexate and cytoxan than were younger patients, they reported no more treatment-related symptoms than did younger patients. Indeed, older patients reported significantly fewer symptoms of psychological distress than did younger patients.

Little comparable information is available for toxicity related to radiation treatment. Glicksman did a study of matched patients over and under 65 who received radiation to the pelvis for colorectal, bladder and uterine cancer, to compare the rate of haematological and other toxicity. He found no statistically significant difference between elderly and younger patients in terms of tolerance to the treatments delivered, on any of the parameters measured (A. S. Glicksman, unpublished data 1984).

Summary

In the coming decades the number of elderly patients confronting the medical-care system with diagnoses of cancer will increase dramatically. While the age-adjusted incidence rates remain largely constant, growth in the elderly population in the United States as well as in all other industrialized nations will greatly influence the disease profile seen by medical practitioners. The old biases cannot be maintained if the advances in early diagnostic techniques as well as public education efforts are to be effective in reducing cancer mortality rates. Advances in treatment must also reach the elderly population, rather than being reserved for the younger patient population.

Since chronological age as such does not appear to be an important determinant of treatment-related toxicity, patients should not be excluded from receiving new treatments. However, biases appear to operate among physicians, and in society at large, in making referrals for treatment. The type of treatment patients receive after diagnosis reflects the physician's recommendation, as well as the patient's and family's ability to accept it and follow through with it. When we control for the patient's clinical condition, the differences in the types of treatments that older and younger patients receive can be seen as reflecting a bias. It may be the physician's, the patient's, the family's, or a combination of all three. Regardless of the source of the bias, it can be seen as reflecting a general cultural value system.

Nonetheless, just as chronological age should not exclusively determine treatment, survival expectations should be kept in mind, since current treatments are costly, both financially and physically, and may reduce an older person's quality-adjusted survival. Treatments with high expected complications from toxicity, but only limited benefits in terms of survival, should be carefully considered before proceeding with very old patients.

Acknowledgements

Supported in part by HHS/NCI Grant No. 36560. I should like to acknowledge the Rhode Island hospitals, physicians and patients whose participation has made the

Brown University Cancer and Aging Study possible, and particularly the study co-investigators, Drs Arvin Glicksman, Francis Cummings, Alan Weitberg, Rebecca Silliman, Edward Guadagnoli and Marsha Fretwell.

References

Allen C, Cox EB, Manton KG, Cohen HJ 1986 Breast cancer in the elderly: current patterns of care. J Am Geriatr Soc 34:637–642

Begg CB, Cohen JL, Ellerton J 1980 Are the elderly predisposed to toxicity from cancer chemotherapy? Cancer Clin Trials 3:369–374

Carbone PP, Begg CB, Jensen L, Moorman J 1983 Oncology perspective on breast cancer in the elderly. In: Yancik R (ed) Perspectives on prevention and treatment of cancer in the elderly. Raven Press, New York, vol 24:63–71

Chu J, Diehr P, Fiegl P et al 1987 The effect of age on the care of women with breast cancer in community hospitals. J Gerontol 42:185–190

Donegan WL 1983 Treatment of breast cancer in the elderly. In: Yancik R (ed) Perspectives on prevention and treatment of cancer in the elderly. Raven Press, New York, vol 24:83–96

Feldman AR, Kessler L, Myers MH, Naughton MD 1986 The prevalence of cancer: estimates based on the Connecticut Tumor Registry. N Engl J Med 315:1394–1397

Goodwin JS, Samet JM, Key CR, Humble C, Kutvirt D, Hunt C 1986 Stage at diagnosis of cancer varies with the age of the patient. J Am Geriatr Soc 34:20–26

Greenfield S, Blanco DM, Elashoff RM, Ganz PA 1987 Patterns of care related to age of breast cancer patients. JAMA (J Am Med Assoc) 257:2766–2770

Holmes FF, Hearne III E 1981 Cancer stage-to-age relationship: implications for cancer screening in the elderly. J Am Geriatr Soc 29:55–57

Janerich DT 1984 Forecasting cancer trends to optimize control strategies. J Natl Cancer Inst 72:1317–1321

Masterson-Allen S, Mor V, Kaufmann R 1986 Health promotion campaign impact on the old old. Gerontologist 26:21A (abstr)

Mor V, Masterson-Allen S, Goldberg RJ, Cummings FJ, Glicksman AS, Fretwell MD 1985 The relationship between age at diagnosis and treatments received by cancer patients. J Am Geriatr Soc 33:585–589

Mor V, Guadagnoli E, Glicksman AS et al 1986 Lung, breast, and colorectal cancer: the relationship between disease stage and age at initial diagnosis. Gerontologist 26:217A (abstr)

Mueller CB, Ames F, Anderson GD 1978 Breast cancer in 3558 women: age as a significant determinant in the rate of dying and causes of death. Surgery (St Louis) 83:123–132

National Center for Health Statistics 1986a Advance report of annual mortality statistics, 1984. Monthly Vital Statistics Report, vol 35 no 6 suppl 2. DHHS Publication No. (PHS) 86–1120

National Center for Health Statistics (Thornberry OT, Wilson RW, Golden PM) 1986b Health promotion data for the 1990 objectives. Estimates from the national health interview survey of health promotion and disease prevention, United States, 1985. Advance data from vital and health statistics No. 126. DHHS Publication No. (PHS) 86–1250. Public Health Service, Hyattsville, Maryland, September 19

Nerenz DR, Love RR, Leventhal H, Easterling DV 1986 Psychosocial consequences of cancer chemotherapy for elderly patients. Health Services Research part II 20:961–976

Oncology News/Update 1987 Survey on breast cancer therapy yields surprising results. Curr Trends Oncol 2:1–2

Patterson WB 1983 Oncology perspective on colorectal cancer in the geriatric patient. In: Yancik R (ed) Perspectives on prevention and treatment of cancer in the elderly. Raven Press, New York, vol 24:105–112

Samet J, Hunt WC, Key C, Humble CG, Goodwin JS 1986 Choice of cancer therapy varies with age of patient. JAMA (J Am Med Assoc) 255:3385–3390

Satariano WA, Belle SH, Swanson GM 1986 The severity of breast cancer at diagnosis: a comparison of age and extent of disease in black and white women. Am J Public Health 76:779–782

Ward-Hinds M, Kolonel LN, Nomura AMY, Lee J 1982 Stage-specific breast cancer incidence rates by age among Japanese and Caucasian women in Hawaii, 1960–1979. Br J Cancer 45:118–123

Wilkinson GS, Edgerton F, Wallace HJ et al 1979 Stage of disease and survival from breast cancer. J Chronic Dis 32:365–373

Yancik R 1983 Frame of reference: old age as the context for the prevention and treatment of cancer. In: Yancik R (ed) Perspectives on prevention and treatment of cancer in the elderly. Raven Press, New York, vol 24:5–17

DISCUSSION

T.F. Williams: I have the impression from the limited age-specific data available that the incidence of at least some cancers begins to decrease in people in their late 80s or 90s.

Mor: That is so for some cancers. Lung cancer incidence peaks between 70 and 74, falling thereafter; breast cancer incidence appears to fall after age 85. Colorectal cancer incidence continues to go up even in people in their nineties.

Fox: Presumably the increasing *prevalence* of cancers in the oldest age groups reflects the fact that patients with cancers like breast cancer have long survival times, and therefore the prevalence will include many women who have had breast cancer earlier and are now surviving to older ages. Do your figures include skin cancers?

Mor: No; the Feldman data do not include skin cancer and I did not bring in skin cancers from the SEERS data. Colorectal, testicular and cervical cancers also have a relatively long natural course, depending on the stage at diagnosis.

Katzman: To what extent is the claim that we are 'losing the war against cancer' (Bailar & Smith 1986) the result of failing to take into account the reduction in deaths from myocardial infarction that you mentioned, which means that a large older population is more at risk of cancer?

Mor: That study used age-adjusted data, so there was no possibility of confounding competing risks. The important point made was that total age-adjusted cancer mortality has not gone down, even though certain reductions have occurred, particularly in stomach cancer—and no one really understands the stomach cancer reduction. It was emphasized that there are sufficient vagaries in the coding of death certificates and the diagnostic process to serve as a competing explanation. Remember that if one does not now develop stomach cancer at the age of 55, colorectal cancer may be identified at 72.

Hollander: You have stated that it is a myth that cancer of the aged runs a more benign course, and I entirely support this view. This idea of the more benign course was held very firmly in medical schools and is extremely difficult to eradicate.

Mor: My view, from talking with people who are familiar with this issue in the literature, is that on the basis of tumour morphology and the rate of progression (controlling for the kind of treatment provided), cancer does not appear to have either a more or a less virulent course in the elderly.

Hollander: One surely has to treat cancer just as aggressively in older people as at other ages, but taking into account the quality of life that remains, as you emphasized.

Mor: You probably should do that for younger persons as well!

Fries: I would like to raise a potential challenge to your thesis, Dr Mor. You are saying that there are older people who are receiving less care than younger patients, although the courses of treatment as used are no more toxic. Therefore they should have been receiving the same more aggressive treatment as someone diagnosed at an earlier age; they are being neglected at present. A decision analyst wouldn't like that reasoning, because he would say that the decision whether to treat vigorously or not is a function of comparing the 'expected value' of the two forms of treatment. Expected value is computed using many other factors besides the toxicity of the treatment regimen, which you might term the 'bad time'. The bad time might be the same for younger and older, but if 'good time' (the period after chemotherapy and prior to death) is reduced in older patients, the decision might appropriately be shifted towards a less vigorous approach. We see this decision behaviour in patients when they say that if the treatment will make them feel ill for most of the rest of their lives, they don't want to have it. I would suggest that this might be an appropriate judgement of the older patient and his or her physician, and not necessarily indicative of neglect.

Mor: I think that's true. Researchers at Harvard and McMaster Universities have been examining the concept and role of quality-adjusted life years (QUA-LYs) (Beck et al 1982, Torrence 1986). This is an important consideration. It has not always been my experience that the patient takes an active role in making those choices, however. The choice is a subtle process that permeates the interaction between patient, family and physician. It is not necessarily anything conscious in terms of the 'decision tree' that should be offered. It seems to be important that patients should make explicit decisions, rather than having them implicitly imposed.

Wenger: What is the role of the patient's family, Dr Mor? Do you have any way of telling, in your data, whether the patient made the initial decision to come for evaluation, or whether a family member helped in that decision? Likewise, for the initiation of therapy, is this the patient's decision or a joint family decision? Sometimes these features may be very different and it may be important to see whose judgement initiated the process.

Mor: We did ask, as part of the symptom recognition process, whether a family member or some other person told the patient to go to the doctor. From the patients' own reports there was a fairly low proportion of those who recognized their symptoms but had to be urged by someone else to seek a definitive diagnosis. I have found it to be extremely difficult to disentangle the decision-making processes in another area—the choice to go into an institution for elderly patients. The process of asking questions of patients and families retrospectively about how a decision was made affects the quality of the answers. It might be possible to control for such 'measurement artifacts' of recall bias if this were the object of a study. I am not sure how one would do that in this instance, but I agree that it is important to be aware of and to understand the decision-making process.

T.F. Williams: What about the origins of cancer in older people? Is it a process of the accumulation of oncogenes that are turned on by the progressive effects of secondary factors, and therefore it makes sense that the longer you live, the greater chance you have to turn on the relevant oncogenes? Is there a cohesive theory about the accumulating risk of cancer as you get older?

Fox: The arguments about a cohesive theory tend to focus on the relationships between cancers and exposures to carcinogens. In general there is a high correlation between age and the duration of exposure. For some cancers, such as breast cancer, the incidence tails off at older ages. It is thought that, in this case, exposure to oestrogens ceases after the menopause, and that women do not have the same exposure to a factor that may be influencing the progress of the disease at younger ages. With many other cancers, exposure continues throughout life and therefore one will see an increase in incidence right up to the oldest age groups.

Fries: That is consistent with the way I have looked at these figures. The change in lung cancer incidence at the older ages, where incidence does fall off, fits the exposure model perfectly (Fries 1987). The people who are now 85 were not a heavy-smoking cohort, compared with those who are now 65 or 75; the major adverse effects of smoking were yet to come. So the apparent decline at older ages is probably a consequence of lesser exposure to carcinogens.

Mor: Yes; that relates to the selective survival of those 85-year-old people.

References

Bailar III JC, Smith EM 1986 Progress against cancer? N Engl J Med 314:1226–1232
Beck JR, Pauker SG, Gottlieb JG, Klein K, Kassirer JP 1982 A convenient approximation of life expectancy (the 'DEALE'). II. Use in medical decision making. Am J Med 73:889–897
Fries JF 1987 Aging, illness, and health policy: implications of the compression of morbidity. Perspect Biol Med, in press
Torrence GW 1986 Measurement of health state utilities for economic appraisal. J Health Econ 5:1–30

Longitudinal insights into the ageing population

A. J. Fox

Social Statistics Research Unit, The City University, Northampton Square, London EC1V 0HB, UK

Abstract. In several countries the fraction of the population who are very old is increasing dramatically. Interest in this phenomenon in part reflects concern about the burdens this section of the community will place on younger people. Views of the elderly are generally based on cross-sectional data on generations who 'aged' in quite different circumstances to those who will be old in 20 or 40 years time. This paper describes recent findings relevant to the changing experiences of older men and women during the 1970s and early 1980s from the Office of Population Censuses and Surveys Longitudinal Study. This is a new source which enables researchers to study the sociodemographic histories of a representative sample of the population of England and Wales. The period after retirement from formal employment is one which sees men and women experience more changes to their domestic circumstances than is commonly appreciated. Many of these changes are related to earlier socioeconomic circumstances which also influence people's abilities to cope with change and their need for support.

1988 Research and the ageing population. Wiley, Chichester (Ciba Foundation Symposium 134) p 177–192

Much of the existing research in ageing populations derives from stereotypes of the old based on experiences of elderly populations of the present and recent past. The elderly in the future are likely to be different, in the main part because of sociodemographic differences during their working life. Compared with earlier generations some may have accumulated more wealth and possessions, may have led more varied and healthier lives, and may have been subject to less stress. Others will enter old age after prolonged unemployment or early retirement have impoverished them and with a welfare system incapable of coping with the size of the elderly population. Therefore, in order to obtain a more realistic picture of older people in the future, we need to combine our views based on cross-sectional pictures obtained in the past with a perspective on the life course of different generations (Elder 1985).

Interest in the elderly has been increasing to a large extent because they are expected to place burdens on the remainder of the adult population. The later years of life see individuals experience a number of changes. These include retirement from formal, and then voluntary, work; movement from the home in which they had reared a family; loss of spouses and friends with whom they have shared their lives and who have provided psychosocial support; onset of physical disability and loss of physical independence; and, often finally, movement into an institution. These changes lead the elderly, as a group, to call on the community for greater social, physical and medical support. Longitudinal pictures of these changes and factors influencing them will help us appreciate what happens as people age and what factors influence the consequences of various changes.

This paper outlines longitudinal insights on ageing and the changing elderly population in England and Wales provided by a number of different researchers using a single statistical source, the Office of Population Censuses and Surveys (OPCS) Longitudinal Study.

OPCS Longitudinal Study

The OPCS Longitudinal Study (LS) brings together information in England and Wales from a variety of routine data sources for which OPCS has prime responsibility. As has been described in more detail elsewhere (Brown & Fox 1984), these sources currently include the 1971 and 1981 Census records and vital registration records, such as birth, cancer and death records, for the period 1971–1985.

The sample of people born on one of four dates in any single year is a dynamic sample. Initially it included some 530 000 people selected from the 1971 Census on the basis of dates of birth given in the census. Since 1971, some 121 000 people with the same birthdays have been added to the sample as immigrants (17 000) or births (65 000) since the 1971 Census, or because they were subsequently found in the 1981 Census (39 000). Some 115 000 others have been lost through death (59 000), emigration (9000), or because their records were not found in the 1981 Census (46 000). As a result, the sample in 1981 covers approximately 536 000 people. Records are available from both 1971 and 1981 Censuses for over 415 000 people.

In this paper I shall outline longitudinal descriptions of change based on comparisons of circumstances recorded in the 1971 and 1981 Censuses and prospective analyses based on deaths, new cancers, losses of spouses, and entry to long-stay psychiatric hospitals in the period 1971–1981.

Sociodemographic change

Family circumstances

Men die earlier than women and the difference has widened substantially during the middle part of this century. As a result men tend to be married at the time of death whereas women are generally widowed. This has implications for the family support available in periods of chronic ill-health shortly before death.

Those men who survive to older ages are however likely to experience the loss of a spouse, whereas women in the older age groups will already be widowed (Fox & Grundy 1985). There will, therefore, be marked differences between men and women in their family circumstances in the older age groups. More women than men will be left to cope on their own and more still will have to make changes to their domestic arrangements when they are unable to cope. We might expect these differences to increase in the latter part of this century as a consequence of the increased differences in mortality between men and women at younger ages.

Housing

Marital status is particularly important in determining the likelihood of entering or staying in a home for the elderly, or a hospital. Single men and women are more likely to enter such institutions than widowed and married people of the same age (Fox & Goldblatt 1982, p 57).

Although these observations are based on cross-sectional analysis, Table 1 shows that differences between men and women in the proportions found in institutions can be explained by differences in mortality between men and women. There are no differences between the sexes for those who were married in both 1971 and 1981. The table also suggests that there are socioeconomic differences in institutionalization, although these might be explained by socioeconomic differences in mortality leading to different bereavement rates and hence differences in the availability of support.

When we look at family and other non-institutional households we find that, age for age, widows and widowers are more likely to rent and less likely to own their accommodation than are married men and women. This is primarily a function of differences in mortality rates by tenure. Holmans et al (1987) found little evidence to indicate that more owner-occupiers than tenants cease to live as independent households when widowed, or that widowhood leads to movement from owner occupation to renting or to institutions.

Geographic mobility

The 1970s saw the development of a large number of retirement areas in the

TABLE 1   Percentage of people resident in non-private households[a] in England and Wales in 1981, by sex, age and tenure in 1971 and by change in marital status

Age 1971	Men		Tenure 1971		Women		Tenure 1971	
	All	Married in 1971 & 1981	Owner occupier	Local authority tenant[b]	All	Married in 1971 & 1981	Owner occupier	Local authority tenant[b]
50–	1.4	0.1	0.1	0.3	1.3	0.1	0.3	0.2
55–	1.8	0.2	0.4	0.4	1.4	0.2	0.4	0.5
60–	2.5	0.3	0.8	0.7	2.5	0.3	0.9	0.9
65–	3.8	0.8	1.2	2.0	5.2	0.7	2.9	3.3
70–	7.1	1.5	3.3	4.5	9.9	1.6	5.6	7.8
75–	11.3	2.8	8.3	5.8	16.2	4.9	12.0	13.1
80–	18.3	11.5	12.3	12.8	27.3	12.5	18.8	25.0
85+	27.7	(0.0)	8.0	(60.0)	35.0	(14.3)	27.6	26.2

(), N less than 20.

[a] Non-private households includes old people's homes and psychiatric and other hospitals.

[b] Local authority tenants are those in council housing other than old people's homes or other institutions run by the council.

UK. Grundy (1987a) has shown that net shifts in the elderly population as a result of retirement-age migration, 1971–1981, were considerable; six counties experienced gains or losses of 15% or more in the number of elderly people resident. London was the chief loser of population while southern counties on the coast predominated among those gaining population.

Migration in the retirement age group was less in the early 1980s than in the early 1970s. However, housing tenure, economic position and social class were all associated with the rate of migration, particularly between counties (that is, over longer distances), in both the early 1970s and 1980s. The drop in retirement migration was greatest among the younger retired and owner-occupiers (Grundy 1985, 1987a).

Grundy suggests that lack of support from immediate family may present a problem in the receiving areas. Women who moved longer distances tended to have fewer children to fall back on than those who moved locally or who did not move. At least a quarter of those moving between counties in 1971–1981 had no living children. A third of married women who moved between counties in 1970–1971 and who in 1981 were 70–74 years old were no longer married in 1981; a quarter of those five years younger who moved no longer married in 1981.

Long-distance migration was associated with low mortality in the first few years after the move (Fox & Goldblatt 1982, Fox et al 1982; see later). On the assumption that lower mortality reflects the better health of migrants, Grundy (1987a) argues that areas such as London which lose substantial proportions of their elderly population through migration may as a consequence need to spend more per capita on services for those remaining. In contrast, the chief destination areas, which may need to expand services in line with the growth in number of elderly people, benefit, in the initial period after arrival, from lower per capita use of resources associated with the health and wealth advantages of those migrating into these areas. The smaller family size of the 'in-migrants' and greater geographic distance from relatives may influence the demand for support in receiving areas after the initial health selection has worn off. The importance of this will become clearer once we have looked more carefully at distance from relatives and at patterns of subsequent moves for distance migrants.

Differences in mortality at older ages

Differences based on marital status and institution type

It has long been believed that married men and women have lower death rates, age for age, than the single, widowed and divorced. The Longitudinal Study leads us to question this finding for women at older ages. Fox & Goldblatt (1982, p 42–46) found little difference in mortality between single and married women, and only a hint that widows have slightly raised death rates at age 65 and over. The differences were not statistically significant.

Support for the conclusion that the traditional findings may be wrong comes from a comparison between successive censuses which highlights the magnitude of 'errors' in marital status reporting (Fox & Grundy 1985). Analyses of survival from bereavement also suggest that widows have increased mortality rates only for a short time after the death of their husbands (see next section).

Differences between the widowed and the married in mortality at older ages affect projections of the family and household structure of the population, which in turn have implications for projections of housing needs and of demand from the elderly for residential homes and hospitals.

Since institutions provide care for the sickest and most disabled members of society, we expect the mortality of people in institutions to be raised. Fox & Goldblatt (1982) and Moser & Goldblatt (1984) show that differences in mortality are a function of the type of institution, the duration of the stay, and the length of follow-up, as well as the age and marital status of people in institutions. Different patterns were found for different causes of death.

In the period immediately after the 1971 census the highest standardized mortality ratios were observed for 'visitors'* to non-psychiatric hospitals, a group which would include those with acute problems. The mortality of people in non-psychiatric hospitals was higher than that for those in psychiatric hospitals, which in turn was higher than that for people in homes for the elderly. As follow-up increased, the standardized mortality ratios of all institutional populations declined, irrespective of the type of institution. This reflects the earlier deaths of people with acute problems and the longer survival of those with chronic or less severe conditions. These differences were most marked at working ages and shortly after retirement, when only a small fraction of people are institutionalized. The excess mortality tended to be more for respiratory diseases and for cerebral, arterial and venous diseases than for heart disease and neoplasms.

Fox & Goldblatt (1982, p 54–60) show marked differences between the married, single and widowed in the proportions enumerated in different types of institutions, as well as differences in mortality according to marital status, within those institutions. Single men and women are several times as likely as the married to be enumerated in homes and communal establishments or as 'residents' in hospitals (that is, as chronically sick patients). However, married men and women in each type of institution have much higher death rates. Both in entry and survival the widowed lie between the single and the married. This reflects the support in the community available to the married

---

* 'Visitors' is the term used in the UK censuses to describe people who were not usually resident in the place where they were enumerated. For people enumerated in institutions a six-month rule applied.

from partners and children and to the widowed from children; single men and women enter, or are kept in, institutions for lesser health problems, presumably in part because of lack of support at home.

Differences between socioeconomic groups

The traditional decennial supplements on occupational mortality (OPCS 1978, 1986) suffered from inadequate reporting of occupations by the retired. As a consequence there has, until recently, been no information on differences between socioeconomic groups in mortality at older ages. Analyses of mortality for men of working age suggested that differences between socioeconomic groups diminish with age. It came as a surprise therefore when we (Fox et al 1985) found evidence that differences between social classes were nearly as wide for men aged over 80, classified on the basis of their pre-retirement job, as for men in their fifties.

In the earlier part of this century a high proportion of women did not pursue careers outside the home. As socioeconomic status was usually assessed in terms of occupational position, data on differences in mortality between women in different socioeconomic groups were only available for married women classified according to their husbands' occupations. Moser & Goldblatt (1985) have recently demonstrated how household and housing characteristics, such as household tenure and access to cars, can be used to compare women in different socioeconomic circumstances. Again, differences are found to persist into the oldest age groups. There are signs, particularly when access to cars is used as the socioeconomic indicator, that differences among women may decrease with age, but these could be artefacts of the classifications used.

Geographic mobility and mortality

As already indicated, old age is a time of substantial change. Fox & Goldblatt (1982) showed that the pattern of geographical movement was clearly related to health. Long-distance migration is concentrated in the few years after retirement, whereas local migration is more a feature of the changes made by the very old. Age for age, people who moved short distances had higher mortality rates than those who did not move and those who moved longer distances had the lowest mortality of all. On balance the first group, which probably reflects people moving to live with family or into homes and other institutions, outweighs the last group.

I have already discussed some of the implications of relationships between geographic mobility and health. Grundy (1987b) shows how geographic movement, the likelihood of entering an institution and mortality are closely linked to socioeconomic factors. Women in owner-occupied housing in 1971 were more likely than those in rented accommodation to migrate longer distances in the period 1971–1981. Even when account is taken of their age and marital status, they were also less likely than tenants to enter an institution and were more likely to survive the decade.

Antecedents and consequences of bereavement

The loss of a partner with whom one has shared one's life is increasingly concentrated in older age groups (Anderson 1983). The growing literature on relationships between life stress and chronic disease (McQueen & Siegrist 1982) leads us to question who is affected most by the loss of a partner and to check whether we can observe an effect of bereavement on health and on changes in circumstances.

Studies of mortality after bereavement enable us to investigate the immediate consequences of bereavement for the health of the bereaved. As has been observed in a number of other studies, Jones & Goldblatt (1987) found raised overall mortality in the period shortly after widow(er)hood. Increases in the very short term were more marked for widows than for widowers, with for example a doubling of mortality from all causes in the first month after widowhood. Marked peaks in deaths from accidents and violence were seen for both sexes. In subsequent months the mortality in widowers, but not in widows, was about 10% greater than that in all members of the LS sample.

Differences in post-bereavement mortality were observed according to socioeconomic status, but Jones & Goldblatt (1986) found little evidence that social or familial support, as measured by household structure and numbers of children, affected the probability of surviving.

These findings have also been used to address questions about the role of stress in heart disease (Jones 1986) and cancer (Jones et al 1984, Jones & Goldblatt 1986, Jones 1987). In each case the evidence has been inconclusive, suggesting that if there are associations they are likely to be relatively weak. Jones & Goldblatt (1987) also found little evidence to support arguments for concordance in causes of death between widow(er)s and their spouses.

I have already discussed some of the relationships between marital status and sociodemographic change in 1971–1981. However, the importance of ties between factors influencing mortality and factors influencing changes in circumstances may not be fully appreciated. Socioeconomic differences in mortality imply that men and women from the poorer sections of the community will lose a partner at younger ages than will those who are better-off. The narrowing, with increased age, of differences in mortality between women (but not men) in different socioeconomic groups suggests that women from poorer backgrounds will tend to spend a higher proportion of their lives alone and without immediate family support and, as a result, will be more likely than those from more affluent circumstances to be institutionalized. The association between socioeconomic circumstances and institutionalization may be even stronger than suggested by Grundy (1987b). As was shown by Holmans et al (1987), differences between the proportions of married and unmarried people in owner-occupied, privately rented and local authority accommodation are a function of differences in survival between different tenure groups. These differences in distribution can therefore be seen as a reflection of the socioeconomic circumstances implied by the type of housing.

Brief discussion

I have outlined some of the longitudinal insights to the ageing population currently being provided by researchers using a national record linkage study based on routine information. In their introduction to a special issue of the *Milbank Memorial Fund Quarterly* on the 'oldest old', Suzman & Riley (1985) commented:

> 'the mounting number of the very old . . . is so new a phenomenon that there is little in historical experience to help in interpreting it. Not only are the older living longer, but they are also growing older in markedly different ways from their predecessors. The work at hand, still partial and tentative, indicates that the oldest old can no longer remain invisible in the economy, the polity, the health care system, or the statistical records.'

Whereas old age is popularly conceptualized as a time for rest and stability, the period after official retirement age is found to involve many changes to one's household and family circumstances. It is important that we improve our understanding of the factors influencing changes so that we can better plan the resources that will be required to meet any changing demand arising from the ageing population. This should enable future generations of very old people to maximize the opportunities that will enable them, and the remainder of society, to properly adjust to their changing and differential needs.

Acknowledgements

The author has drawn on the work of a number of colleagues who have at some point worked in the Social Statistics Research Unit, City University, using the OPCS Longitudinal Study. These colleagues were funded by grants from the Medical Research Council, the Economic and Social Research Council and the Cancer Research Campaign. Of course, none of this would be possible without the considerable support provided by OPCS staff.

References

Anderson M 1983 What is new about the modern family: an historical perspective. In: The family. Occasional Paper 31, Office of Population Censuses and Surveys, London

Brown A, Fox AJ 1984 OPCS Longitudinal Study: ten years on. Population Trends 37:20–22. HMSO, London

Elder GH 1985 Life course dynamics: trajectories and transitions 1968–1980. Cornell University Press, Ithaca, New York

Fox AJ, Grundy EMD 1985 A longitudinal perspective on recent socio-demographic change. In: Measuring socio-demographic change. Occasional Paper 34, Office of Population Censuses and Surveys, London

Fox AJ, Goldblatt PO 1982 Socio-demographic mortality differentials, Longitudinal Study 1971–1975, Series LS no. 1. HMSO, London

Fox AJ, Goldblatt PO, Adelstein AM 1982 Selection and mortality differentials. J Epidemiol Community Health 36:69–79

Fox AJ, Goldblatt PO, Jones DR 1985 Social class mortality differentials: artefact, selection or life circumstances? J Epidemiol Community Health 39:1–8

Grundy MED 1985 Divorce, widowhood, remarriage and geographic mobility among women. J Biosoc Sci 17:415–435

Grundy EMD 1987a Retirement migration and its consequences in England and Wales. Ageing & Society 7:59–82

Grundy EMD 1987b Ageing: age related change in later life. In: Murphy M, Hobcraft JN (eds) Population research in Britain. Oxford University Press, London

Holmans AE, Nandy S, Brown AC 1987 Household formation and dissolution and housing tenure: a longitudinal perspective. In: Social Trends 17. HMSO, London

Jones DR 1986 Heart disease mortality following widowhood: some results from the OPCS Longitudinal Study. In: Does stress cause heart attacks? The Coronary Prevention Group, London

Jones DR 1987 Cancer mortality following widow(er)hood in the OPCS Longitudinal Study. In: Proceedings of the first International Symposium on Primary Prevention of Cancer, Antwerp, 1986, in press

Jones DR, Goldblatt PO 1986 Cancer mortality following widow(er)hood: some further results from the OPCS Longitudinal Study. Stress Medicine 2:129–140

Jones DR, Goldblatt PO 1987 Cause of death in widow(er)s and spouses. J Biosoc Sci 19:107–121

Jones DR, Goldblatt PO, Leon DA 1984 Bereavement and cancer: some data on deaths of spouses from the longitudinal study of Office of Population Censuses and Surveys. Br Med J 289:461–464

McQueen DV, Siegrist J 1982 Social factors in the aetiology of chronic disease: an overview. Soc Sci Med 16:353–367

Moser KA, Goldblatt PO 1984 Mortality of women in institutions and private households using data from the OPCS Longitudinal Study. Social Statistics Research Unit LS Working Paper no 14, City University, London

Moser KA, Goldblatt PO 1985 Mortality of women in the OPCS Longitudinal Study: differentials by owner occupation and household and housing characteristics. Social Statistics Research Unit LS Working Paper no 26, City University, London

OPCS 1978 Occupational Mortality 1970–1972 Decennial Supplement, Series DS no 1, HMSO, London

OPCS 1986 Occupational Mortality 1979–1980, 1982–1983 Decennial Supplement, Series DS no 6, HMSO, London

Suzman R, Riley MW 1985 Introducing the 'oldest old'. Milbank Mem Fund Q 63(2):177–186

DISCUSSION

Andrews: It occurs to me that your approach could be undertaken on a cross-national basis, in countries with comparable census collections and the capacity to collect data. Has this been duplicated elsewhere?

Fox: This type of study is now being duplicated. At a conference in Mexico in 1979 organized by WHO and the UN on the causes and consequences of socioeconomic differences in mortality it became clear that there were virtually no international data, collected using similar techniques that would allow one to make direct comparisons between countries. One of the recommendations was that such data should be collected in industrialized countries. Since that conference, a group of European demographers have met regularly. The Scandinavians were the first to produce such data using their powerful record-linkage systems. We now have studies based on Finland, Norway and Denmark, and there are data from Sweden as well. France has a similar study; Italy already has data for Turin and is developing data for the country as a whole; Austria is also developing a similar study. In the USA the National Center for Health Statistics has used the current population survey as the basis of a mortality follow-up study.

Maeda: I am very impressed by your well-designed, large-scale longitudinal study. In Japan we have not done such a big longitudinal study, but in my Institute we are doing a small-scale longitudinal study on the medical and socio-behavioural background of ageing in one of the suburban cities of Tokyo. This study was started 11 years ago, in 1976. Last year we carried out the 'third wave' survey. The longitudinal data obtained from three surveys covering 10 years are now being analysed by a multidisciplinary research team that includes physicians, psychiatrists, nurses, psychologists and sociologists.

I would like to back up what you told us about the importance of the effect of socioeconomic factors on the mortality rate of older people. In connection with our longitudinal study we compared the age-adjusted mortality rate (including all ages) of all administrative wards and cities in Tokyo Metropolitan area (Koganei City Government & Tokyo Metropolitan Institute of Gerontology 1986). The results were remarkable. Localities in the western part of Tokyo, where the proportion of highly educated persons is much greater than in other areas of Tokyo, invariably show significantly lower mortality rates. (In Japan we usually measure socioeconomic status by the length of the formal education received—most Japanese sociologists believe that this is the only way to measure socioeconomic status in Japan.)

The length of formal education also has a significant effect on the level of activity of older people. In our study (Maeda 1984), the length of formal education in Japan has a statistically significant influence on the level of activity, with three related variables (sex, the level of ADL, or activities of daily living, and the level of mental ability, measured by Benton's Visual Image

Retention Test) being held constant. We also found that if the effect of socioeconomic status (measured by the length of education in this study) is held constant, there is no statistically significant difference in the level of activity between older men and women.

Fox: I am interested to learn how you measure socioeconomic differences in mortality for women. Until recently in the UK, data for women have mainly been based on analysis according to the husband's social class. We were not able to look at other classifications of women's socioeconomic circumstances. We have now used education, which is of limited value because in the UK educational system a large fraction of the population leave school at the minimum school-leaving age, which is now 16 years. As a result one is not able to separate out reasonably sized socioeconomic groups for analysis. We turned to housing measures because they are powerful discriminators between a variety of different outcome measures. It is very striking, for example, that the differences in mortality between owners (who are 50–60% of the population) and local authority tenants (who are 30% of the population) are almost as large as the differences between social classes I and II (which make up 25% of the population) and social classes IV and V (which are 25%). We are effectively splitting the population into two groups and getting large differences in mortality. Also, type of tenure applies to men and women almost equally, to children and to the retired. It is therefore much easier to use.

Katzman: Are there other differences between those two groups, such as ethnic differences?

Fox: Only very minor ones. Our minority populations in the UK are relatively smaller and younger than those in the USA, so they will not be major factors in explaining socioeconomic differences in mortality.

Fries: Two trends in the USA that will influence these kinds of data in the future and should probably be included in predictive models are, first, that the gap in life expectancy from birth between men and women is now narrowing. It reached a maximum of about 8.4 years in 1982; it is now 7.9, and falling. The likely causes of a continued decline are further reductions in cardiovascular disease rates, in lung cancer rates in males, and in accident rates, which are influenced by the use of seatbelts in cars. The gap will thus probably continue to close over the next decade or so (Fries 1987).

The second trend is an adverse one and has to do with changes in habits relating to health by social class. Here, from current trends, we expect to see a widening difference in terms of social, and social class, influence, in the USA. Changes in terms of more exercise, giving up cigarette smoking and dietary manipulation are occurring in a very class-conscious way in the USA; the people who already have good health are those who have changed their habits for the better. Those who already have the worst health, in the lowest socioeconomic classes, have made almost no changes at all. So one would predict that the gap in health between rich and poor may widen.

Fox: The same downturn in sex differences in mortality has been seen in the UK. I don't know when that will start to affect the proportions of each sex who are surviving to older ages. It will not have an immediate effect because, as you say, some of the effect is because of fewer accidents, and some is the changing patterns of cardiovascular disease and lung cancer.

Wallack: You use housing, and also employment, as proxies for income or wealth. Do you also have direct measures of those? It is hard to get that information for the elderly. Also, in the USA at least, many elderly people, although they may be retiring earlier, seem to have more money now, from private pensions, social security, housing and so on.

Fox: We haven't got data on incomes. Although the elderly as a group are increasing in wealth, they are increasingly divided in the UK. There is a large core of people who own their own homes and therefore will have assets; their homes will be the major asset they take into their old age. A second asset will be occupational pensions, and then other kinds of savings. Other groups of elderly people have not benefited from these forms of saving; they have lived through-out their lives in local authority housing and have no assets in terms of housing; nor will they have occupational pensions. They are also the group who have experienced disproportionally shortened working lives as a result of an in-creased likelihood of prolonged unemployment during the recent recession.

T.F. Williams: The figures in the USA show that widows and the very old are quite poverty stricken. Most elderly widows at present don't receive pensions, in the USA; with heightened awareness of this problem, spouses are now beginning to be included in the retirement and annuity plans of many em-ployers.

Hollander: We cannot be over-optimistic about the influence of pensions on health. The pension system is not an insurance system but a direct turnover of the assets of the working part of the population; but with the change in demographic composition it will be difficult to see whether income will increase for the elderly in the future, or decrease.

Wenger: Dr Fox, are there systems in other countries where there is a different availability of health care at age 62 or 65, as we have in the USA with our Medicare health insurance plan? Different health-care schemes and diffe-rent health-care costs may contribute significantly to the impoverishment of sick elderly people in some societies, an outcome that may not occur with some form of national health insurance, although the latter may administratively limit the availability of resources.

Fox: I presume that differential access shouldn't arise in the UK, although one trend is now the increasing reliance on private health insurance, which is changing attitudes towards the national health service. The extent to which that trend may become important is unclear; it has already had an effect in the UK in the area of access to different types of old age homes, for instance.

Arie: There is a bimodal picture there; very poor people can enter privately run old people's homes more easily than people in the middle income band, and very rich people can afford to do so. The people in the middle are not funded by the State, as the very poor are.

Let me also comment on the relationship between unemployment and poverty. Unemployment will probably be with us on a large scale in all Western countries for a long time. In the past, 'not working' has most commonly been an attribute of being retired, and therefore of being aged. The fact that large numbers of the non-aged are not working may blur the distinction between the aged and the young; it is something they have in common. But of course John Fox has emphasized that being unemployed during one's working years impedes one's capacity to accumulate resources for old age, when one is most vulnerable. What we may see is a compounding of the effect which now exists in industrialized countries like ours, whereby the aged are already relatively disadvantaged in all sorts of material ways (access to transport, to telephones, to consumer durables, to central heating). The long-term unemployed will move into old age further impoverished not only in income, but also through having failed to accumulate the material possessions which are needed most in old age; and this is going to be a very sad story.

T.F. Williams: This is a profound societal issue; I can't see anyone wanting a world that doesn't in one way or another achieve essentially full employment. The employment figures in the USA may go the other way, however, simply because of the low birthrate in the 1960s and 1970s. The projections are that even at present productivity levels, we shall actually need old people to be the employed people in our economy by about 2000 or 2010. We won't have enough people to do the work unless we extend employment into the later years.

Grimley Evans: The emergence of a powerful social-class difference in mortality in old age is extremely interesting. One has always interpreted an apparent narrowing of social class differences in mortality with age as due to errors in the data, although there has always been the possibility that the lower social classes are under more powerful selective survival pressures and so mortality rates might converge in old age. What is your interpretation of your findings? Is it simply that you have better data, or has another risk factor for mortality in later life emerged which previously operated only at younger ages?

Fox: There are two aspects. In the past we had a picture of social class differences in mortality at ages 15–64, and we were using that to ask what would happen after age 64. So we were taking the narrowing of differences in the latter period of working life and saying that differences would continue to narrow at older ages. We probably still have the narrowing of differences during working life, and that principally reflects occupational and other accidents which show wide differences between social groups at young ages. In contrast, the chronic diseases, which influence specific mortality rates at ages

45–64 (heart disease and the cancers, basically), also affect mortality at older ages.

We have argued elsewhere (Fox 1985) that the selection hypothesis doesn't hold at these older ages. This hypothesis would suggest that the difference between social classes in mortality is a consequence of those who are going up to the higher social classes being healthy and those coming down being less healthy. If this were the case you would expect the difference between classes in a prospective study to narrow with the duration of follow-up. This doesn't happen; the gradients diverge over time.

This same question has been raised about studies on the mortality of the unemployed. Those who were seeking work straight after the census had an SMR of about 130; that figure increases over time, instead of falling, as it would if the unemployed were selected on ill-health grounds. In this case we have taken out of the unemployed those people who reported themselves as temporarily or permanently sick. This illustrates how one can try to pick out such a selection process by looking at the trend over time. On those arguments, I don't think the differences in mortality between social classes are due to selective mobility. I don't think they are due to an artefact, either.

T.F. Williams: Could one use the type of figures you are getting to identify populations or groups at special risk? Thinking preventively, one might look at it in terms of major disease conditions, or other deleterious circumstances that could be related back to the initial characteristics of the populations involved. If one is trying to organize a national health service, one could take such data and target groups at greatest risks for certain conditions, and intervene to try to minimize the risk.

Fox: One reason I like to use housing tenure as an indicator of social group is that it identifies groups who are already targeted for social policy purposes. We talk about subsidizing, for example by tax relief, those who are owner-occupiers, and also, in other ways, those living in local authority housing. So, where such marked differences in mortality are observed, you have groups to whom you can direct policy. I haven't yet seen such groups identified as the basis for preventive campaigns or screening campaigns. A student of mine is involved in trying different approaches to persuading women to come forward for cervical cancer screening. One approach is to direct effort to women through those responsible for the administration of local authority housing. In the UK, the housing system offers a way in which to change policies, to reach the different groups. For each issue there will be different policy implications.

Mor: Dr Fox, did you find that the effect of bereavement on mortality appeared to be attenuated with increasing age?

Fox: The effect diminished as the period after bereavement increased. There was little evidence that the effect was stronger among young than among older widows and widowers.

Mor: The shape of the curve resembles data reported on depression rates over the first year of bereavement, using repeated measurements of depression (Kane et al 1986).

Fox: The problem is that there are very small numbers of widows and widowers at the younger ages, so we can't really test the differences. However, if we look at prospective mortality rates for widowed people, the differences between them and married people appear to be wider at younger ages than at older ages.

Mor: That is consistent with the hypothesis that accidental or unexpected deaths cause more disruptive bereavement consequences than do expected deaths.

Fox: Yes.

References

Fox AJ, Goldblatt PO, Jones DR 1985 Social class mortality differentials: artefact, selection or life circumstances? J Epidemiol Community Health 39:1–8

Fries JF 1987 Aging, illness, and health policy: implications of the compression of morbidity. Perspect Biol Med, in press

Kane RL, Klein SJ, Bernstein L, Rothenberg R 1986 The role of hospice in reducing the impact of bereavement. J Chron Dis 39:735–742

Koganei City Government & Tokyo Metropolitan Institute of Gerontology 1986 Zusetu: Koganeino Otoshiyori (The elderly in Koganei City—illustrated). Social Welfare Section of Koganei City Government, Tokyo, Japan

Maeda D 1984 Change in activity level in old age (in Japanese). Shakai Rounengaku (J Soc Gerontol) 21:47–61

The nature and causes of ageing

T.B.L. Kirkwood

National Institute for Medical Research, The Ridgeway, Mill Hill, London NW7 1AA, UK

Abstract. Ageing is a process where the end result is obvious but the mechanism remains obstinately obscure. The phenomenology of senescence is rich in the abundance of model systems that it offers for the experimental study of ageing. The field is also rich in the theories to account for ageing in terms of specific changes noted or postulated to occur as organisms grow older. Since neither models nor theories are scarce, the slowness of progress to date may therefore be due at least partly to inadequate cross-referencing between the two. Both in the choice of a model organism or cell system and in the selection of a specific mechanism to study, it is important to have in mind the nature and role of ageing at the organism level. Recent evolutionary insights into ageing suggest that senescence occurs because through natural selection a strategy is favoured in which organisms invest fewer resources in the maintenance and repair of somatic cells and tissues than are necessary for indefinite survival of the individual. This 'disposable soma' theory provides a broad predictive framework within which to assess the relevance of models with which to investigate specific mechanisms of ageing.

1988 Research and the ageing population. Wiley, Chichester (Ciba Foundation Symposium 134) p 193–207

Physical deterioration associated with old age is responsible for a large and still growing fraction of the health problems in human populations. Clinical and biological studies have provided a substantial body of knowledge on the nature and progress of specific age-related disorders. Yet, despite more than a century of research into the basic biology of senescence (Kirkwood & Cremer 1982), gerontologists still cannot identify with assurance any specific mechanism by which ageing is caused.

The problems of gerontology stem not from a shortage of possible experimental models in which to study ageing processes, but from an excess. Almost any character in any of a very wide range of animal species may be observed to undergo some alteration with age. In consequence, the diversity of research in ageing is so great as to be almost bewildering, and unrelated pursuit of separate theories postulating often highly specific causative mechanisms is commonplace. This fragmented approach is particularly unsuited to a field where the crucial issue may be to identify which of the many age-related changes are causes rather than mere consequences of senescence. In this paper, the broad conceptual problems of gerontology are examined and a theoretical framework is outlined which offers a unification of diverse observations and hypotheses about the biology of ageing and which also sets out clear predictions amenable to experimental test.

There are three principal questions to be addressed about the biology of ageing: What is ageing? Why does ageing occur? How is ageing caused? The first and second of these questions are concerned with the nature and role of ageing at the organism level, while the third is concerned mainly with mechanisms of ageing at the cell and molecular level. If we are to understand ageing fully, we need not only to answer each question in its own right but also to relate the answers to one another.

Definition of ageing

The question 'What is ageing?' can be answered in at least two ways. First, we may attempt to describe the physical changes that take place in individuals as they grow older. These are manifested mainly as a decline in a variety of body functions. We find, however, that although the general features of ageing are common within a population, the specific details vary quite considerably from one individual to another. More seriously, this approach is really a description rather than a definition of ageing, as we may apply it only when we are already agreed that ageing takes place in the population or species in question. The second definition, which is more basic and serves better to compare different species with respect to the presence or absence of intrinsic senescent processes (see Kirkwood 1985), concerns the net effect of age-related changes on the ability of the organism to survive.

At the population level, the pattern of mortality experienced by human populations serves to illustrate what is generally agreed to be definitive of ageing (Fig. 1). Following the attainment of sexual maturity and a peak of vitality which occurs early in adulthood, a long period of progressive deterioration takes place during which individuals become increasingly likely to die. Eventually, the age-specific mortality rate becomes so great that an effective upper limit is imposed on the duration of an individual lifespan.

This definition of ageing in terms of a mortality pattern showing progressive increase in age-specific mortality allows comparisons to be made even among species where the detailed features of senescence may differ markedly. There are however some qualifications which must be noted. First, it is not necessarily the case that all age-related changes are deleterious in terms of survival (see Medawar 1955, Lamb 1977). Second, the survival curve is highly susceptible to modification by extrinsic factors, so that many populations in the wild may show little or no sign of any intrinsic process of senescence (Lack 1954, Kirkwood 1985). Third, species to which the definition is applied both should have a clear distinction within individual organisms between germ line and somatic tissue, and should also be capable of repeated reproduction

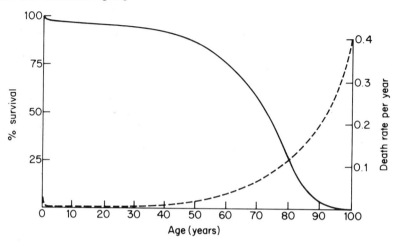

FIG. 1. Age-specific patterns of survival (continuous curve) and mortality (broken curve) which typify a population in which ageing occurs. The example is of a human population with well-developed social and medical care (from Kirkwood & Holliday 1986 by permission of Cambridge University Press). A high level of mortality due to environmental causes unrelated to age will tend to mask these patterns, which may then become apparent only when the population is transferred to a protected environment.

during the adult lifespan. Where there is no clear distinction between germ line and somatic tissue, it is usually possible to generate one individual from another by vegetative growth. The concept of individual survivorship is correspondingly imprecise and the problem of arriving at a satisfactory definition of ageing is complex (Kirkwood 1981, Kirkwood & Cremer 1982). For semelparous species which reproduce once only and die soon afterwards, death and reproduction are often intimately connected and the nature and biological significance of post-reproductive death in such species is probably quite different from the more gradual decline of repeatedly reproducing organisms whose life histories could, in principle, extend indefinitely (Kirkwood 1981, 1985). In this paper, we will restrict attention to species, like humans, in which sex offers the only means of reproduction and individuals are capable of reproducing repeatedly during their lifespan.

Evolution of ageing

The question 'Why does ageing occur?' addresses the role of ageing from an evolutionary point of view. At first sight, the evolution of ageing may seem to have little relevance to the immediate problems of research into the causes of senescence in present-day species. Ageing presumably evolved very many years ago and any future evolutionary change is likely to come about only on a very extended time scale. In practice, however, an examination of why and how ageing has been shaped under the action of natural selection may aid considerably in clarifying the general nature of the causative processes which need to be investigated. For instance, should one look for genes and gene products which bring about senescence in a controlled and coordinated way, similar to development, or should one look for extrinsic or intrinsic sources of damage which cause loss of viability in a random, progressive manner?

Probably the most widespread explanation for the evolution of ageing is that senescence provides a mechanism to limit the survival of individual organisms in order to prevent overcrowding and thus to provide living space for newcomers to the species (see, for example, Beutler 1986). A similar idea is that senescence serves to shorten the intergeneration time and so promote evolutionary progress. These ideas suggest a positive, *adaptive* role for ageing and they support the notion that senescence is a programmed process under its own strict genetic control.

Despite the popularity of the adaptive view of ageing, there are compelling reasons why it is generally unsound. First, as pointed out by Medawar (1952), the mortality in wild populations is usually so great that individuals seldom survive long enough to show clear signs of senescence. If ageing is not normally seen in the wild there can be neither need nor opportunity for an adaptive ageing mechanism to evolve. Second, for ageing to have arisen adaptively would have required that selection for advantage to the species or kin group was more effective than selection among individuals for the repro-ductive advantages of a longer life. This would have occurred only under special circumstances (see Maynard Smith 1976 for a general discussion on the limitations of group selection) and therefore cannot explain the wide-spread occurrence of ageing among animal species.

If ageing is not adaptive, then its evolution must be explained indirectly by means of a *non-adaptive* theory. The two principal types of non-adaptive theories are: (i) ageing occurs because natural selection is unable to prevent the deterioration of older organisms; or (ii) ageing is a by-product of selection for some other beneficial trait.

Underlying all non-adaptive theories is the principle, first clearly stated by Medawar (1952) and later refined by others (Williams 1957, Hamilton 1966, Charlesworth 1980), that the force of natural selection — that is, its ability to discriminate between alternative genotypes — weakens with age. The essen-tial point is that because selection acts through the differential effects of genes on reproductive fitness, the force of natural selection must decline in propor-tion to the decline in the remaining fraction of the organism's total lifetime expectation of reproduction. If a gene effect is expressed early in life, it will influence the reproductive success of a much larger proportion of individuals bearing that gene than if it is expressed late, when many individuals will already have died. This principle is the basis of the first type of non-adaptive theory of ageing, which proposes simply that deleterious genes with late age-specific effects occurring at ages beyond the normal range of survivorship in the wild environment could accumulate in the genotype subject to little or no effective counter-selection (Medawar 1952). In a protected environment, however, individuals would on average live longer, since they would be exposed to fewer hazards, and senescence would occur as the result of the combined expression of these late-acting deleterious genes.

That a simple accumulation of late-acting deleterious genes is a sufficient explanation for the evolution of ageing has been questioned, however, in more recent experimental and theoretical studies (Rose & Charlesworth 1980, Kirkwood 1977, Kirkwood & Holliday 1979). The alternative type of non-adaptive theory similarly recognizes the attenuation in the force of natural selection that occurs with age, but it goes further to suggest that ageing is the late deleterious by-product of processes which are beneficial to the organism during the earlier and, in terms of natural selection, more important stages of its lifespan (Williams 1957). One particular process is the optimization of the life history with regard to the allocation of resources among the various metabolic tasks that the organism needs to perform.

At a fundamental level of biological thinking, an organism may be regarded as an entity which takes up resources, primarily in the form of nutrients, from its environment, and ultimately converts these resources into its progeny. Of the resources taken in only a fraction is allocated directly to reproduction, however, the rest being divided among activities such as growth, foraging, and defence, as well as, in particular, the maintenance and repair of non-reproductive, or *somatic*, parts of the body. The greater the fraction allocated to one particular activity, the less is available for the others. As the following argument reveals, the optimum allocation of resources involves a smaller investment in somatic maintenance and repair than would be required for the soma to last indefinitely.

Given the continual hazard of accidental death, to which no species can be entirely immune, each individual soma can have only a finite expectation of life, even if it were not subject to senescence. When the soma dies, the resources invested in its maintenance are lost. Too low an investment in the prevention and repair of somatic damage is obviously unsatisfactory because then the soma may disintegrate before it can reproduce. However, too high an investment in these activities is also wasteful because there is no advantage in maintaining the soma better than is necessary for it to survive its expected lifetime in the wild environment in reasonably sound condition. Fitness in the latter case would actually be enhanced by reducing the investment in somatic maintenance and channelling the extra resources into, for example, greater reproductive output or more rapid growth. Fitness is therefore maximized at a level of maintenance and repair which is less than would be required for indefinite somatic survival. This conclusion has been termed the *disposable soma* theory (Kirkwood 1977, 1981, Kirkwood & Holliday 1979) for its obvious analogy with the manufacture of disposable goods where little is invested in their long-term durability.

The precise optimum level of investment in somatic maintenance will depend on the species' ecological niche. If the level of environmental mortality is high, the individual can expect to survive only a short time and there is little point in investing much in somatic maintenance and repair. In consequence, when the organism is removed to a protected environment senescence should be found to occur early. Conversely, if the level of environmental mortality is low, survivorship in the natural environment will be enhanced and there may be advantage in investing more heavily in somatic maintenance and repair so that the organism does not die of senescence before it has realized its potential for a longer life. This argument can be formalized in mathematical models of life-history optimization (Kirkwood & Holliday 1986).

Mechanisms of ageing

The disposable soma theory lends strong support to the various hypotheses which suggest that slow accretion of random defects will result ultimately in loss of function in so large a proportion of somatic cells that the organism senesces and dies. Some of these hypotheses postulate rather specific sources of damage, for example, cross-linkage between macromolecules, accumulation of toxic metabolic wastes, racemization of amino acids, damage by oxidative free radicals, damage to cell membranes, and so on. Whilst each of these sources of damage may be likely to contribute some part of the general spectrum of degeneration observed during senescence, it is unlikely that any one of them in isolation is the main cause of ageing. On empirical grounds there is no clear indication that a single type of cellular damage is conspicuous in ageing tissues. Also, on general theoretical grounds the selection process which underlies the disposable soma theory can be expected to produce more or less synchronous accumulation of heterogeneous types of damage. Nonetheless, it is possible that defects arising in the more fundamental cellular processes may provide a common source of distinct classes of cellular malfunction. The existence of a relatively small number of primary cell maintenance functions capable of determining the overall rates of accumulation of cell damage would also make it easier to explain the divergence of species' lifespans.

A common denominator of all cellular functions is the molecular machinery for replicating, maintaining and translating genetic information. These enzymic processes operate with exquisite fidelity, but mistakes do nevertheless occur (see Kirkwood et al 1986). The cost of proofreading each step of DNA, RNA and protein synthesis is considerable and some trade-off between cost and accuracy seems likely. Errors in DNA and in protein synthesis have been the basis of two distinct theories of cell ageing. The somatic mutation theory attributes ageing to the gradual accumulation of multiple errors in DNA. The protein error theory attributes ageing to the cyclic propagation of errors in the cellular translation process, which can be independent of gene mutations. In fact, there is reason to believe that somatic mutation should be considered together with the protein error theory as part of a more general error theory in which errors in all pathways of intracellular information transfer and in the control of gene expression can participate and interact (see Holliday 1986). Such a theory could account for the accumulation of almost all forms of somatic defect, since a breakdown in the fidelity of molecular processes would result in progressive impairment of all cellular functions.

Prospects for research

Research into the biology of ageing has produced much information on the course of the ageing process (see, for example, Finch & Schneider 1985). Nonetheless, the causes of ageing remain unknown. This may simply reflect the multi-faceted complexity of senescence. Comfort (1979), however, has suggested that an excess of theory may be to blame:

> 'Throughout its history the study of ageing . . . has been ruinously obscured by theory, and particularly theory of a type which begets no experimental work'.

The multiplicity of ageing theories, together with the multiplicity of experimental model systems, has generated a body of knowledge which is conspicuous for the looseness of its connections. In this paper, an attempt has been made to address basic conceptual issues of gerontology in the belief that research effort may be guided more effectively if it is conducted within a unified theoretical framework, which may serve not only to order existing knowledge into more coherent patterns, but also to stimulate pertinent experimental tests. In particular, careful reference to the two basic questions 'What is ageing?' and 'Why does ageing occur?' may prove valuable in selecting appropriate model systems with which to address the ultimate question: 'How is ageing caused?'

A first requirement is to ensure that a model organism's life history is taken into account when considering what is meant by the term ageing. Species selected as models for studying the biology of human ageing should be species which are obligate users of sexual reproduction (i.e. have a distinct soma and germ line) and should be capable of repeated reproduction during the adult lifespan. In this context it is apparent that some confusion concerns the phenomenon of the menopause in human females; for instance, it has been suggested that post-menopausal life in humans is analogous to post-reproductive survival in semelparous animals, such as marsupial mice, and may be an example of programmed senescence (Diamond 1982). This suggestion is misleading (Kirkwood 1985). The best explanation for the evolution of the menopause is that humans are unique both in the very slow development of children and in the extent to which senescence occurs in the 'wild' (Medawar 1952). As a woman grows older, the hazards of a further pregnancy increase and, beyond 40–50 yeras of age, it may be more advantageous for a woman to cease reproduction while she is bringing up her later children. It is probable therefore that in evolutionary terms the menopause is a comparatively recent adaptation which reflects the extent to which social and cultural evolution has reduced human environmental hazards and exposed us increasingly to the ravages of senescence (see Kirkwood & Holliday 1986).

An appreciation of the nature and role of ageing at the organism level is also highly relevant in selecting the broad types of ageing mechanisms which should be prime candidates for intensive study. The widely held view that senescence is a programmed means of limiting the duration of life has for too long provided false support to the idea that specific genetically determined processes may be the major cause of death. The serious weaknesses of the adaptive theories of ageing, and the relative strengths of the non-adaptive theories, need to be more generally appreciated. In particular, the disposable soma theory provides a strong theoretical justification for the view that the principal causes of senescence are to be found in the many intrinsic and extrinsic sources of damage to which all living systems are exposed (see also Sacher 1978, Cutler 1978).

Mechanisms of ageing involving random damage present, however, some special difficulties for experimental study. First, many types of damage may arise and each may contribute only partially to the overall process of senescence. This will make it difficult to establish a clear causative role for each particular type. Second, defects arising at random may be heterogeneous in frequency, in extent, and in the specific cellular targets affected. There may therefore be some difficulty in measuring them. Third, the rate of accumulation of defects *in vivo* may be quite low, presenting additional problems of measurement. Depending on the type of damage involved, quite low levels of accumulated defects may produce quite marked effects, especially when interactions between different types of damage may occur. Thus, the obvious senescent effects may depend upon much less obvious physical causes.

One particularly promising line for further experimental study may be the comparative study of mechanisms for somatic maintenance and repair in species which have different lifespans (see, for example, Sacher & Hart 1978). The disposable soma theory predicts that the efficiency of these mechanisms should in general be positively correlated with longevity. By systematic comparative study it may be possible not only to test this prediction, but also, if it is correct, to identify mechanisms which show the clearest correlations with lifespan; these would then be candidates for mechanisms which play a primary role in regulating the duration of life.

References

Beutler E 1986 Planned obsolescence in humans and in other biosystems. Perspect Biol Med 29:175–179

Charlesworth B 1980 Evolution in age-structured populations. Cambridge University Press, Cambridge

Comfort A 1979 The biology of senescence, 3rd edn. Churchill Livingstone, Edinburgh

Cutler RG 1978 Evolutionary biology of senescence. In: Behnke JA et al (eds) The biology of aging. Plenum Press, New York, p 311–360

Diamond JM 1982 Big-bang reproduction and ageing in male marsupial mice. Nature (Lond) 298:115–116

Finch CE, Schneider EL (eds) 1985 Handbook of the biology of aging, 2nd edn. Van Nostrand Reinhold. New York

Hamilton WD 1966 The moulding of senescence by natural selection. J Theor Biol 7:1–16

Holliday R 1986 Genes, proteins and cellular ageing. Van Nostrand Reinhold. New York

Kirkwood TBL 1977 Evolution of ageing. Nature (Lond) 270:301–304

Kirkwood TBL 1981 Repair and its evolution: survival versus reproduction. In: Townsend CR, Calow P (eds) Physiological ecology: an evolutionary approach to resource use. Blackwell Scientific Publications. Oxford, p 165–189

Kirkwood TBL 1985 Comparative and evolutionary aspects of longevity. In: Finch CE, Schneider EL (eds) Handbook of the biology of aging, 2nd edn. Van Nostrand Reinhold, New York, p 27–44

Kirkwood TBL, Cremer T 1982 Cytogerontology since 1881: a reappraisal of August Weismann and a review of modern progress. Hum Genet 60:101–121

Kirkwood TBL, Holliday R 1979 The evolution of ageing and longevity. Proc R Soc Lond B Biol Sci 205:531–546

Kirkwood TBL, Holliday R 1986 Ageing as a consequence of natural selection. In: Bittles AH, Collins KJ (eds) The biology of human ageing. Cambridge University Press, Cambridge, p 1–16

Kirkwood TBL, Rosenberger RF, Galas DJ 1986 Accuracy in molecular processes: its control and relevance to living systems. Chapman & Hall, London

Lack D 1954 The natural regulation of animal numbers. Clarendon Press, Oxford

Lamb MJ 1977 Biology of ageing. Blackie, London

Maynard Smith J 1976 Group selection. Q Rev Biol 51:277–283

Medawar PB 1952 An unsolved problem of biology. HK Lewis, London

Medawar PB 1955 The definition and measurement of senescence. In: Ciba Foundation Colloquia on Aging 1. Churchill, London p 4–15

Rose MR, Charlesworth B 1980 A test of evolutionary theories of senescence. Nature (Lond) 287:141–142

Sacher GA 1978 Evolution of longevity and survival characteristics in mammals. In: Schneider EL (ed) The genetics of aging. Plenum Press, New York, p 151–167

Sacher GA, Hart RW 1978 Longevity, aging and comparative cellular and molecular biology of the house mouse, *Mus musculus*, and the white-footed mouse, *Peromyscus leucopus*. In: Bergsma D, Harrison DE (eds) Genetic effects on aging. Alan R Liss, New York, p 71–96
Williams GC 1957 Pleiotropy, natural selection, and the evolution of senescence. Evolution 11:398–411

DISCUSSION

Katzman: Investigators have looked for increased errors in DNA as a function of lifespan; have they found that relationship?

Kirkwood: Studies pioneered by Hart & Setlow (1974) showed a correlation between longevity and the efficiency of DNA repair after ultraviolet radiation of mammalian fibroblasts that was remarkably close to the theoretical one. Other studies attempting to correlate levels of errors with longevity have been bedevilled by the problems of measuring these errors. Better techniques must be developed.

Riggs: Is it possible that in certain species adaptive mechanisms might operate, as well as the non-adaptive mechanisms? Specifically, it seems important to understand why human beings have a lifespan approximately three times longer than all the great apes, with whom we share 90% of our genes. Anthropologists feel that part of the answer lies in our prolonged childhood, which has advantages in that it allows us to impart culture to our children, as well as allowing for continued postnatal growth of the brain. Since brain size, intelligence and culture are related, the extension of the lifespan in humans compared to that of other primates would seem to be adaptive.

Kirkwood: In the disposable soma theory it is only ageing itself which is seen as non-adaptive. If a species acquires adaptations such as greater intelligence and social organization, which will combine to reduce environmental mortality, there very well may be selection pressure to increase the investment in repair and maintenance. We would expect to see increased longevity as a consequence of that process, and in humans the factors you point out are likely to have been very significant in this regard. To put this another way, the theory suggests that ageing *per se* has come about non-adaptively as a by-product of optimizing the amount to be invested in the repair and maintenance of the individual. However, for each species in its individual ecological niche there will be an adaptive fine tuning of how much to invest in the maintenance, and hence longevity, of the 'disposable' soma.

Lints: Does your disposable soma theory apply only to mammals? You refer to the Hart & Setlow study; I am surprised that no other mammalian studies have been done. The next step would surely be to look at repair mechanisms in the great apes, by comparison with man. There was a second study, by Woodhead et al (1980), with the long-lived turtle, the rainbow trout and the Amazon molly, where there was no relation at all between repair mechanisms and life expectancy.

Kirkwood: The original study by Hart & Setlow has been repeated by several groups and with one exception these studies indicate the same general correlation for mammals. I don't know the study by Woodhead et al. It would be interesting to see whether this finding extends to non-mammalian species. The theory covers any species with distinct germ line and soma and with a life history that incorporates repeated reproduction. In fact, the principle of optimizing how resources should be invested in repair and maintenance of the soma should extend even to species which reproduce only once. I excluded such species from my paper because they are so different from our own, and we are primarily concerned here with ageing in human societies. In a species which reproduces only a single time, once the commitment to reproduction has been made, every resource should be put into maximizing the number of viable progeny produced, even if this means neglecting the soma to such an extent that death is a consequence of the reproductive act. This is what we seem to see in species such as the Pacific salmon.

Hollander: Hart & Setlow (1974) measured only one aspect of DNA repair, namely excision repair. Secondly, if you accept their correlation between species, you should also assume that it has a predictive value within a species and would pick out those individuals who are ageing more rapidly than others. This isn't so in the rat (Vijg 1987). Perhaps the methods are not sensitive enough here.

Kirkwood: I am not appealing to Hart & Setlow's data to derive any of the disposable soma theory, which is founded on *a priori* theoretical argument. Their data are, however, consistent with the prediction. This suggests that, if the theory is right, DNA excision repair is one system for repair and maintenance which correlates with longevity and therefore may be important in determining how long individuals live.

The more important conclusion is that the theory predicts that if we do systematic comparative studies against this background, we may be able to relate findings from distinct physiological systems to a unifying theoretical framework. It is a predictive theory, rather than one established by the data.

A. Williams: There is a remarkable analogy between your model and the conceptualization of health which economists have been using for about 15 years now (see, for example, Grossman 1982, Muurinen 1982, Muurinen & Le Grand 1985, Wagstaff 1986). The notion is that health is a capital stock of which each of us has a variable inheritance. This capital stock is subject to two kinds of depreciation—a use-related and a time-related depreciation. This rate of depreciation can be decreased by various activities (regular patterns of sleep, good nutrition and medical care, among other things). The stock can also be depreciated more rapidly by smoking or drinking and so on. The value of this capital stock is measured by the quality-adjusted life expectancy of an individual at any one time. People can convert their health, in those terms, into money or other resources. For example, they can work too hard, at the expense of their health; they will then fall ill, but when medical care is given to them they may choose to use up the good results of that medical care—their health capital—to make even more money. So (within limits) one can convert health into money (and vice versa). You can use money to improve your health: rich people on the whole live longer than poorer ones. This is equivalent to the energy input in your model. It raises questions about what the system is optimizing. In your system you are optimizing some rate of population growth, effectively; but in human beings there is a trade-off between overall population growth and the quality and length of life of the individual. I suspect that the formal analogies between the system that economists are using (to optimize investments in health between length of life and quality of life) and the model you use would be very close. I find the similarities remarkable, because they appear to be the result of quite independent intellectual developments.

Kirkwood: That is a very interesting observation. An economist has also pointed out to me that the problem of the optimal allocation of resources is a well-recognized economic problem. I agree that it is attractive to draw these parallels, but we must remember too that there may be important distinctions. The values assigned by natural selection need not correspond to the values we ourselves would attach to the various options.

T.F. Williams: The point about length and quality of life interests me. There is a distinction to be made between lifespan or longevity as a goal of a species, or of any one individual, and 'non-ageing'; given a relatively fixed lifespan, 'non-ageing' might be good-quality life. You are talking about how much to invest in 'non-ageing', or minimizing ageing; in other words, not length of life but the quality of life as long as it goes on.

Kirkwood: I am not sure that I agree with the distinction you draw between quality and length of life, except for the rather special case of human populations. For most animal populations, in their natural environments, the great majority of individuals do not show any clear signs of senescence. In other words, death occurs while the animal is reasonably vigorous and its quality of life is still high.

T.F. Williams: The laggard in the herd, for example, is picked off by the lion or tiger—the weaker member of the species is caught first. He is aged, in that sense.

White: That suggests that a condition such as arthritis, that puts the individual at the back of the herd, constitutes a selective pressure; and we do see osteoarthritis as a disease of ageing. Lens opacities must make an animal less able to see a predator, and that is also something we think of as ageing. Likewise, a reduction in pulmonary vital capacity would also put individuals at the back of the herd; we certainly think of that in terms of ageing. These are changes that reduce survival in the wild animal, and that influence the quality of life in humans.

Kirkwood: It is true that any individual weakened by senescence is likely to be picked off by natural causes first. But this is where humans are so different from the animal populations that one has in mind when considering the evolution of ageing. Through our social organization we have means to keep individuals alive when their vitality, or quality of life, has been seriously compromised. By contrast, for wild mice or rabbits, for example, the earliest signs of physical deterioration, or loss of quality of life, would be likely to result in death. A further problem is that if, say, lens opacity were to contribute to the mortality of an animal in the wild, and one takes lens opacity as being associated with ageing, we would expect to see, in wild populations, an increase in age-specific mortality. The available data on populations in the wild are admittedly scant but they do suggest that for the majority of vertebrate species, particularly small species such as rodents and small birds, there is no marked increase in age-specific mortality in natural conditions.

Phair: I am also intrigued by your theory. There is evidence that if a young female rat is fed well, reproductive maturity comes on early, and longevity is reduced. In contrast, in the undernourished rat, reproduction does not begin till much later and longevity is increased. This seems to go along with your idea of a balance of repair with reproductive life and fecundity; if puberty is earlier, in theory you have more chance to reproduce. So the input side may influence what happens.

Mor: Would the organism's devotion to repair and maintenance lead to an associated reduction in the number of offspring born in a population at any given time, in your theory? If so, might that difference be observed when human populations in developed and underdeveloped countries are compared? Are there animal models that extend to that situation?

Kirkwood: These are interesting points, but the theory deals primarily with differences between species, rather than plasticity within a species and the ability, in a species, to respond to varying events in the life of an individual. It is not necessarily valid to extend the argument to a comparison of individual organisms within a species, because that will be governed by the extent to which life history flexibility exists in that species. For instance, one could argue that an individual that produces fewer offspring than the average has potentially more resources available for somatic repair and maintenance; but it may not be possible, physiologically, to convert those resources into greater repair and maintenance if the amount invested in the latter is determined by things set within the genome that are not responsive to individual variations in life history. So one cannot predict in general what one would see if one made those kinds of studies in a given population. Some species may have evolved to have greater plasticity and to respond in the ways suggested, but this would not necessarily be the case.

Wise: Your theory states that one option is to optimize repair. Since the environments in which different species live are so different, would you expect the mechanisms of repair to be the same from species to species? If not, is it valid to choose one animal model and expect the results to apply to any other animal species, much less to humans?

Kirkwood: That is a very good question. One would expect species in different ecological niches to place different priorities on the various possible repair systems. We cannot study the biology of ageing very effectively in humans, except perhaps in human cells in tissue culture. In selecting systems for study we need therefore to choose species with a similar life history to our own, because only in those species can we expect evolutionary forces to have operated in the way I suggest. We also need to study species with a broadly similar physiology, because the repair and maintenance processes that will be most relevant to us are more likely to be operating in the same ways in species with roughly similar physiological processes. Again, since many of the processes, for instance relating to DNA repair and the accuracy with which macromolecules are assembled, have to be studied in cells, we must also consider the relationship of the cells studied to the organisms as a whole, and choose cell systems which exhibit an age-related deterioration which is likely to be involved in a causative way in the deterioration seen in the whole individual.

Fries: One of your assumptions troubles me. You almost seem to imply that if a species devoted enough of its resources, an organism could actually achieve immortality; there is no reason why cell division couldn't go on for ever. It would be nice to work out a way to deploy more resources so that the events that we call ageing do not happen, but there is no information in any area of medicine to suggest that this particular leap of faith is justified.

Kirkwood: The suggestion is merely that it is in principle possible to invest enough in repair and maintenance processes to survive in a physiologically steady state, as appears to be the case in some simple animals, such as sea anemones. If selection pressure were strong enough, nearly all types of damage should be repairable or preventable. The disposable soma theory suggests why, in the case of species such as our own, evolution has not followed this course. It may thus help us to understand not only the nature, but also the causes of ageing. The issue of whether or not it is actually possible, given the present-day make-up of our bodies, to adjust the levels of repair and maintenance so that we could live indefinitely is something we cannot properly address until the causative mechanisms of ageing have been identified.

References

Hart RW, Setlow RB 1974 Correlation beween deoxyribonucleic acid excision-repair and lifespan in a number of mammalian species. Proc Natl Acad Sci USA 71:2169–2173

Grossman M 1982 The demand for health after a decade. J Health Econ 1(1):1–4

Muurinen JM 1982 Demand for health: a generalised Grossman model. J Health Econ 1(1):5–28

Muurinen JM, Le Grand J 1985 The economic analysis of inequalities in health. Soc Sci Med 20:1029–1035

Vijg J 1987 DNA repair and the aging process. Publication of the TNO Institute for Experimental Gerontology, P.O. Box 5815, 2280 HV Rijswijk, The Netherlands

Wagstaff A 1986 The demand for health: theory and applications. J Epidemiol Community Health 40:1–11

Woodhead AD, Setlow RB, Grist E 1980 DNA repair and longevity in three species of cold-blooded vertebrates. Exp Gerontol 15:301–304

Changing health needs of the ageing population

Jacob A. Brody

Office of the Dean, School of Public Health, University of Illinois at Chicago, P.O. Box 6998, Chicago, Illinois 60680, USA

Abstract. The drama unfolding in this century can be viewed in terms of the age at which people are now dying. Most medical needs, attention and costs occur in the last years of life. At the turn of the century about 25% of people survived age 65. In the developed countries at least 70% of the population now survive beyond this age and 30–40% of deaths are at age 80 or over. Entirely different diseases, conditions and social structures are involved when most people survive to these late ages. Increasing longevity raises the issue of net gain in active functional years versus total years of disability and dysfunction. The available evidence gives rise to pessimism: at present for each active functional year gained we add about 3.5 compromised years. The need for long-term care will continue to grow. Improvements in long-term care involve economic considerations, political will and better mechanisms for the delivery and acceptance of this labour-intensive practice. The education and preparation of the ageing population in terms of normal realities and expectations are even more important. Health-care givers, politicians, and other decision makers are increasingly likely to have first-hand exposure to the good and bad realities of an ageing society, and thereby to perceive the realities of ageing more clearly than ever before. A new political will for more creative and equitable responses to the needs of the elderly and their families is rapidly emerging. The greater our familiarity with the problems of old age, the greater the likelihood for us to find means for improvement.

1988 Research and the ageing population. Wiley, Chichester (Ciba Foundation Symposium 134) p 208–220

The social drama unfolding in this century can be viewed insightfully in terms of the age at which people are now dying. Most medical needs, attention and costs occur in the last years of life. At the turn of the century, about 25% of people survived the age of 65. In the developed countries at least 70% of the population now survives this age and between 30% and 40% of deaths occur in those aged 80 and over. Entirely different diseases, conditions and social structures are involved when the vast majority of people survive to these late ages. New needs and solutions will be understood slowly and falteringly, largely through trial and error, with the hope than an empirical body of

knowledge will instruct us. Humankind has no experience with this population phenomenon, so our greatest efforts must be directed toward monitoring
and describing the baffling transitions and reactions in order to be in a
position to take useful and successful actions.

The third of the Ashley–Perry statistical axioms states 'skill in manipulating
numbers is a talent, not evidence of divine guidance' (Dickson 1978). One
need not be particularly talented or divine to recognize that when the absolute numbers and percentage of the population aged 65 and over are increasing and, at the same time, when life expectancy for people age 65 and above is
increasing, startling events are at hand. I cannot predict when these growth
trends and patterns will diminish, but I do accept that life is finite and some
diminution is inevitable.

A central issue raised by increasing longevity is the net gain in active
functional years, as compared to the total years of disability and dysfunction.
This is the arena in which our data are weakest but, so far, the bulk of the
available evidence gives rise to pessimism (Brody 1985, Schneider & Brody
1983). Since we are living longer, we obviously are healthier at each age, but
since we are living into increasingly old ages, we pay the price of the multiple
social and medical risks incurred with extended ageing. Wilkins & Adams
(1983), comparing Canadian life tables for 1951 and 1978, noted an increase
of 1.3 years (males) and 1.4 years (females) for disability-free life out of a
total increase of 4.5 and 7.5 years, respectively. At present, then, it appears
that for each active functional year gained, we have added about 3.5 compromised years. Our statistical measurements are sparse and crude, leaving us
with gaps and guesses about how well or badly we are living during our
increased years. The crucial data we need are age-specific incidence rates for
those conditions which affect the elderly, such as hip fracture, blindness,
deafness, dementia, or the loss of spouse or caregivers. Unless we can
postpone the onset of diseases and disabilities, we are committed to an
ever-increasing burden of illness with increasing age.

I have been looking for data which would indicate a critical shift in age-
specific occurrences. The data are scanty, confusing and vulnerable to cohort
and period effects. For example, the European data indicate that the age-
specific incidence of hip (proximal femur) fracture is increasing whereas, in
the United States, mechanisms for collecting such data are weak, but notice-
able increases have not been documented (Zetterberg et al 1984, Boyce &
Vessey 1985, Melton et al 1982). Deaths from acute myocardial infarction
seem to have commenced early in this century and in many countries are now
declining rapidly (Brody 1987). Older women are increasingly entering or
remaining in the work force while, in the United States, men are still retiring
at earlier ages. The number and duration of hospitalizations are declining for
all ages, including the vulnerable elderly. I know of no indication that the age
at menopause is increasing, although women are living much longer. Life

expectancy for men is considerably less than for women, but active life expectancy is almost equal for the two sexes (Guralnik et al 1987).

The need for long-term care as a major component of continuing care will surely increase in the foreseeable future. Our approaches to improvement in long-term care must involve economic considerations, political will and better mechanisms for the delivery, as well as the acceptance of this extraordinarily labour-intensive practice. Even more important than the need for improved long-term care is the education of the ageing population in terms of normal realities and expectations, since most of the elderly will be healthy but potentially subject to systems and processes that ensure survival and subsistence but leave them with many healthy but inwardly unsatisfying years.

Population

Many of the population data that I shall mention here will emphasize the experience in the United States, which differs somewhat from that of other industrialized nations. Because of the enormous increase in birth rate following World War II (the baby boom), only about 11.5% of the US population is age 65 and over, in contrast with countries in northern Europe, where rates for those aged 65 and over are in the neighbourhood of 15%. In all developed countries, it is anticipated that approximately 20% of the population will be 65 and over within the next 25 or 30 years (Siegel & Davidson 1984). Most impressive in the United States is the increasing percentage of older segments of the elderly population. Thus, among those 65 and over in 1980, 61% were 65 to 74 and 9% were 85 and over, while, by 2000, those aged 65 to 74 will be approximately 50% and those 85 and over will be 14%. In 1920, life expectancy of females in the United States was less than two years greater than for males, but, by 1984, this had increased to over seven years. This difference increases at the oldest age groups and, by age 85, there are only 41 men per 100 women. The ratio of elderly males to females is expected to remain constant for the next 25 or 30 years.

Family composition and living arrangements are strongly influenced by the differential mortality of men and women. Overall, the most common living arrangement for elderly persons is to reside with one's spouse in a household with no other person. This, of course, varies greatly by age and sex. In 1980, 74% of older men and 36% of older women had a spouse present in the household, while, at age 75 and over, 65% of men, but only 19% of women had a spouse present in the household. Currently, over age 65, there are about 1.5 million men and six million women in the United States living alone (Brody et al 1987).

The 'oldest old', here defined as those aged 85 and over, represent a segment of our population with the highest per capita needs for medical and social services. The future growth of this segment will have an exaggerated impact on our ability to provide adequately for the needs of the elderly. While the US population increased by 26% between 1960 and 1980, the population age 85 and over increased by 126%. In actual numbers, the oldest old are expected to increase from 2.2 million in 1980 to 4.9 million by 2000 and to 7.1 million by 2020 (Guralink et al 1987).

In the United States, life expectancy at age 65 and over was virtually unchanged between 1900 and 1940. Since 1940, however, there has been an increase of four years. Approximately 70% of all deaths among those 65 and over are from cardiovascular disease, cerebrovascular disease and cancer. Cardiovascular and cerebrovascular disease account for about half the deaths over age 65 and about 70% of deaths over age 80. Cancer, on the other hand, is considerably less common, accounting for about 20% of deaths above age 65 and 12% above age 80 (Brody 1982). Remarkable declines have occurred during the past 20 years for cardiovascular disease and over an even longer period for cerebrovascular disease. It is estimated that half the decline in mortality seen since 1968 can be attributed to decreases in these diseases. Cancer is the only major disease which has increased during this time, but the size of this increase is small and decelerates with age. Thus, it is likely that cardiovascular disease and cerebrovascular disease will remain the dominant causes of mortality in future years.

Morbidity and disability

Although cause-specific mortality data are widely available and extremely useful for assessing trends of various diseases and conditions that affect the elderly population, no national data system is available to assess morbidity and disability. A most useful data set is derived from the National Center for Health Statistics' National Health Interview Survey. In their most recent published data on causes of morbidity, as reported through interviews with household members, only three of the top ten causes listed also appear among the ten leading causes of mortality: hypertension, heart disease and diabetes (DHHS 1985). Thus, most morbidity is non-fatal, but clearly detracts greatly from the comfort and quality of life among the elderly. Arthritis is the leading cause of disability; other important conditions mentioned are hearing impairment, deformity or orthopaedic impairment, and visual impairment. The nature of the survey does not provide critical estimates of the impact of dementia and mental disease.

As the population ages, chronic conditions will, of course, become more numerous and will present increasing problems in care and management. They are complex, frequently interrelated and, perhaps, the arena in which basic research into cause and prevention is most lacking and most difficult.

Since the functional impact of a disease on a person is, in a practical sense, more important than the specific disease pathology, various methods for measuring functional status have been developed. One such measurement describes the ability to perform certain activities of daily living (walking, bathing, dressing, eating, getting in and out of bed, and using the toilet). Other 'surrogate' measures are the frequency of visits to a physician, and the number of days a person must remain in bed. It is likely that better refined and more easily conducted and communicated mechanisms for functional assessment will evolve.

Limitations of the activities of daily living increase rapidly with age. This rise is paralleled by the rise in age-specific institutionalization in nursing homes, and undoubtedly these observations are related. Between age 65 and 74, fewer than 2% of the elderly are in nursing homes while, at age 85 and over, no fewer than 25% reside in nursing homes.

Expenditure

The United States currently spends more than 3% of its gross national product on health services for the elderly. Personal health care for those age 65 and over was estimated to be $120 billion in 1984, or more then $4000 per person. Medicare pays half of the total health-care costs for the aged, while Medicaid and other government programmes, including the Veterans Administration, provide about 18% of the bill. Private health insurance covers $9 billion, leaving $30 billion paid by individuals and their families (Waldo & Lazenby 1984). To state the obvious, the needs for more money will increase as the size and age of the population increase. Various countries in the developed world are approaching expenditures differently, but all are rapidly reaching crisis levels in national and personal costs.

While each nation will attempt to solve its problems in its own way, the mechanisms used in the United States will probably remain pragmatic, rather than an attempt at a sweeping single nationally imposed solution. Recent efforts to standardize and regulate health-care expenditures by reimbursement based on 'diagnostic related groups' (DRGs, a system for grouping medical conditions on the basis of average costs) will be under scrutiny and will be frequently changed and updated. The ability of private insurers to accept a greater portion of the burden of long-term care costs will depend on the willingness of healthy middle-aged people to begin to pay increased premiums earlier in life.

Because of the 'capping' of Federal health expenditures, new health industries, such as home health care, respite care, and hospice care, are expanding, as is the traditional nursing home. These will all require regulation and a concerted effort to maintain professionalism in the rapidly emerging world of commercial enterprise. To this end, at the University of Illinois at Chicago, we have developed a gerontology programme which confers a Masters degree in Public Health and a Masters in Business Administration. There is an urgent need, and a deep responsibility, to use professionally trained administrators in guiding these entrepreneurial health-related ventures.

Finally, there is a great need for Medicare and other government health spending to be taken out of the budgetary cycle within the United States and placed in a non-political and sheltered category, as is Social Security. It is necessary that citizens force congressional action in order to preserve the sense of security and well-being in our growing elderly and ageing population.

Conclusions

The word 'needs' is ambiguous, but useful. We shall surely have more older people, they will surely be living more years, and their needs will be greater than those of older people in past years. Thus, we are placing more people in the high need/high risk/high utilization category. The phenomenon of having more people living longer, and of the elderly themselves experiencing an increase in life expectancy, has not been witnessed before in the history of humankind. Measurements of trends in health among the elderly have produced, at best, equivocal data. It is not logical that people would be living longer if, at each given age, they were not healthier in some way. This, however, begs the critical quantitative question: are we providing enough years of healthy, active life expectancy to offset the increased years of compromised health? It appears that there has been a modest improvement, or at least a stationary pattern, in terms of health trends, but the quality of life shows no dramatic increase in improved years late in life. Variability among older people must be recognized, and it is clear that the majority of people live actively and independently into their ninth and tenth decades, while simultaneously an increasing percentage of people are surviving prolonged periods of disability and loss of autonomy. Since the elderly are getting older and more numerous, and major breakthroughs are not apparent, the needs of this population will increase and will be confounded by the fact that the family size is shrinking and the usual support-givers, particularly women, are now in the work force. Between 1940 and 1979, the proportion of employed married women rose from 11 to over 55% (Brody & Schoonover 1986).

With Dr Schneider, I have described a dichotomy in diseases associated with ageing (Brody & Schneider 1986). Many diseases and conditions are what we define as age related, in that they occur at a specific time in life but are not dependent on the progressive ageing of the subject. These diseases include multiple sclerosis, amyotrophic lateral sclerosis, schizophrenia, and probably most cancers. They occur at a certain age in life and, therefore, if you survive the critical years, you will not contract that particular age-related disease or disorder. Age-dependent diseases appear to be more closely related to the specific ageing of the individual and these diseases continue to increase exponentially with age, as does mortality. Such diseases include cardiovascular disease, cerebrovascular disease, type II diabetes, hip fracture, blindness, deafness, arthritis, and probably Alzheimer's disease and related disorders. Medical research will gradually move us through the age-related conditions and diseases and, increasingly, we shall be suffering and dying from age-dependent diseases and conditions.

Age-dependent diseases are the result of gradually diminishing organ, cellular or bodily functions and, hence, specific cures and treatment offer limited promise. We shall be in an arena where age and multiple diseases and conditions predominate and where postponement of morbidity by interventions by research methods intended to delay body ageing, or by modification of health habits and diet, will be our great allies. The need, therefore, is to identify those age-dependent diseases and conditions which produce the greatest hardship and cost and pursue them from the point of view of postponement and palliation rather than cure.

Trends in health care are in a dynamic and transitional phase. Financial limits are being imposed and we certainly lack a clearly formulated national health policy. I do not find this alarming in an historic sense, and perhaps it actually leaves us in a position of greater flexibility than is found in other developed countries for seeking intelligent and just solutions. I say this because, in the US, we are not doing badly, relative to the rest of the world, in the measurable aspects of the health and well-being of elderly populations. Data available up to 1980 (we are attempting to collect newer data) indicate that, in the US, life expectancy at age 65 is greater for women than for any other country in the world and, for men, is exceeded only by Norway, Sweden and Israel (Siegel & Davidson 1984). While this could easily change, the elderly in the US are at least comparable with those of other industrial nations. Thus, there is no simple government policy or intervention which produces markedly better results. Our need is to determine the best practical steps to take in each situation.

There is little doubt that we are rapidly producing a new political will for more creative and equitable decisions affecting the mental and physical health of the elderly. This new energy is derived from the fact that health-care givers, politicians, and indeed, most decision makers now have first-hand (and will increasingly have more first-hand) exposure to the good and bad involved in an increasingly ageing society. The greater our familiarity with problems such as arthritis and dementia, and the anxieties of living alone, and the filling out of forms to secure payment and quality care, the greater becomes the likelihood that we shall find better solutions.

References

Boyce WJ, Vessey MP 1985 Rising incidence of fracture of the proximal femur. Lancet 1:150–151

Brody EM, Schoonover MA 1986 Patterns of parent-care when adult daughters work and when they do not. Gerontologist 26:372–381

Brody JA 1982 An epidemiologist views senile dementia — facts and fragments. Am J Epidemiol 115:155–163

Brody JA 1985 Prospects for an ageing population. Nature (Lond) 315:463–466

Brody JA 1987 The best of times/the worst of times: aging and dependency in the 21st century. In: Ingman SR, Engelhart HT Jr (eds) Philosophy and medicine. D Reidel Publishing, Boston, Mass./Dordrecht, Holland

Brody JA, Schneider EL 1986 Diseases and disorders of aging: an hypothesis. J Chronic Dis 39:871–876

Brody JA, Brock DB, Williams TF 1987 Trends in the health of the elderly population. Annu Rev Public Health 8

DHHS 1985 Current estimates from the national interview survey, United States, 1982. In: National Center for Health Statistics, DHHS Publication No. (PHS) 85–1578. US Government Printing Office, Washington DC

Dickson P 1978 The official rules. Dell Publishing Co, New York

Guralnik JM, Brock DB, Brody JA 1987 The changing demography of the elderly in the United States. In: Carid FI, Evans JG (eds) Topics in advanced geriatric medicine. John Wright, Bristol, UK

Melton LJ, Ilstrup DM, Riggs BL, Beckenbaugh RD 1982 Fifty-year trend in hip fracture incidence. Clin Orthop 162:144–149

Schneider EL, Brody JA 1983 Aging, natural death and the compression of morbidity: another view. N Engl J Med 309:854–856

Siegel JS, Davidson M 1984 Current population reports: demographic socioeconomic aspects of aging in the United States. Bureau of the Census, US Dept of Commerce, Series P-23 No. 138, Washington DC

Waldo DR, Lazenby HC 1984 Demographic characteristics and health care use and expenditures by the aged in the United States: 1977–1984. Health Care Financing Review 6:1–20

Wilkins R, Adams OB 1983 Health expectancy in Canada, late 1970s: demographic, regional, and social dimensions. Am J Public Health 73:1073–1080

Zetterberg C, Elmerson S, Anderson GBJ 1984 Epidemiology of hip fractures in Göteborg, Sweden, 1940–1983. Clin Orthop 191:43–52

DISCUSSION*

Svanborg: The methodology of making comparisons of longevity is sometimes complicated. A few years ago, in collaboration with Japanese epidemiologists and gerontologists, we compared Japan and Sweden and confirmed what others had shown, namely that the registration of stillborn children is not the same in the two countries. In Japan a considerably higher proportion of stillborn children are reported than in Sweden. If a child takes just a few

---

* Dr Brody's paper was presented by Dr L. R. White, in Dr Brody's absence through illness.

breaths after birth, it is registered as having been born alive in Sweden, but apparently not always so in Japan. In order to compare the effect of this difference in birth recording we calculated the 'extreme' effects of such a registration difference. If the total infant mortality for boys in Sweden were reduced to zero, male longevity would have increased by only 0.6 years. From such calculations we concluded that although there is a difference in the registration of stillborn children, the Japanese have indeed passed Sweden in longevity.

Let me also comment on the estimation of further life expectancy. Further life expectancy in old age obviously reflects mortality earlier in the life of the cohort. More and more people are allowed to live a long life. During the past years in Sweden, three out of four women who died were 73 years old or more, and three of four men dying were 67 or more. This also implies that more and more frail people approach old age, which must have a negative effect on further life expectancy. Earlier they would have died before, say, age 70; now they are helped, through medical resources, to live further and beyond that age. It is fascinating to see that although this group of frail individuals is within the cohorts of 70-year-olds, the further life expectancy at age 70 and 75 is generally increasing in Sweden, in both men and women.

T.F. Williams: A concept that, at least in the USA, has been accepted very rapidly is the distinction between 'active' and 'dependent' life expectancy. However, there are problems in defining this difference in a reproducibly useable way. I wonder whether people in other countries see it as a major issue to distinguish for how much of our later years we will be dependent, imposing a burden of care on others. There is much debate here, but virtually no evidence, on what direction this trend is taking. The pessimistic view is that with more people, and no likely change in 'dependent life expectancy', we shall have more people with longer periods of dependence. Others say that we shall reduce that dependency by means of advances in science and medicine.

Fries: The question is whether we are able to increase the age at which morbidity begins to occur more rapidly than life expectancy increases. It is useful here to look at absolute figures for changes in life expectancy from different ages. It is illuminating to know that above age 100, for example, over the last 20 years in the USA we have had only a three-month increase in life expectancy, whereas from about age 60 the increase has been around 30 months (Fries 1987).

Let me reiterate my earlier point on the change that probably happened in most developed countries around 1975–1980, when large decreases in the major morbid events (cardiovascular disease, lung cancer) began to occur. It is therefore difficult to speak meaningfully about the present situation using data which end in 1979 or 1981. The current data will be the interesting ones, but they are obviously not yet available.

Two lines of evidence are relevant here. One has to do with the question of whether changes in, say, lung cancer and cardiovascular disease mortality have been changes in the incidence of the diseases or changes in survival. All the data show that the change mostly has been in incidence, so the disease is occurring later, both for myocardial infarction and for lung cancer.

The second point is that evidence from the randomized controlled trials which have looked prospectively for what we could accomplish by lifestyle interventions demonstrates that we will get better results in terms of improved morbidity, rather than mortality (for example, in the LRC or MRFIT studies: Fries 1987). This suggests to me that present and future trends (as we are coming around some kind of a corner) will be positive ones in terms of morbidity.

Katzman: Of the diseases we have discussed, osteoporosis and hip fracture seem to be the most likely to follow cardiovascular disease in declining incidence rate. If we hypothesize that the rate of, say, hip fracture will fall by 50% as a result of preventive measures, is it possible to project the effect that this will have both on life expectancy as such, and on *active* life expectancy?

Riggs: With the best medical care, hip fracture has a 12–20% mortality, whereas with poorer care, it increases to 50%, so there is the potential for an absolute increase in lifespan. The major effect of the successful prevention of osteoporosis, however, will be on morbidity. So often, a hip fracture turns a self-sufficient woman into a woman confined to a nursing home and dependent upon others. While there will be some reduction in mortality if osteoporosis is prevented, I expect the major benefit to be a reduction of morbidity.

Wenger: One factor to consider as we investigate dependent and independent life expectancy will be societal differences. We can expect to see differences among countries, and also differences between urban and rural communities, in what constitutes the ability to live alone or to live with one's family; or the choice of whether the elderly return as part of the family unit, or remain independent. This will vary among different societal patterns, so that comparability in numbers may not be true comparability, simply because of different patterns of relationships of the elderly to younger groups.

My major concern is that we have done the same things for the elderly as we have for other populations, and that very little of the planning derives from the elderly population in question. So many recommendations, plans and perceptions are ours, rather than being the perceptions and choices of the affected population. In the USA, at least, surveys have not gone beyond reporting what is the case to reporting what the individuals concerned would personally like to have be the case. I am uncertain that we are correct in our projections of what should be done for an elderly population; certainly there are many elderly individuals in the very active, the moderately active, and the semi-dependent but still alert groups, from whom we should determine what each of these populations want. Otherwise we risk imposing our value system on a population who may have a relatively different set of values.

Mor: When the Older Americans Resource Survey was designed (Fillenbaum & Smyer 1981), one aim was to take successive cross-sectional random samples of elderly people over the decades and to see whether there is a shift in the distribution of functional disabilities or dependencies. It is now increasingly possible to do this, despite the problems of definitions. My suspicion is that random sample surveys of the elderly today, age-adjusted to those of 1975, might reveal less functional impairment per age group than previously. It is now possible to examine this.

Andrews: It seems to me that longevity is a very rich area for comparative studies, particularly between developing countries, where the greatest changes may be taking place in life expectancy. Getting 'a fix' on that and on morbidity and dependency in such circumstances could teach us a great deal. As an aside, I was startled to see, from the officially recorded figures for Pakistan, that this is the one country where it appears that males enjoy a greater life expectancy at birth than females. That may however reflect a problem in the way the figures are collected, rather than any inherent factor.

Svanborg: As a methodological comment, when we make international comparisons we have to be aware that age groups may differ in their average age. In our comparison of 70–75-year-olds in Japan and Sweden, we found that Japanese 70–75-year-olds were significantly younger than the 70–75-year-old Swedes. In some comparisons (Mellström et al 1982) we had to go down below one-year age groups in order to eliminate differences in chronological age.

T.F. Williams: Dr Brody and Dr Schneider (1986) have distinguished between age-related and age-dependent diseases, where the age-dependent group includes some of the most common diseases, such as cardiovascular disease and dementia. It seems to me that their concept of age-related disease is rather sensible, but do we want to consider these other conditions as age dependent?

Fries: I agree with that distinction. I call them the 'Gompertzian' and the 'non-Gompertzian' diseases, which is basically the same distinction (Fries 1984). Conditions like rheumatoid arthritis, Hodgkin's disease and multiple sclerosis are mid-life diseases which are not Gompertzian in their incidence patterns, although they sometimes are in their mortality patterns. That is, their incidence rates do not increase exponentially with age. By contrast, all the solid tumours, atherosclerosis and osteoarthritis are Gompertzian and incidence increases exponentially. The distinction I make is that the 'medical' model of disease is more likely to hold for the non-Gompertzian, age-related diseases. In other words, these are not universal diseases; people appear to 'catch' them; they probably have causative pathogens or environmental precipitants of some kind. To me, the research 'imperative' for the non-Gompertzian diseases is much like that for acute diseases, whereas the imperative for the age-dependent diseases is prevention, because they have long presymptomatic periods where one might affect the rate of accumulation of pathology.

Grimley Evans: I am dubious about Schneider & Brody's distinction, because it seems to be the dichotomy between ageing and disease re-emerging under other names. My objections are, first, that the concept of 'age-related' diseases postulates that they have something to do with specific exposures. However, Burch (1968) showed that you can construct several models which give that type of 'rising and falling' curve, including the 'using up' of a genetically susceptible group. I am also not sure how bimodal diseases, like chronic inflammatory bowel disease and Guillain-Barré syndrome, would be accommodated in an age-related model.

I also wonder about the distinction between Gompertzian and non-Gompertzian diseases. Adult cancers do not follow an exponential (Gompertzian) incidence curve; they follow a power law curve (Doll 1971). If you consider mortality, you have two components, an incidence effect and a fatality effect, which determine the final pattern. So I fear that the models based on mortality may mislead us.

White: It seems to me that the distinction noted by Schneider and Brody between age-related and age-dependent diseases is both conceptually interesting and operationally useful. Even as a tautology, the idea has value for organizing our thoughts. It also has operational value in terms of how we do research. In cardiovascular disease, most of the epidemiological research has focused on end-points, such as angina or myocardial infarction; that is, specific precipitated events. But we have been looking mostly at risk factors which are more directly associated with the continuous underlying disease process, the accumulation of atherosclerotic lesions in the vessels. In arthritis the continuous underlying process is an accumulation of damage to cartilage. In the lens it is the accumulation of cross-linked proteins that fail to transmit light. Perhaps the classification of diseases in late life proposed by Schneider and Brody serves to focus our attention on these diseases which are primarily the result of such continuous and relentless processes; and perhaps this focus will lead us to a better understanding of how different diseases of ageing may be related one to another.

This line of thought leads me to conclude that the research epidemiologist interested in the diseases of ageing must develop better methods for the study of such disease processes. We need to deal with the onset and slope of the curve which eventually takes us to the point when a disease event becomes highly probable. Depending on the disease, the curve may reflect a continuous loss of neuronal cells, or of cartilaginous elasticity, or of the elasticity of the aorta, or light transmission through the lens, or bone mineralization. When we have methods to define these slopes in people who are 35, 45 or 50 as end-points in epidemiological research, perhaps we can develop methods that bear directly on the pathogeneses of these 'age-dependent' diseases in a way which will lead to more rational preventive measures.

References

Brody JA, Schneider EL 1986 Diseases and disorders of aging: an hypothesis. J Chronic Dis 39:871–876

Burch PRJ 1968 An inquiry concerning growth, disease and ageing. Oliver & Boyd, Edinburgh

Doll R 1971 The age distribution of cancer: implications for models of carcinogenesis. J R Statist Soc Ser A 134:133–155

Fillenbaum GG, Smyer MA 1981 The development, validity and reliability of the OARS multidimensional functional assessment questionnaire. J Gerontol 36:428–434

Fries JF 1984 The compression of morbidity, Benjamin Gompertz, the two types of chronic disease, and health policy. In: Forum Proc; Exploring new frontiers of US health policy. UMDNJ–Rutgers Medical School, New Jersey

Fries JF 1987 Aging, illness, and health policy: implications of the compression of morbidity. Perspect Biol Med, in press

Mellström D, Nilsson Å, Odén A, Rundgren Å, Svanborg A 1982 Mortality among the widowed in Sweden. Scand J Soc Med 10:33–41

Planning for health services for the elderly

Carel F. Hollander* and Henk A. Becker†

*Department of Safety Assessment, Centre de Recherche, Laboratoires Merck, Sharp & Dohme-Chibret, B.P. 134, 63200 Riom Cédex, France and †Department of Social Science, Research Unit on Planning and Policymaking, University of Utrecht, 1 Heidelberglaan, 3508 TC Utrecht, The Netherlands

Abstract. In order to create health services that effectively respond to the changing picture of health, governments should try to anticipate the health needs for the future. The scenarios for the elderly that are briefly discussed in this paper are approximations of developments that are largely autonomous if considered from the position of the individuals and organizations responsible for policies on health and health services. The three contextual scenarios developed are based on the forecasts, explorations and speculations to be found in the literature and also on the outcome of discussions with groups of experts in the fields of medical, biological and technological research and practice. The following variables have been incorporated in the study preparing the scenarios: demographic developments, the health status of the elderly, health services for the elderly, developments in medical, biological and technological fields, and societal developments, both economic and social. These scenarios provide policy makers with a learning environment in which they can test the strategies that are considered to answer the questions that they face, and evaluate the particular circumstances in which these strategies might be feasible.

1988 Research and the ageing population. Wiley, Chichester (Ciba Foundation Symposium 134) p 221–234

Health and disease by the year 2000 will be quite different from health and disease in 1984 or 1985. In order to create health services that respond effectively to the changing picture of health, governments should try to anticipate the health needs of the future.

In the Netherlands there is current interest in applying the context scenario technique (Becker et al 1986, Schnaars 1987) to the long-term planning for health services up to the year 2000. For this purpose the Steering Committee on Future Health Scenarios (STG) was set up in 1983 by the State Secretary of Welfare, Health and Cultural Affairs. The Committee's chief task is to create alternative pictures of possible and desirable developments in the field of public health and health care. An important part of its work is to complete 'scenarios'.

The scenarios for the elderly to be briefly discussed here have been pub-lished in the report 'Growing Old in the Future' (1987) and are approxima-tions of developments that are to a large degree autonomous, if considered from the position of individuals and organizations that are responsible for policies on health and the health services in the Netherlands. They have been developed by the Scenario Committee on Ageing. The Chairman and its members are appointed by the STG in a personal capacity. Attached to the Committee is a research team consisting of experts in the relevant fields as well as experts in scenario research.

Methodology

The idea of compiling scenarios as a method of forecasting future develop-ments was first developed in California in the early 1950s by the Rand Corporation and similar think-tanks for military strategic purposes.

The Scenario Committee on Ageing consists of eight experts in the areas of health services for the aged, health economics, epidemiology, sociology and medical–biological research on ageing. The assisting research team consists of members of the Department of Social Science, Research Unit on Planning and Policymaking, Universty of Utrecht.

The two main questions addressed were the following:

What (future) developments will exert most influence on the health of the elderly in the Netherlands in the period 1984–2000?

In view of the future health situation of the elderly and their increasing share in the population in the Netherlands, what are the possible patterns of (health) care services in the period 1984–2000?

The first question relates to developments which to a large extent take place autonomously in present-day health care. The second question also serves to define the limits of the project.

A scenario is defined as 'a description of the present situation of the society (or part of it), of possible or desirable future situations of this society, as well as of series of events deriving from the present situation which could bring about those future situations'. The scenarios presented focus on 'possible future situations'. They are the most important possible 'contexts' within which (health) care services will be realized in the Netherlands until the year 2000.

The areas in which autonomous changes to be anticipated can be summa-rized in the diagram shown in Fig. 1. As can be seen, not only demographic (population) changes but also future changes in health and disease will exert influences on 'demand'. On the other side, when dealing with the problems of the elderly, one has also to take into consideration future changes in health

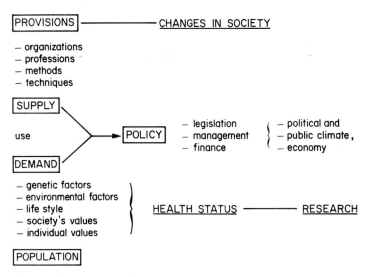

FIG. 1.   Areas of autonomous developments incorporated into the context scenarios presented to policy makers. (Modified from van Duyne 1984.)

service provisions (i.e., organizations, professions, methods and techniques) as well as social changes. Also, future economic profiles cannot be omitted. The arrow in the diagram depicts the flow of information to be incorporated into the context scenarios to be presented to the policy makers for use in their exercise in preparing long-term health strategies for dealing with the problems of the elderly.

Results and discussion

After several rounds of designing, adapting and redesigning, three context scenarios were developed (Growing Old in the Future 1987):

A reference scenario containing developments resulting in about the same pressure on health services for the elderly as at present. In this scenario, the situation of 1984 is extrapolated towards 2000. With regard to the economic aspects, 0.6% economic growth per year is assumed, and if associated with a financial redistribution in the public sector will permit a continuation of the budgets for health services at the level of 1984. This scenario is so designed that the other two scenarios can be contrasted with it.

A scenario containing developments resulting in more pressure on health services — that is, a growth scenario. This scenario presents a development in which demand for health services grows more than could be expected on the basis of the calculations in the reference scenario. The health situation of the elderly will be affected by the increasing pressure on the health services. Professional and commercial assistance may improve, especially for the well-to-do elderly. Self-reliance is poor, however, and social isolation predominant. In this scenario the developments are seen as characteristic of a type of society in which achievement, labour productivity and attachment to material assets are central values.

A scenario containing developments resulting in less pressure on health services — that is, a 'shrinkage' scenario. This scenario is characterized by a decrease in the demand for health services as a result of a change in attitudes toward health and disease, lifestyles and socioeconomic position. The most important trend which in this scenario determines the decreasing pressure on services is thus not the (improved) state of health of the elderly, but changes in the conception of care.

The scenarios show some degree of deliberate over-emphasis of characteristic aspects which is typical of the scenario technique.

After consultations with 30 specialists in the fields of medicine, biomedical and technical research, it was decided to keep these areas identical to all three scenarios, because a period of 15 years or so is thought to be too short to envisage any major breakthroughs in these areas that will have a major impact on both health and health services. However, consideration has been given to issues such as the influence on the health status of the elderly of developments in medicine which will cure or prevent diseases at a younger age, as well as the influence of the so-called 'double greying' — that is, the increase in the proportion of the 'old elderly' (80 years or above). Furthermore, future changes in lifestyle may well have a dramatic influence. For instance, if the lung cancer incidence rate in women continues to rise in future as it has in recent years (Janerich 1984), and is associated with a decline in mortality from cardiac disease in males and a possible increase in females (The Heart of the Future 1987), the result would be a diminution in the difference in life expectancy which exists between females and males. This, in turn, would have an important influence on the health service provisions. A major question addressed is the extent to which chronic diseases will be curable in the 1990s and beyond, or whether society will be faced with an increasing proportion of disabled, dependent elderly people. Also, the long-term consequences of future developments in modern (bio)electronics, which may enable us to deal more effectively and efficiently with some of the handicaps of the elderly, have been addressed. Developments in the pharmaceutical industry and their possible influence have been scrutinized. As already mentioned, because no further breakthroughs in medical science are envisaged in the immediate future by the relevant experts, it was decided not to formulate alternatives for the variables 'medicine, biomedical and technical research' in the scenarios, but to treat them as a single unvarying context.

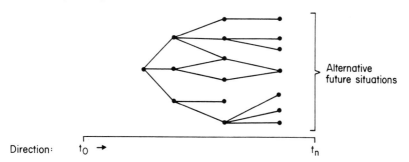

FIG. 2. Exploratory or context scenario development, starting from the present situation (to the left).

Two disturbing developments, namely the potential impact of a postponement of the onset of senile dementia of the Alzheimer type and of a further decrease in inter-generational solidarity, with the result that children are no longer prepared to care for elderly parents, have been added to enhance the realism of the 'learning environment'. In both instances an estimate has been made of the resulting increase or decrease in the demand for facilities if these developments should come about. Also, the cross-impact of the autonomous developments described in the three scenarios, and three potential patterns of health services, has been analysed. These are: maintaining the present course; 'top' care in a strictly medical and medical-technological sense; and moving towards a reciprocal-aid society — that is, a society in which the elderly are stimulated to manage for themselves, to keep themselves occupied, as well as to assist each other and participate actively in society. In the last situation, health-care facilities shift their priorities in such a way that 'care' receives somewhat more attention than at present. The third option would stand a chance if the state of the art of planned social changes were taken seriously, and if a major effort were made, on the basis of the knowledge available, to induce changes in the social conditions of the elderly.

Context scenarios, as described here, provide management decision makers with 'a learning environment' in which to test their strategies for the future. By confronting decision makers or policy makers with alternative future situations (Fig. 2) which are more or less favourable, it is easier to foresee the effects of a new policy, especially if decision makers use the target-setting scenario technique (Fig. 3), in which one begins with the desired future objectives.

The impact of the 'scenario study on ageing' on policy developments since the publication of its preliminary and final reports (in Dutch) can be summarized as follows. Two policy memoranda have been published since the scenario study's preliminary report was issued. These memoranda show that the study has had a major impact, but it is still too early to know whether or

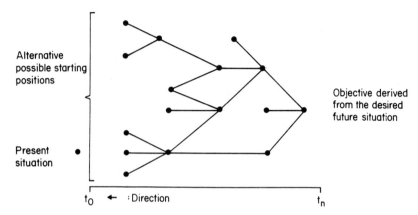

FIG. 3.   Target-setting scenario development, establishing the objectives to be obtained (to the right) and starting from alternative possible positions, including the
present situation (to the left). This technique provides clues for making decisions and
clarifying the consequences of alternatives.

not its recommendations will be taken up. In this context it is worth noting
that there is a difference in the application of the scenario technique in the
health field and in industry. Generally speaking, industry has well-defined
targets in the form of a concern with profits and a unitary power structure
within management, and the variables involved are fewer. Among other
things, this makes the implementation of the outcome of scenario studies in
industry easier than in the health field, where there are more actors involved
(including government, politicians, and organizations of professionals and of
patients). However, it is felt that much can be learned from the way scenario
techniques are currently being used in industry, as discussed at the STG/
WHO Workshop 'Scenarios and methods to support long-term health planning' held in Noordwijk, The Netherlands, in October 1986 (unpublished).

Conclusions

The scenarios for the elderly have made clear that the health (care) policy of
the Netherlands will have to be prepared for a wide range of autonomous
developments. Only in a few areas — especially demographic developments
— is it possible to make forecasts which are sufficiently reliable and precise to
serve as an unambiguous basis for policy. The expected autonomous developments call for a strategy which can survive reversals and leaves scope for the
necessary adjustments in the course of implementation until the year 2000. In
order to obtain such a flexible policy, a system of monitoring — following
developments with the aid of social indicators — and an 'early warning

system' — the early recognition of reversals or new trends in the autonomous developments — have recently been installed. The scenarios do not provide an unambiguous recommendation on the choice of a pattern of health-care facilities for the elderly. However, they provide clues for making these choices and they clarify the consequences of alternatives. It is believed that they will assist in establishing the long-term strategy for health care for the elderly.

It should be stressed that the emphasis of this scenario project was on delineating different possible futures rather than on predicting what the future course of events should be, and that a key component was thus a careful consideration of likely or possible future developments that were not reflected in the present situation or in past trends. It is still too early to evaluate the outcome of this project. However, it seems to be extremely important that good relationships between planning and management and between the planning process and the political decision-making process exist. It is also too early to assess the transferability of methods and results between countries. This aspect should be addressed in the future. In the workshop held in Noordwijk, it was felt that the World Health Organization could play a useful role in this field.

Acknowledgements

The authors are respectively chairman (C.F.H.) of the Scenario Committee on Ageing and co-ordinator (H.A.B.) of the Research Team; however, this article has been written in a personal capacity. The authors wish to thank their colleagues in the Committee and Research Team for their valuable discussions and Miss G. Pouyet for preparing the manuscript. Dr Ch.O. Pannenborg has kindly provided Figs. 2 and 3.

References

Becker HA, Klaassen-van den Berg Jeths A, Kraan-Jetten A, van Rijsselt R 1986 Contextual scenarios on the elderly and their health in the Netherlands. In: Becker HA, Porter AL (eds) Methods and experiences in impact assessment. Impact Assessment Bulletin vol 4 no. 3/4:15–48

Growing Old in the Future. Scenarios on health and ageing 1984–2000 1987 Hollander CF, Becker HA (eds) Martinus Nijhoff Publishers, Dordrecht, Boston & Amsterdam

Janerich DT 1984 Forecasting cancer trends to optimize control strategies. J Natl Cancer Inst 72:1317–1321

Schnaars SP 1987 How to develop and use scenarios. Long Range Planning 20:122–131

The Heart of the Future. The Future of the Heart. Scenarios on Cardiovascular Diseases 1985–2010 1987 Volume 1. Scenario-report 1986. Dunning AJ, Wils WIM (eds) Martinus Nijhoff Publishers, Dordrecht, Boston & Amsterdam

van Duyne WMJ 1984 Gezondheidszorg vergt meer wetenschappelijk onderzoek. TNO-project 12, p 52–53

DISCUSSION

T.F. Williams: The National Institute on Aging, working with other Federal agencies, is taking a somewhat similar approach to yours in a report to the US Congress on needs for personnel for the care of older people to the year 2020. We have taken in effect three different scenarios, based on assumptions about health-care needs over this period. One is a straight-line projection in relation to what we already know will be the population changes. We have also taken a projection based on optimistic views of what could be accomplished by improving people's health, and a pessimistic course, and have tried to estimate what the needs for health personnel will be in all three cases. All this is based on assumptions, but it seems to me that we have obligations to try to develop such alternative views.

Wenger: Dr Hollander's approach is a fascinating one. In the public response to the scenarios, were particular segments of the public over-represented or under-represented—or could you tell?

Hollander: The problem is that the elderly themselves are under-represented in the response. In the Netherlands, moreover, they are usually represented by the 'elderly organizations' and by young staff members, usually with a background in areas such as sociology. One can ask how well the young can speak for elderly people. Also, the elderly are not a homogeneous group. There were indeed elderly people, of a better educational level, who expressed their views on the scenarios very strongly.

Andrews: There is a fundamental problem with the representation of elderly people in these debates, because if we are considering the year 2020, say, the views of the elderly today are not really relevant, in terms of their attitudes, aspirations and desires. Then there is a question of whether those who will be elderly in 2020 are capable now of expressing a valid view about what their needs are likely to be by then. I don't know any simple solution to that problem. You probably need to have a mix of views across a range of ages, and to recognize that it isn't possible to obtain a valid consumer perspective.

Hollander: You are right. This is one reason, also, why scenarios tend to over-emphasize certain points, in order to provoke responses.

A. Williams: I have had experience of similar exercises to your scenarios. One important point is how scenarios are used. If they are used in a mechanical way, and one of the scenarios is chosen as 'the target', and the indicated steps in it are taken as 'a plan', that is disastrous. We don't know enough about the world to be able to operate like that! The correct use of scenarios is to identify those features which, on almost any scenario, are going to give trouble; these need to be worked on for 5–10 years, because it takes a long time to bring about any change, monitoring change as you go along. Often the scenarios will also lead you to see what you need to monitor more carefully, because the usual problem is that the information needed isn't there and you are guessing wildly about things which should have been known. So the scenarios direct attention to the need to monitor more closely certain trends in society that would not otherwise have been given much attention.

Picking up Gary Andrews' point, this isn't so much a problem for the elderly; it's a problem for the whole society. It is a mistake to concentrate on the views of the elderly, because how much of our resources will be made available for them depends on the attitudes of the *other* members of society. Although some representation of the views of elderly people is obviously required, it is a matter for the whole of the society to think through.

Hollander: This is right. The Dutch government is trying to evaluate the different scenarios, but people then have to make their choices. It is also true that the present elderly will be phasing out in this period, and the future elderly, from whom we need to get responses, generally don't want to look ahead in that way.

Mor: Today's elderly may reflect some of the attitudes of what tomorrow's elderly might be, because those who will be old in 2010 may have different attitudes from those they currently hold, 20 or 30 years from now, precisely as a function of ageing.

Wallack: As a general point, it strikes me that we are all struggling with the large, long-term trends that Dr Hollander discussed, and whether they will make sense when they play out over time. Our willingness to accept the scenarios requires believable behavioural assumptions and the inclusion of adjustments to unacceptable trends or outcomes. It's analogous to the decline of Keynesian economics. Keynes pointed out the importance of investment driving the overall level of economic activity, but he had no explanation at the individual level of what really determined investment. As a result, Keynesian macroeconomic theory fell into disrepute in the USA. That is, the theory failed because of this inability to link macro and microeconomics. This comes back to the behavioural relationships that we don't understand. Yet, if we don't understand them, we are likely to make bad mistakes in the development of scenarios.

I helped make projections for the US government on, for example, the needs for physicians, nurses, and hospital beds. We were always seriously off in our projections, because we lacked good behavioural models. It is interesting to analyse our surplus estimates for nurses of a few years ago in relation to the shortage of nurses that we are now facing. The significant shift from a large surplus to a large deficit occurred because we didn't build into the projection of nursing supply an understanding of their response to relative wage rates, of expanding opportunities, and so on. Therefore, it is crucial, as we explore these scenarios, to identify the key behavioural relationships that lie behind them. If not, your projections are likely to be in error. Models need to build in adjustments as well.

Hollander: This is why the exercise was not terminated when the first scenario project was published. It is being continuously monitored, for changes in societal values, and for autonomous developments—such as in health, salaries and wages.

Arie: I would like to mention two extreme scenarios which we should consider. I would like to know how far their potential effects have been calculated.

One scenario is the abandonment of cigarette smoking, which seems to me to be possible now. There could be major shifts in political will that would drastically reduce or even eliminate smoking. And of course, unlike many of the risk factors that we have discussed, tobacco smoking is an adventitious activity that could go out even as it came in; for much of the history of the human race, it wasn't there. This is different from alcohol, for drinking fermented liquors is an almost universal part of human behaviour, except where there are specific religious vetos. If smoking went out as a habit, what would this mean for mortality and morbidity for the elderly, in the present context? We might even expect some deleterious effects, in that it has been suggested that smoking may even protect against some diseases, for instance Parkinson's disease. Has anyone made those calculations?

The other scenario to be considered seriously is that the AIDS epidemic gets totally out of hand. These two seem to be extreme scenarios that could be realized. What thinking has been done about them?

A. Williams: Joy Townsend (1987) observed that in Britain between 1980 and 1984 the price of cigarettes rose by 26% in *real* terms, while consumption of cigarettes fell by 20% in volume terms (of which about half was due to the price increase), yet government revenue from tobacco taxes rose by 10%. And as the tobacco industry is relatively capital intensive, employing only 22 000 people in the UK, there is unlikely to be a major problem absorbing the workforce as it slowly becomes redundant. The companies themselves are already widely diversified into other sectors. Other studies have suggested that the higher pension costs due to the greater longevity associated with less cigarette smoking are more or less offset by the reduction in morbidity costs. So, all in all, the economic and financial consequences are minor, and quite sustainable. It is the health consequences that should dominate the discussion.

White: Predictions of the public health benefits that will follow a change in the rates of exposure to something like smoking involve calculations of age-specific attributable risk. The results may be expressed in terms of reductions in pulmonary and cardiovascular mortality. Sometimes the predicted reductions are large; more often they seem disappointingly small.

Fries: Dorothy Rice has made an economic analysis of the impact of smoking (Rice et al 1986). Smoking appears to account for about 1.2 years of life expectancy, and all cardiovascular diseases perhaps 2–3 years. The estimates depends on the 'competing-risk' model used, and even these estimates are probably high, because there is no 'senescence' term in the usual competing-risk models and such a term will provide a certain amount of additional mortality in the prediction.

Svanborg: The World Health Organization has published figures on lung cancer and the increased risk of myocardial infarction associated with smoking. We also have evidence that smoking accelerates the rate of ageing and has other general consequences for functional performance and the need for health care.

Katzman: This relates to what I was asking about hip fracture. Supposing that we did eliminate smoking and that there were fewer heart attacks and fewer cases of lung cancer, one could draw up a scenario in which people would have a longer life expectancy, there would be many more elderly people developing dementia, so you would need a vastly increased number of nursing-home beds. Has this kind of calculation been done?

Arie: This is exactly what I am asking!

T.F. Williams: Dementia is certainly an epidemic of comparable proportions to AIDS, posing as much of a major public health problem.

Hollander: We considered the postponement of the onset of Alzheimer's disease by a couple of years, and re-calculated all the data for health-care provisions. We found that these did not change much.

Svanborg: We need to be aware of the difficulty of differentiating clearly between different forms of organic brain disorder. We know that multi-infarction dementia patients have considerably shorter lives than the rest of the population, but our experience and that of others indicates that those with an Alzheimer type of dementia live much longer than those with multi-infarction dementia. Before we can make realistic scenarios in this field we need to know more about the differentiation of Alzheimer's dementia, multi-infarction dementia, brain damage due to alcohol abuse, and so on.

Hollander: In the Netherlands we lack good data on the incidence of Alzheimer's disease. If one uses the best data available and calculates the effects of a postponement by five years, one finds that part of the population shifts from a nursing home for the psychiatrically disturbed elderly to a nursing home for the somatically disabled elderly, and that partly clouds any gain anticipated in saving health guilders. We came to the conclusion that playing with separate disease entities, eradicating them, in our scenarios, doesn't change much, in the sense of planning for health provision.

Arie: The fact that no one has taken up the possibility of a 'doomsday' scenario for the spread of AIDS suggests that denial is operating here!

A. Williams: I am particularly interested in people's attitudes to their own health. We did a survey of 400 randomly selected members of the general public (so this is cross-sectional data), asking them to tell us about their current health and about the best possible health that they expected. Actual reported health was elicited by giving the respondents a visual analogue scale on which to draw a point somewhere between 'poor' and 'excellent'. Reported current health reached its lowest for the age group 55–64 and then rose. The last part of that rise is probably an artefact, because these were people in private house-holds, drawn from the electoral register; it therefore does not include the institutionalized population.

The interesting result was that the respondents' expectations about their best possible health were falling continually; they begin to fall from an early age. We then asked how satisfied people were with their health. Satisfaction was clearly related not to their actual current health, but to the gap between this and their expectations about what their health ought to be at their particular age. Where there was little discrepancy between the two, people are 'doing fine'; where the discrepancy increases, they 'do' much worse. Satisfaction with health conse-quently rises very sharply for the oldest group (over 74 years). It is not that they are fitter, but they are so pleased still to be here!

We separated out those who had never smoked, those who were ex-smokers and those who were current smokers. Remarkably different patterns of ex-pectation emerged. Among the current smokers, expectations about their health aren't much different from anybody else's, initially. Around age 35–44, expectations begin to diverge: by 45–54 they are significantly lower among current smokers, and they continue to fall. In old age, the people who are still smoking (of whom there are now relatively few) have very pessimistic views about their own future, and their reported health isn't good at that point, either.

So current smokers show a steady decline in expectations. The people who never smoked begin with high expectations, but these fall sharply after 55-64. Why should that be? This is in fact the age when people retire in the UK. There is a sharp drop then in expectations about their health which is not correlated with current health. It seems that retirement is a traumatic event in relation to expectations about what future health will be. That is something we perhaps need to work on. Employment is said to be an important source of self-esteem; it also seems to be important as an element in formulating one's expectations about health.

I regret that we didn't question the ex-smokers more than we did. We didn't ask why they gave up smoking, or how long ago it was; both pieces of informa-tion would have been useful. The ex-smokers have much the same expectations as the 'never smokers', until 45–54. In the next period, ex-smokers suffer a sharp drop in their expectations about their future best possible health, maybe because that is when smoking catches up with them; ten years before they are due to retire perhaps they begin to suffer ill health related to past smoking. The ex-smokers at later ages are much closer in their expectations to the 'never' smokers than to the current smokers; so the ex-smokers among the oldest age group have high expectations of their future health.

Andrews: Are those figures available separately for men and women?

A. Williams: Yes. Women who never smoked tail off much more steadily in the age range 45–74, and this is a good clue to the retirement element, because women don't retire in such a traumatic way (indeed some housewives might say they don't retire at all!).

Fox: If we compare the 1971 and 1981 censuses for England and Wales, there was in each case a simple question: 'were you working last week, and if not why not?' The categories of 'why not' included: temporarily sick but intending to seek work; seeking work; retired; permanently sick; housewife; student; and other. The proportion in the 'permanently sick' category trebled between 1971 and 1981. The level of unemployment in the UK was also three times as high in 1981. This suggests that the proportion of people referring to themselves as 'permanently sick' who previously would have been employed, even though they may have been in sheltered employment, in part fits in with the change you are seeing in people's perceptions of their health before and after retirement.

A. Williams: I have one other piece of information, which ties in with earlier discussion. We were anxious to find out at what stages in people's lives they value health most, because we must not assume that old age is the only time when there are health problems. We asked people to select the time in their lives when it was most important to be guaranteed good health, specifying various stages of life (infancy, starting school, starting work, setting up home for the first time, bringing up young children, the peak of one's earning power, looking after elderly relatives, having just retired from work, coping with the death of a husband or wife, and when getting very old). This recalls Tom Kirkwood's 'repair and maintenance' expenditures. In other words, our question might be seen as concerning the stage at which people should invest in repair and maintenance. The interesting point about the choices is that the most frequent first choice was 'when bringing up young children'; and this was the predominant reply at any age, and from both sexes. So it isn't a matter of self-interest. The interesting point was that 'when getting very old' was not the highest priority.

Arie: There must be considerable differences in the ranking of choices between different age groups of respondents?

A. Williams: There was a slight bias towards a self-interested response, but not very much, on that question. We asked a second question: 'when would *you* like most to be guaranteed good health?' The choice was usually an event in the decade they were in, or the next decade.

Wenger: Did you differentiate between those who were currently well and those who were ill?

A. Williams: No, but very few were ill, because they were all at home and able to answer the questionnaire.

Wenger: You might perhaps obtain a different response if you questioned a population that was not well, at different ages; this would sample their current experience, rather than their distant perceptions.

References

Rice DP, Hodgson TA, Sinsheimer P, Browner W, Kopstein AN 1986 The economic costs of the health effects of smoking. Milbank Mem Fund Q 64:489–547
Townsend J 1987 Economic and health consequences of smoking. In: Williams A (ed) Health and economics. Macmillan, London

The costs of long-term care: distribution and responsibility

Stanley S. Wallack and Marc A. Cohen

Bigel Institute for Health Policy, Heller Graduate School, Brandeis University, Waltham, Massachusetts, 02254, USA

Abstract. Long-term care costs will result in financial hardship for millions of elderly Americans and their families. The growing number of elderly people has focused public attention on the catastrophic problem of coverage for long-term care. Social insurance is unlikely to emerge as a solution in the USA. One reason is that the expected total cost is viewed as an unmanageable burden by both Federal and State governments. To others, it is the uncertainty surrounding the projected costs. This paper reports on the results of a double-decrement life-table analysis, based on a national survey of the elderly taken in early 1977 and one year later, that estimated the distribution and total lifetime nursing-home costs of the elderly. Combining the probability of nursing-home entry and length of stay, a 65-year-old faces a 43% chance of entering a nursing home and spending about $11 000 (1980 dollars). The distribution of lifetime costs is however very skewed with 13% of the elderly consuming 90% of the resources. Thus, while the costs of nursing-home care can be catastrophic for an individual, spread across a group they are not unmanageable. Given the distribution of income and assets among the elderly, a sizeable proportion could readily afford the necessary premiums of different emerging insurance and delivery programmes. Alternative private and public models of long-term care must be evaluated in terms of the goals of a finance and delivery system for long-term care.

1988 Research and the ageing population. Wiley, Chichester (Ciba Foundation Symposium 134) p 235–253

It is over 20 years since the US Congress enacted the Medicare and Medicaid programmes in 1965 to meet the challenge of providing medical assistance to the elderly and to specific groups of low-income individuals and families. While coverage for acute care is fairly comprehensive, long-term care coverage is lacking. Thus, it is not surprising that even with these programmes, 25% of the health-care costs of the elderly are paid out-of-pocket. The largest out-of-pocket expense faced by the elderly is nursing-home care.

Generally, there are two levels of care provided in nursing homes in the United States: skilled and custodial. Skilled nursing care is most often provided for elderly people in need of short-term recuperative care, whereas custodial care is provided to those in need of long-term maintenance care as a result of disabling chronic conditions. In 1984, more than $34 billion was spent on nursing-home care, of which the elderly and their families paid about $17 billion and Medicaid, the major public payer of nursing-home care, paid most of the remainder. Of particular concern to policymakers in the USA is the rate at which Medicaid expenditures are growing. Medicaid is the fastest growing component of State spending and its historical growth has been about 25% higher than State revenues (Rymer et al 1979).

Medicaid will pay for the nursing-home bills of someone who qualifies on the basis of low income or impoverishment resulting from excessive health-care costs. Becoming impoverished in a nursing home is not uncommon. About 50% of those elderly people who receive Medicaid reimbursement enter the nursing home as private paying patients and 'spend down' to Medicaid eligibility (Gornick et al 1985). An individual with average levels of income and assets can expect to spend down to Medicaid eligibility within seven months of entering a nursing home. The implication of this is that, with respect to long-term nursing-home care, the Medicaid programme reimburses services for many elderly people who, after spending their own resources to finance the initial months of care, become impoverished by a long nursing-home stay. Most of these elderly are from the middle class. Furthermore, because care is paid for in a nursing home but not generally in the community, there is consistent evidence of inappropriate placement of people into nursing homes.

What to do for this group, which represents the mainstream of elderly persons, is a critical issue facing policy makers. There is a developing consensus that alternatives to the current system of reimbursement and delivery are desirable and feasible. If we are to move forward, however, a number of key issues must be examined. First, we must determine the current distribution of long-term care costs among the elderly. The way such costs are distributed has implications for the development of new models for the financing and delivery of care. Second, we need to focus attention on the financial capacity of society and of the elderly to pay for long-term care or, alternatively, to pay for new models of care that emphasize community and home-care services and cover these costs. Finally, we must examine the implications of adopting a public, private or mixed strategy for addressing the problem of catastrophic long-term care costs.

The distribution of long-term care costs

Nursing-home care is only one service among a continuum of home, community and institutionally based long-term care services. In dollar terms, however, nursing-home care is the largest component of long-term care costs. Although a great deal of research has been done on the topic, there is no clear consensus on the actual chance of an individual entering a nursing home. Estimates for the lifetime risk of entering a nursing home range from 25% to

TABLE 1   Lifetime risk of entering a nursing home

Age category	Total population	Men	Women
65–69	43.1%	30.5%	51.9%
70–74	44.7%	30.6%	53.4%
75–79	47.7%	29.7%	57.4%
80–84	47.6%	27.6%	57.3%
85+	43.0%	22.9%	52.0%

60% (Kastenbaum & Candy 1973, Palmore 1976, Wershow 1976, Lesnoff-Caravaglia 1978–1979, Vicente et al 1979, McConnel 1984). The inability to develop more precise estimates derives from the lack of longitudinal data on nursing-home utilization. Thus, researchers are left with trying to make longitudinal inferences from cross-sectional data. Few have been successful at this.

Using double-decrement life-table analysis, we took cross-sectional data from the 1977 Current Medicare Survey and made longitudinal inferences about the lifetime risk of nursing-home entry among a cohort of elderly people of 65 and over (Cohen et al 1986). To calculate the lifetime risk rate, a hypothetical cohort was 'aged'. At each age interval, those alive faced the twin risks of either dying (not having entered a nursing home) or entering an institution. These incidence risks were derived from age- and sex-specific mortality tables as well as from annual nursing-home entry rates taken from the Current Medicare Survey. The number of people who had either died or entered an institution at specific ages was substracted from the initial population and the procedure was applied to the survivors repeatedly until the entire cohort had expired. The number of persons who entered a nursing home across the age categories was then summed and divided by the number in the original cohort. In this way the proportion of people who actually entered a nursing home was determined. Table 1 shows the lifetime risk of nursing-home entry at various ages.

In 1977, a 65-year-old person faced a 43% chance of entering a nursing home at least once before death. The risk increases until about age 85, where it actually begins to fall. This is because, after the age of 85, a person is more likely to die before entering a nursing home. At all ages, women are about twice as likely to enter a nursing home as men. These figures should be qualified in two ways. First, given the smaller sample size for people in the older age groups, the 95% confidence intervals around the point estimates are larger. For example, while the point estimate for the lifetime risk of nursing-home entry of 85-year-olds is 43.9%, the 95% confidence interval is from 36.0% to 50.0%. Second, these numbers may be somewhat high since they do not account for the impact of repeated nursing-home use, or medical relapse. Many nursing-home residents enter a long-term care facility more than once

TABLE 2   Expected lifetime cost of nursing-home care by age cohort

| Age cohort | Expected lifetime costs | | |
	Total population	Men	Women
65–69	$11 500	$8100	$13 800
70–74	$11 900	$8200	$14 200
75–79	$13 600	$8500	$16 400
80–84	$13 600	$7900	$16 400
85+	$10 500	$5600	$12 800
Average	$12 000	$8000	$14 580

and this can confound incidence rates derived from cross-sectional data (McConnel 1984). If we assume, for example, that 30% of entrants into nursing homes have entered an institution at least once before at an earlier age interval, then, by allowing for repeat use, the lifetime risk for a 65-year-old is reduced to 34%.

Identifying 'risk' is only one factor in understanding the distribution of costs among the elderly. Most of the literature on nursing-home use looks at the issues of risk and cost separately. We use the risk estimates to project the expected lifetime costs of nursing-home care for an elderly entrant as well as for all the elderly. We combine risk estimates with length of stay data from the 1976 National Nursing Home Discharge Survey. Assuming an average daily rate of $55.00 in 1977, the average costs *per entrant* are between $24 500 and $28 000. Using risk data, we can estimate the expected lifetime costs for all members of an age cohort. Table 2 shows these costs. As indicated, the expected lifetime costs of nursing-home care across all ages in the late 1970s was between $10 500 and $13 600. The costs for women are nearly twice as high as for men. The range for females across all age groups is between $12 800 and $16 400, whereas for men the range is from $5600 to $8200. The age cohort with the highest expected costs is the 75- to 84-year-olds. Those over age 85 have the lowest expected costs. This is because fewer of them enter nursing homes and those who do so stay for shorter periods of time.

The distribution of expected costs is especially interesting. For most nursing-home entrants, the lifetime costs are much less than $10 000. A very small percentage of entrants consume about two-thirds of all nursing-home expenditures. This is explainable by the high degree of variance in the length-of-stay patterns among those entering nursing homes. The majority of nursing-home entrants (75%) stay less than a year, and one-third to one-half of all who enter stay less than three months. About one-quarter of all entrants stay beyond one year and very few (14% to 17%) stay more than three years (Liu & Manton 1983, 1984, Liu & Palesch 1981, Keeler et al 1981, Shapiro & Webster 1984).

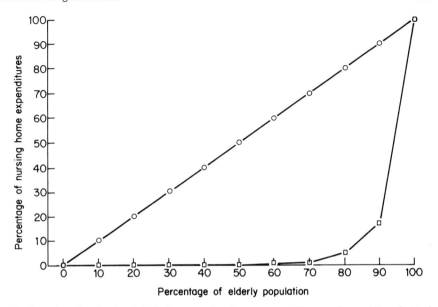

FIG. 1.   The distribution of lifetime nursing-home expenditures. Curved line (– □ –) actual distribution (a bowed line means a more unequal distribution); 45-degree line (– ○ –) line of equality.

When nursing-home expenditures across the entire elderly cohort are examined, we find that approximately 3.6% of all elderly people use about 43% of all nursing-home resources; another 6% use 40% of total nursing-home resources. Alternatively, roughly 90% of all the elderly account for somewhat less than 13% of all nursing-home expenditures. Compared to the distribution of hospital resources across the elderly population, nursing-home expenditures are distributed much more unequally (Zook & Moore 1980). Thus, most of the costs of care are in the tail of the distribution. Fig. 1 shows the percentage of nursing-home expenditures attributable to different proportions of the elderly population.

Given the distribution of costs, nursing-home care is an ideal candidate for risk sharing. There is a relatively small probability of incurring a large expense. While individual costs can be extremely high, group per capita costs are rather low. If each individual contributed the rather small average value of expected use, the group as a whole could be insured. This is because close to one-half of all elderly people will not enter nursing homes, in the USA.

We also estimate the total nursing-home resource costs for a particular age cohort by multiplying the number of people in the cohort by the expected lifetime costs per person. For example, in 1982, there were 16.0 million Americans aged 65 to 74. These people will consume between $131.8 and

TABLE 3   Total lifetime cost of nursing-home care by age cohort

	Total cohort costs (billions)		
Age cohort	1982	2000	2020
65–74	$188.4	$207.7	$349.4
75–84	$112.4	$166.5	$194.8
85 and over	$ 25.8	$ 54.2	$ 77.4

$188.4 billion in nursing-home resources, depending on the extent of repeated stays after age 74. Table 3 summarizes the estimated cohort costs of nursing-home use for the years 1982, 2000 and 2020.

Given current life-expectancy figures, the expected annual cost per person, over age 65, is less than $1000 for long-term nursing-home care. This should not be an unmanageable burden on society's resources. The estimated annual liability represents about 23% of per capita personal health-care expenditures on the elderly. Moreover, such costs represent less than 10% of the total health bill in the United States (Liu & Manton 1984). These figures point to the feasibility of long-term care risk-sharing arrangements among the elderly. These arrangements might be made at the national level; alternatively, private initiatives, such as long-term care insurance, Life Care Communities, and other models, may offer the elderly a way to protect themselves against the catastrophic costs of long-term care.

Public insurance in the form of a 'Medicare Part C' has a number of strengths. First, since everybody in the USA over age 65 would be covered, there would not be a problem of adverse selection into the risk pool. (Adverse selection refers to a general problem in insurance whereby people most likely to be in need of benefits are also the most likely to seek insurance. If only these people purchase insurance, there will be no healthy group over which to spread costs.) Second, universal coverage would assure that, regardless of level of income, those people who require long stays in a nursing home would not need to become impoverished to cover their stay. Finally, because the size of the risk pool would be so large, the law of large numbers would assure that slight changes in morbidity and mortality would not threaten the financial integrity of the pool of funds available to those insured.

Although on a societal level, social insurance for long-term care costs is affordable and desirable, such universal insurance is not likely to emerge as the single solution of the problem of long-term care in the USA. This assessment is based on the political reality that the Federal government is moving in exactly the opposite direction—relying on private markets and State initiatives to solve many social problems. Given current budgetary deficits, this trend is likely to continue into the foreseeable future. Thus, it is important to explore the feasibility and desirability of private models for the financing and delivery of long-term care.

The financial capacity to pay for long-term care costs

The pooling of risk is of most benefit to the middle-income group — precisely the group most likely to face heavy long-term care expenditures. Except in very rare instances, most wealthy older Americans can pay for their own care, even when facing a long stay in a nursing home. On the other hand, Medicaid pays the nursing-home bills for the poor who, in most cases, do not have the money to finance their own care for even a short time. Similarly, they are unlikely to be able to pay the premiums for different insurance programmes. For older middle-class people, risk-pooling programmes are desirable because they would keep the middle-income elderly and their spouses off welfare; long-term care costs would be spread across a premium-paying group. Also, the benefits to the State Medicaid programmes may be significant, especially in terms of potentially reduced Medicaid outlays. Medicaid expenditures are inversely related to the ability of elderly *users* of nursing-home services to finance their own care. However, the resources that *non-users* of nursing-home services might be willing to spend to protect themselves against catastrophic expenses are not available for use by Medicaid. That is, the willingness of these people to spend money to insure themselves cannot be tapped by the Medicaid programme (as it is currently constituted) to reduce total outlays. To the extent that people participating in programmes that insure long-term care costs through risk-pooling do not 'spend down' to Medicaid eligibility, Medicaid will experience reduced direct (reimbursement for services) and indirect (administering estate recovery) costs. Given the distribution of risk and costs for nursing-home care, the Medicaid costs of caring for an individual who has insurance covering up to three years in a nursing home are between 25% and 40% lower than the costs of a similar non-insured individual.

A key question is: how much insurance is affordable? There are two aspects to this issue that need to be explored. First, we must assess the private capacity to insure for long-term care. Second, we need to evaluate the public willingness to pay for long-term care.

We considered the financial capacity of the elderly to purchase three newly emerging long-term care options representing different degrees of coverage for long-term care costs. Each of these models has as a central feature the pooling of risk across a group of elderly people. The Social Health Maintenance Organization (S/HMO) is a finance-and-delivery model that provides an integrated package of health and chronic-care services to an elderly population for a fixed premium. It provides less than one year of insurance coverage for nursing-home care and is being demonstrated in four sites that

TABLE 4   The proportion of the elderly who could afford different long-term care models, given a willingness to devote 10% of discretionary resources (1984)

	Monthly premiums for different long-term care models			
	S/HMO: less than 1 year of coverage	LTC insurance: up to 2 years of coverage		Life Care at Home: lifetime coverage
Age	($25–$50)	$50–$100	$100–$150	($125–$150)
65+	57%	50%	19%	23%[a]
65–69	66	60	19	24
70–74	57	51	18	21
75–79	50	43	19	21
80+	47	39	24	26

S/HMO, Social Health Maintenance Organization. LTC, long-term care.

[a] The percentage of elderly that can afford the $125–$150 premium for the Life Care at Home Plan is greater than the percentage that could afford the $100–$150 premium for long-term care insurance. This is because the Life Care at Home Plan eliminates a number of expenses of the elderly, the most important of which is out-of-pocket medical expenses for Medicare Part B and Medigap policies.

have very different sponsor orientations. Long-term care insurance is offered by at least 15 major insurance companies in the USA. These policies provide indemnity benefits that cover up to three years of care. The Life Care at Home Plan provides lifetime insurance against the catastrophic costs of long-term care and provides a case-managed delivery system to ensure access to needed services. (In a case-managed delivery system, social workers or nurses work with the elderly and their families to develop the most appropriate plan of care for the elderly person. The 'case manager' does assessments, develops care plans, arranges for services, and monitors the conditions of the client.) It is being demonstrated in one site, and an additional three sites are being selected as precursors to a national demonstration. The S/HMO costs between $25 and $50 a month and long-term care insurance costs between $50 and $150 a month. The Life Care at Home Plan has a lump-sum entrance fee of about $7500 and monthly premiums of about $150. The three options represent points along a continuum of comprehensiveness of benefit.

Table 4 shows the proportion of elderly persons who could afford these emerging options, given a willingness to devote 10% of their discretionary resources to a purchase. Discretionary resources are defined as the amount of income and financial assets (not including a house) remaining after expenditures on standard necessities have been subtracted from an assessment of the income and assets of the elderly.

Up to one-half of all elderly people in the USA could afford to purchase one of these emerging long-term care models. However, given our assumptions about willingness to pay and the distribution of income and assets among the elderly, many could not afford to purchase one of these insurance coverages. In addition, because asset income comprises 50–70% of discretionary income, how the elderly ultimately choose to spend their assets will in large part determine the size of the market for these products. If the elderly refuse to spend their assets on long-term care purchases the figures for affordability will be substantially lower.

Many elderly people cannot afford to purchase these coverages, given their levels of income and assets after retirement. One alternative is to encourage the pre-funding of benefits so that accumulations throughout one's working years could finance insurance coverage during retirement. Also, pre-funding may offer an alternative way to pay for insurance for elderly people who do not wish to spend their assets. Beginning at age 35, a working individual would need to contribute about 1% of his or her pay to pre-fund the expected lifetime long-term care liability. Convincing people of the need for pre-funding may, however, prove difficult. Most people do not think they will ever need nursing-home care. Furthermore, most retired people think that should they need nursing-home care, Medicare, or Medicare supplemented with a Medigap policy, will cover most of the costs. The lack of information about risks and coverages will make it difficult to persuade employed people to trade-off current wages for uncertain future benefits.

Public and private responsibility

There are many possible solutions to the problem of the financing and delivery of long-term care. Making the appropriate choice between a privately based, publicly based, or mixed system depends on the goals of the system. Clearly, the current Medicaid system is an unacceptable model for care. It forces people into nursing homes and into dependence on welfare payments, and causes many middle-income older people to become bankrupt. Public programmes are possible, and in many ways easier to establish, because of their involuntary nature. A 'Medicare Part C' or enhanced Medicaid programme would solve the problem of coverage in the USA. In fact, if the only goal of the system is to insure people against long-term care costs, then a national programme designed to finance social insurance could meet this objective. Because, however, there are other goals of a long-term care system that relate more to retirement lifestyle, a national finance programme is not sufficient. Most agree that the long-term care system should be designed to meet a number of objectives, including access to high quality care, financial protection against catastrophic long-term care costs, and the provision of home and community services to help maintain dignity and independence and an acceptable lifestyle for elderly people during retirement. Multiple objectives require flexibility in both the finance and the *delivery* of

services. The key challenge is to develop a national financing system that can
work with local delivery systems in a way to ensure maximum flexibility in the
delivery of services. The critical issue facing policy makers in the USA is how
finance at the national level can be integrated with delivery at the State and
local level.

In the short run, it is unlikely that an improved method of national financing integrated with local delivery systems will be implemented. Even in the
acute-care sector, Medicare faces obstacles to becoming something more than
an indemnity programme. The major innovation in integration is making
available to individuals the option of joining Health Maintenance Organizations. An understanding of local delivery systems in the long-term care
sector is particularly important, since there are so many different types of
provider and setting, and there are numerous possibilities for service substitu-
tions leading to efficiencies in delivery. For example, in some cases home-
care services can be provided to elderly people who might otherwise have
been referred for care in a nursing home.

In the long-run, national financing may occur. However, even though in
the short-run this form of financing is not politically feasible, it is important to
encourage the development of local private financing and delivery systems.
Short of establishing a national insurance programme, there are other important roles for the Federal government to play. It could have a role in facilitat-
ing the development of models that share risk. An important action that can
be taken is to educate consumers about the risks and costs of incurring
catastrophic long-term care, the gaps in current coverage for such costs, and
the programmes available to cover the costs. Eliminating misperceptions
about coverage would probably lead to increases in the demand for long-term
care insurance. Another role of Federal government would include providing
incentives to consumers to purchase this form of insurance.

Until now, the greatest obstacle to improving the system of financing and
delivering long-term care has been the perception that the costs are overwhelming. Our research shows that the costs are indeed overwhelming for
individuals, but not for groups. Employers, unions, and/or States could insure
for long-term care through the establishment of risk pools. Medicare protects
individuals against the potentially catastrophic costs of acute care, but it
makes little sense to protect one's savings from acute-care expenses only to
lose them to chronic-care costs. The two major goals of the long-term care
system are to protect people financially, and to help them maintain a lifestyle
characterized by dignity and independence. To meet these goals universally, a
national system of finance is necessary. In the short run, however, it is
important to test out different models of care at the local level and to learn
about them. Such learning will raise the level of discussion about the appropriateness of public, private and mixed systems for the financing and delivery
of long-term care.

Acknowledgements

The authors gratefully acknowledge the assistance and advice of Eileen J. Tell, MPH, of the Bigel Institute for Health Policy.

References

Cohen MA, Tell EJ, Wallack SS 1986 The lifetime risks and costs of nursing home use among the elderly. Med Care 24:1161–1171

Gornick M, Greenberg J, Eggers P, Dobson A 1985 Twenty years of Medicare and Medicaid: covered populations, use of benefits, and program expenditures. Health Care Financing Review, Annual Supplement 59

Kastenbaum RS, Candy SE 1973 The 4 per cent fallacy: a methodological and empirical critique of extended care facility population statistics. Int J Aging Hum Dev 4:15–21

Keeler EB, Kane RL, Solomon DH 1981 Short- and long-term residents of nursing homes. Med Care 19:363–370

Lesnoff-Caravaglia G 1978–1979 The five per cent fallacy. Int J Aging Hum Dev 9:187–192

Liu K, Manton KG 1983 The characteristics and utilization pattern of an admission cohort of nursing home patients. Gerontologist 23:92–98

Liu K, Manton KG 1984 The characteristics and utilization pattern of an admissions cohort of nursing home patients (II). Gerontologist 24:70–76

Liu K, Palesch Y 1981 The nursing home population: different perspectives and implications for policy. Health Care Financing Review 3:15–23

McConnel CE 1984 A note on the lifetime risk of nursing home residency. Gerontologist 24:193–198

Palmore E 1976 Total chance of institutionalization among the aged. Gerontologist 16:504–507

Rymer MP, Conchita G, Bailis L, Ellwood D 1979 Medicaid eligibility: problems and solutions. Westview Press, Boulder, Colorado

Shapiro E, Webster LM 1984 Nursing home utilization patterns for all Manitoba admissions, 1974–1981. Gerontologist 24:610–615

Vicente L, Wiley JA, Carrington RA 1979 The risk of institutionalization before death. Gerontologist 19:361–367

Wershow HJ 1976 The four percent fallacy — some further evidence and policy implications. Gerontologist 16:52–55

Zook CJ, Moore FD 1980 The high-cost users of medical care. N Engl J Med 302:996–1002

DISCUSSION

Wenger: A major concern about the institutional (custodial) care of the elderly is the quality of that care. The worry of most elderly patients, and their families and health-care givers, is that in the supposedly supervised setting of institutional care, where staff are supposed to be caring for the residents, the fact is that the day-to-day care-givers are probably at the lowest level of training and motivation, in part related to the low pay scales and personnel shortages.

The quality of care is often disastrous, so that there is realistic fear, of nursing-home residents, both of their care-givers *per se* and of the quality of care they will receive. What will be the safeguard, what will be the accountability system at home, when care is so dispersed? Who will watch? What assurance will there be of adequate nutrition, medication, activity? The elderly as a group have a fear of violence, of their possessions being stolen, in addition to their fear of inadequate physical care; what will be the interplay? I see the quality, as well as the cost, of residential care as a major problem.

Wallack: There are two separate issues relating to nursing homes in the USA. These institutions are basically funded by Medicaid, a State-directed programme. That Medicaid policies have become the driving force behind the long-term care of the elderly in the USA is a very important factor. When one looks at nursing homes supported by a higher proportion of private financing, they look different, they feel different, they are staffed differently; people are even fed differently. 'Quality' is directly related to the funding.

How does one enforce quality in nursing homes? We try to regulate nursing homes, with staffing and other requirements, but we have not been very successful. A preferred solution would be to integrate nursing homes into broader social systems, such as housing, acute health care, or religious organizations. I don't think we can have quality long-term care for the elderly being delivered by 'free-standing' nursing homes—ones that are isolated both organizationally and physically from the rest of the delivery system and the rest of the social system of individuals.

I have been struck by the much better performance of nursing homes that operate in our Life Care or Continuing Care retirement communities, which are campuses composed of independent housing and nursing homes. The facilities and residents are integrated into the rest of the campus community. People in these communities identify with the nursing homes and visit their friends there regularly. One solution is the re-integration of the elderly into different environments where they are not segregated by age. Separation often leads to disaster, because of the possibilities of abuse. Clearly, we must worry about poor quality as we expand home health care. The organizations responsible for delivering home care will be very important in determining the quality of the programme. Quality is a major problem, in either the home or the institution, but system and financial solutions—not regulation—offer the path to good quality. Regulations can only establish the minimum standards, ones that often have little relationship to the outcome for patients.

T.F. Williams: Dr James Perry, who is president of the Florida State Medical Association, and also an appointee to our National Advisory Council on Aging, has spoken feelingly of the plight of older people, as he sees them as a practising neurologist in an area of the USA where vast numbers of people have retired, initially in reasonably good health. Now that their health is failing they are increasingly isolated; a spouse dies; their income is fixed and therefore relatively falling; great personal tragedies are going on and there is no supportive network. He favours our moving to develop, at the local neighbourhood level, networks of mutual support, as well as the infusion of public support. Dr Perry feels that nursing homes could be one focus of activity, but churches, synagogues, social clubs and other organizations should be foci too. We need a small-scale network at a local level, and that is what the Life Care retirement communities create for those who move into them. The problem is that they cater for a single stratum of society, and become rather sterile in that sense. They are not available to everybody (because of cost), and they have limitations. But the concept is a good one.

Arie: In considering economics, we must not forget those aspects of quality which are not necessarily cost related. It is not too much, I think, to say that one of the great social evils of our time is the misery of old people in long-stay care. This is not because all long-stay care is bad, but because the natural tendency of the communal care of impaired old people is towards unwanted features that one has to strive against. These include the almost total loss of choice; the infantilizing of old people by paternalism or, worse, by authoritarianism; forced apathy and loss of a sense of personal dignity and worth. Such things are difficult to measure, and our regulatory activities tend, therefore, to concentrate on more material aspects, like hygiene, space, fire safety, staffing ratios. It is easy to run away from the less material aspects of the quality of care, but one must not.

A particular problem that concerns me is that much of the direct personal care of old people is given by non-professionals, and these are people often of much goodwill but of little education. We, the professionals, generally offer them little training. Yet this is surely a major responsibility for all of us who are engaged in the care of the elderly. We know a lot about the styles of care in which people seem to work best, and the ways in which one can change styles of care (e.g. Clarke 1978, Baker 1983, Revans 1964); we do not sufficiently apply what we know, let alone break new ground.

T.F. Williams: You are entirely right, and this type of problem is also very pervasive in the Life Care retirement communities in the USA. They set arbitrary requirements that are limiting; for example, in many such communities, 'they' won't permit a resident to enter the dining room in a wheelchair, because they fear that this will convey a sense of un-health, of sickliness, in the environment. So a person living in a retirement community who needs a wheelchair has to eat in his or her room, or move to the nursing home. That is an arbitrary rule and a demeaning one. One can understand the fear-based rationale behind it but it isn't compatible with open living or individual choice. We face this kind of problem even more pervasively in some of the large retirement communities.

On the other hand, I was struck by my visit to Sun City in Phoenix, Arizona, where the older people who have retired there have realized that they have to

be responsible for themselves, because nobody else will be. They have organized an ambitious and imaginative approach to meeting their own needs. So
perhaps, out of necessity, in various areas of health and of society, older people
may be going to lead us all (and we shall all be part of it) to face the issues of old
age that have to be faced. We talk about the needs for holistic care, or
multidisciplinary care; in fact you can't give proper care to older people without
a multidisciplinary approach. This might even help us achieve such a goal in all
our care. You cannot deal with the problems of older people without recognizing the immense variety: some will be in wheelchairs, or on crutches; some will
be in bed, but others are mobile. Approaches have to be developed that are
acceptable to all these people and conditions, and perhaps that will be a gain for
society as a whole.

Svanborg: When we ask people if they would prefer to stay at home or go into
a nursing home if they were ill, we are also asking them indirectly whether they
'want' to be only a little ill, or really very ill in the future. Their answers
obviously also reflect their hope for their state of health in the future. When we
studied the actual need for medical care and then compared the interest of an
individual in staying at home or entering an institution, we of course found the
opposite, namely that those who really are in a dependent situation commonly
ask for a high quality of care, and very commonly the form of care that is
available in our nursing homes.

I would in this context like to emphasize that the elderly understand the term
'nursing home' in different ways. Some of our nursing homes are more like
annexe hospitals, with good facilities and a high quality of care, whereas others
are more like homes for those who can no longer live alone in their own
apartments.

Wallack: I would agree that old people generally like to stay at home,
whether or not that is the appropriate care. The problem I identified is that in
the USA, at present, our systems of financing and delivery are biased towards
putting people into hospitals or nursing homes. So people don't have a choice.
The delivery system doesn't really make the choices available. Patients are in
institutions because that is where the resources are. We need to develop the
delivery systems that allow patients the choice of where to get their long-term
care services. The demonstration project that I mentioned, the Social Health
Maintenance Organization (S/HMO), is an integrated delivery system, encom-
passing acute health care, long-term care and support services. We are keeping
more people out of hospital, and those entering do so for a shorter period of
time. The lower rates are adjusted for health status. We are reducing hospitalization rates by as much as 40%. We are also keeping people out of the nursing
home, so our nursing-home utilization will probably decrease by 10–20%. The
real issue is the appropriate level of care and providing people with real
alternatives. The alternatives only become real when they are accessible
through an organized system, appropriately financed. It is the right balance
that we are trying to arrive at.

Fries: I would suggest that for purposes of analysis you should not simply divide people into those in nursing homes and those in the community, but also divide them into that percentage who are going to live out the current year and those who will die in that year. Life-time medical costs in the USA are around $100 000 for an individual. As you point out, about $14 000 of that total over a 75-year lifetime is spent on long-term care facilities; $18 000 is spent in the last year of life, and $12 000 of that is spent in the last month (Fries 1987). When people are surveyed, even in the last several months of life, and asked what they desire with regard to their own 'heroic' care in the terminal stages, there is a large preference for decreasing expenditures in that area. There is a national movement towards 'living wills' and other ways of decreasing the terminal agonies. Let me stress that we have a 'social waste' of some large fraction of that $12 000 which in the interests of the elderly could be transferred to something that people really want.

Coleman: I am interested in the potential role of so-called 'reverse mortgages' in the whole scheme of health-care finance. You also pointed out a model, Dr Wallack, in which there was a form of 'deductible'. Is there any move toward the deductible health-care insurance, along the lines of a commercial automobile policy, in which the individual bears the initial burden and a private company takes over for longer, larger burdens?

Wallack: This is exactly the type of policy that most private insurance companies are offering. The individual is offered long-term health-care insurance, but has to pay the first six months of care. This was the model that we devised for the Carnegie Commission on College Retirement.

'Reverse mortgages' are a way of using the major assets of elderly people to buy a long-term care policy with extensive benefit. A number of programmes exist in the USA but relatively few people are using this, unless some unexpected event occurs. People don't want to give up or mortgage their homes once again. They do not want to increase the possibility of changing their lifestyle. If the possibility of maintaining their lifestyle is increased by using the equity in their home, the elderly may be more willing to participate in a reverse mortgage programme. We have designed a concept, Life Care at Home, which requires a $5000–10 000 down payment. Reverse mortgages represent a way for people to buy in.

Mor: Anne Scitovsky (1984) has focused on the issue of whether or not, over the past 20–25 years, there has been a major shift in the proportion of health-care costs that are concentrated in the last six to twelve months of life. In fact, there has not been a shift as a result of the high technology; the terminal concentration of costs has existed for 30 years. The real problem of trying to discount terminal-care costs and design a policy to reduce those costs in the last month is that it is difficult to predict who will survive acute exacerbations of underlying chronic conditions. It would be a mistake for the elderly population to trade a long-term care policy for acute care, when the probability of at least short-term success in the acute-care sector for certain illnesses is generally high, unless or until we can predict mortality better in the acute-care sectors.

Macfadyen: The international organization that is concerned about insurance-based health-care systems is the International Social Security Association in Geneva. It did a survey of long-term institutional care in different countries (Davis 1985). The rate of long-term care in the USA is by no means the highest; it is in fact highest in The Netherlands. One of the objectives of the study was to consider how those rates might be reduced. The study took the national nursing survey in the USA, worked out the predicted institutional rate in other countries, and compared these with actual rates. I think this needs to be studied as an international issue, looking at some of the innovations made to try to reduce institutional care, including the innovations mentioned by Dr Wallack. This is a major issue in almost all industrialized countries, and also in countries with currently low rates, like Spain and Greece; how can we stop the trend to greater use of institutional care? We need to share international experience on these issues of quality and cost, and some of the alternatives that are being explored.

Svanborg: Is the age rate adjusted to the proportion of the elderly above 65 in the Dutch population? We have a high proportion of very old people in Sweden and these are of course different in many ways from those at age 65–75.

Macfadyen: These are not my data, but they are reported to be derived from detailed age- and sex-specific use rates.

Fries: Perhaps the countries with the greatest use-rate of long-term care facilities might be those with no price barrier for people to enter those facilities.

Wallack: We have an overall rate of about 5% for those over 65 years of age in the USA, but there is much variation across the country. One of the most important variables that has been identified is the weather! The warmer climates in the USA have much lower rates. The highest rates are in States along the Canadian border, where getting around is more difficult and the chance of accidents is greater. One interesting point is that in the Life Care communities, which are controlled living or campus environments, weather is not very important in determining variation between sites. We have to adjust for environmental factors such as weather and see what kinds of delivery and financing systems reduce these institutional rates down to an appropriate level.

Fries: I gather that you would prefer to see people being as independent as possible—that is, in their homes—and would like to shorten the average period of time spent in a nursing home. What is the impact of long-term care insurance, in terms of fostering demand for more 'dependent' services, and thus working against that goal?

Wallack: It depends on how the system is designed and run. On the insurance side, in the USA we don't have insurance yet; we have a financing programme of direct nursing-home payments. When we develop an insurance programme that pays for long-term care, I think it will keep many people out of nursing homes. For example, the average length of stay in a nursing home is much lower in Life Care communities than in the community at large; and nursing homes in Life Care communities are used very differently, for short-term rather than long-term stays. So the pattern is different in an insured environment. But the management of the system is important as well. If an insurance company were to come into long-term care, providing home-health services, people would want to collect on their policy: once one is insured, one wants to take advantage of that insurance. So you have the problem of over-utilization.

If we finance and deliver long-term care in a managed care system as opposed to an indemnity/insurance approach, I believe the results will be different. In the Social Health Maintenance Organization we found that when we went to the family of an older person and talked to them about the goal of maintaining the individual at home and trying to support the family, the family responded positively. Therefore, I feel that if we manage the long-term care system with a social worker, or a nurse practitioner, over-utilization need not occur. In the S/HMO we are providing home health within the budgets we set up. The way in which you design the benefits, set up the system of insurance, and then manage the programme will determine the use.

Andrews: Discussion of long-term care tends to focus on the options of institutionalization or community care as the only possibilities. We should go beyond that polarization; as Alvar Svanborg implied, there are many ways of providing institutional care, and the notion of the generic nursing home is too limited. Likewise with home care, in South Australia we now have a comprehensive system of domiciliary care, run by the State government. It includes home nursing, home helps, the provision of various aids and 'sitting' services, meals on wheels, laundry, and a whole range of other services for older people in their homes. There are limitations. There is an assessment procedure that the individual has to go through, because the service has to be rationed, because of financial limits. Because the scheme is funded by Federal and State monies there are regulations about what can be provided and what cannot. Matching the available services to the needs of the individual is not always possible. Because the service is provided by paid employees, industrial issues arise over hours of work and conditions of employment.

Two interesting responses have been made to these problems. One is the provision of privately run home-care programmes that are not as rigid as government ones, but are available only to those who can afford them (or maybe, in the future, to those who can insure for them). The other response is a non-profit, locally based 'community options' programme where an individual, the community options officer, who may not be a highly trained social worker or nurse, but who lives locally and is given additional training, receives from the programme a certain amount of money to spend. Then, if a person is on a home-care programme but not receiving all the help needed because the regulations limit help to a certain number of hours a week, or who is getting the available services but the real problem is obtaining help with the garden, and a neighbour will do that for five dollars a week, the community options officer is able to arrange that service, either directly for the person or by giving him or her the money to make the arrangement. The people running those programmes argue that they are able, because of the flexibility and ability to respond directly to the individual's needs and not be bound by regulations and assessment procedures, to maintain people cost-effectively in independence in the community, beyond what can be done with the formal structures of the social services. We have yet to see what happens when this system becomes widely available, and how we then monitor it and keep some sort of control.

Maeda: I would like to reinforce what Dr Wallack told us by describing the results of a study I did on the future cost of nursing-care services for the elderly in Japan (Maeda 1982). The assumptions on which the calculation was made were: (1) the proportion of old people needing institutional care will be 3%, which is considerably smaller than in other developed countries, because even at the beginning of the next century the traditional family care of the impaired elderly will be comparatively well preserved in Japan; (2) the quantitative level of other nursing-care services (for example, the ratio between the number of home helps and the number of old people aged 65 and over) will be similar to the average level of Northern European countries of today; (3) the qualitative level of care (such as the staff–patient ratio) will be the same as that of present services in Japan; and (4) all the services which have been found effective in other developed countries should be implemented in Japan at the same quantitative and qualitative level as in the other developed countries at present.

What prompted me to do this study was the widespread misgiving that the future cost of care services for our rapidly increasing numbers of impaired elderly might exceed the financial capability of Japan in the future. Because of this feeling, local government (which should take direct responsibility in providing such care services) will not embark on the construction of the needed service systems. Unless this negative attitude is changed soon there will be a serious shortage or even absence of needed services for the impaired elderly in the rapidly approaching ageing society of the 21st century.

The result of the calculation showed that in the year 2020, when the aged population of Japan reaches a peak of 23.5%, the total annual public cost of providing nursing-care services, including various home delivery services (for example, home-help service, visiting nurse service, day-care service, respite care service, home-delivery meal service) will be only about one-fifth of the total cost of compulsory education at present, and less than twice the amount that is now spent on public assistance. So this is not such a vast amount of money; it is quite affordable by Japan as a nation.

Wallack: I agree; this is exactly the point I was making for the USA.

A. Williams: We have heard much about the financial burden of the elderly, but that needs to be distinguished from the economic burden: these are two different issues. Whether we finance services publicly or privately is a tactical, political and cultural matter for each country to decide in the light of its history.

But whether financed privately or publicly, there is an economic problem of transferring resources from the working population to the non-working population, by whatever mechanism you choose to follow. It is important to distinguish these problems. But, to put the second problem in perspective, those countries that have seen increases in the unemployment rates in the last decade from around 2–3% of the working population to around 10–15% have already placed on themselves a burden far greater than anything they could ever face with the ageing of the population. We should not be frightened off by talk about the economic burden of the aged; we could cope with it readily, simply by reducing unemployment rates at a steady rate.

Wenger: One pervasive problem that none of the various care systems have addressed, and one that has surfaced many times during this symposium, is loneliness. A feature we have not considered in many of these settings, whether residential or not, is the complaint of loneliness by the elderly that often results from their limited mobility, which in turn is typically illness related. So much attention is paid to the specifically physical problems of illness that we have not considered the concomitant emotional problems that relate to change. Many people can maintain control in their familiar setting, but that degree of maintenance of control is often not enough to accommodate the problem of change of setting. We have not addressed this issue in most of the care systems, yet it may prove to be one of the more serious problems of getting old and becoming limited in one's mobility.

References

Baker DE 1983 Care in the geriatric ward. An account of two styles of nursing. In: Barnet JW (ed) Ten studies of geriatric care. Wiley, Chichester

Clarke M 1978 Getting through the work. In: Dingwall R, McIntosh J (eds) Readings in the sociology of nursing. Churchill Livingstone, Edinburgh

Davis CK 1985 Preliminary report: long term care provided within the framework of health care schemes. International Social Security Association, Geneva

Fries JF 1987 Aging, illness, and health policy: implications of the compression of morbidity. Perspect Biol Med, in press

Maeda D 1982 Gerontology and the services for the elderly at the year 2001—level and costs of services for the impaired elderly (in Japanese). Rounen Shakaikagaku (Jpn J Gerontol) 4:23–34

Revans RW 1964 Standards for morale: cause and effect in hospitals. Oxford University Press, London

Scitovsky AA 1984 The high cost of dying: what do the data show? Milbank Mem Fund Q 62:591–608

Summing-up

T. Franklin Williams

National Institute on Aging, National Institutes of Health, Building 31, Room 2C02, Bethesda, Maryland 20892, USA

Let me recapitulate some of the major issues that we have highlighted, although not resolved during the symposium, in the hope that it might stimulate us and others to address them further. One, certainly, is the issue of ageing versus disease, and what we mean by these terms. We have expressed different perspectives on this, and we have not reached agreement among ourselves about how to use these words.

There is the question of length of life versus quality of life, and what enters into the processes of determining longevity on the one hand and quality of life on the other. Longevity seems to come out of evolution, and the whole of the society of a given species; quality of life becomes very individual and personal. Our problem is how to rationalize or interrelate these two aspects.

We have been dealing with the issues of health in the context of society. We haven't dealt very much with some of the societal issues, but we have had to come back to them repeatedly as they make an impact on health and interact with it. There are many fundamental issues of the characteristics of disease processes, especially chronic disease processes, that we are just beginning to be able to understand. Thus, for me, it has been a very useful symposium, and the publication should stimulate new ideas and new work in many people.

Index of contributors

Subject index